pharmacology

The National Medical Series for Independent Study

pharmacology

EDITOR

Leonard S. Jacob, M.D., Ph.D.

Research Associate Professor of Pharmacology
Medical College of Pennsylvania
Vice-President Clinical Research and Development, North America
Smith Kline & French Laboratories
Philadelphia, Pennsylvania

ASSOCIATE EDITORS

John S. Lazo, Ph.D.

Associate Professor of Pharmacology
Yale University School of Medicine
New Haven, Connecticut

Edward Hawrot, Ph.D.

Assistant Professor of Pharmacology
Yale University School of Medicine
New Haven, Connecticut

A WILEY MEDICAL PUBLICATION
JOHN WILEY & SONS
New York • Chichester • Brisbane • Toronto • Singapore

Harwal Publishing Company, Media, Pa.

Efforts have been made by the authors and editors of this book to ensure accuracy and immediacy in drug dosage schedules. However, *Pharmacology* is not intended as a guide to drug therapy. It is urged that the readers consult the manufacturer's package insert to ascertain the recommended drug dosage, administration, and contraindications, especially relative to new and seldom-used drugs.

Library of Congress Cataloging in Publication Data

Main entry under title:
Pharmacology.

(The National Medical series for independent study)
(A Wiley Medical publication)
Includes index.
1. Pharmacology—Examinations, questions, etc.
I. Jacob, Leonard S. II. Lazo, John S. III. Hawrot, Edward. IV. Series. V. Series: Wiley Medical publication.
[DNLM: 1. Pharmacology—Examination questions. QV 18 P5363]
RM105.P47 1984 615'.1'076 84-7301
ISBN 0-471-09626-1

10 9 8 7 6 5 4 3

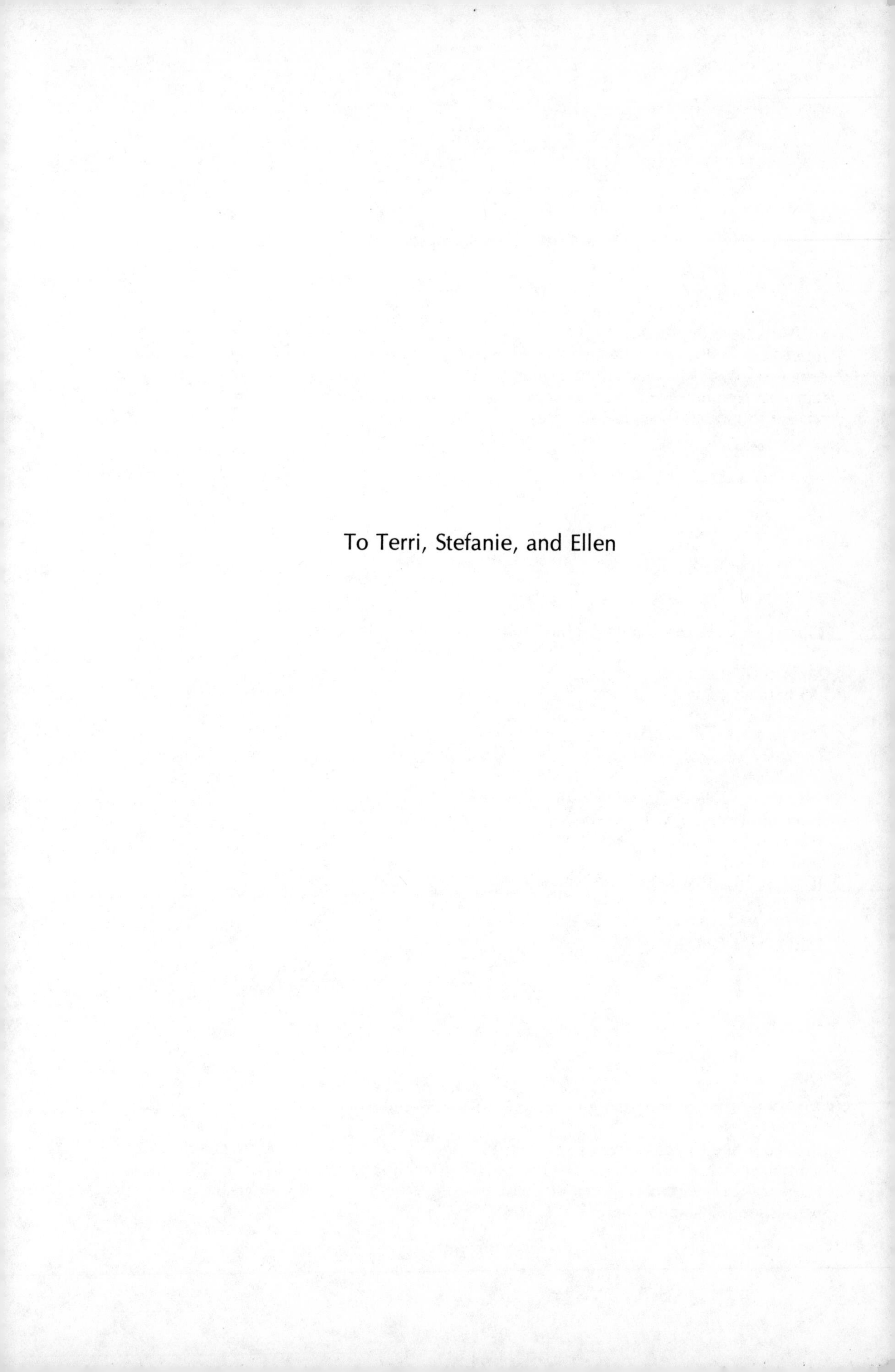

To Terri, Stefanie, and Ellen

Contents

	Preface	ix
	Acknowledgments	xi
	Publisher's Note	xii
	Introduction	xiii
	Pretest	1
1	General Pharmacologic Principles	13
2	Drugs Affecting Peripheral Neurohumoral Transmission	29
3	Agents Acting on the Central Nervous System	48
4	Anesthetic Agents	77
5	Cardiovascular Agents	89
6	Diuretic Agents	115
7	Drugs Affecting Hematopoiesis and Hemostasis	123
8	Autacoids and Their Antagonists	133
9	Non-Narcotic Analgesics, Nonsteroidal Anti-Inflammatory Drugs, and Drugs Used in the Treatment of Gout	145
10	Agents Affecting Endocrine Function	159
11	Cancer Chemotherapy	177
12	Anti-Infective Agents	199
13	Principles of Drug Interactions	229
14	Poisons and Antidotes	237
	Post-test	247
	Appendix: Drug Interactions	263
	Index	267

Preface

In the expanding world of science and medicine it is impossible to be "truly" up-to-date in any defined area. Pharmacology is no exception. In any pharmacology course, the student is confronted with a new language to which many additions will occur. New agents, their mechanisms of action, and untoward effects must be continually added to the already overburdened core knowledge of pharmacology. Understanding this new language is not easy because it is predicated on a thorough understanding of the basic medical sciences, including physiology and biochemistry.

I have personally gone through this educational process in the last 10 years, and although it has been rewarding, it has often been confusing. Most standard major textbooks of pharmacology provide an abundance of detail, which precludes the student from ever reading the book within the confined period of a 24- to 36-week course. Additionally, preparing for the National Boards requires the student to distill an extraordinary amount of information. The large number of drug groups has made it difficult to decipher which agent is or is not important. *Pharmacology* is designed as a *review* textbook, which attempts to present to the student numerous drug groups in an organized fashion.

National Board–type questions are presented, and detailed answers are provided. This is done not only to determine the extent of the preparation that might still be needed prior to taking this very important exam but additionally to reinforce important concepts presented in this textbook. It is important to stress that *Pharmacology* should not serve as a replacement for the major textbooks when detailed references are needed but instead should provide the information necessary for preparing for the pharmacology section of the National Medical Boards.

Leonard S. Jacob

Preface

Leonard S. Jacob

Acknowledgments

The writing and editing of this textbook has been extraordinarily difficult. We are grateful to Bruce Pitt, Ph.D., and Priscilla Dannies, Ph.D., of Yale University for reviewing many chapters. Paul D. DeRenzi, a Yale medical student, has also provided many helpful comments and suggestions. The editors at Harwal Publishing Company have been many, including Gloria Hamilton, Mary Ann Sheldon, and Jane Edwards. All were constructive, and Ms. Edwards in particular was patient in accommodating our busy schedules. Finally, our thanks are extended to Joseph Uri, M.D., Ph.D., a colleague and friend, who ensured that the "final product" met our goals in both accuracy and quality.

Publisher's Note

The objective of the *National Medical Series* is to present an extraordinarily large amount of information in an easily retrievable form. The outline format was selected for this purpose of reducing to the essentials the medical information needed by today's student and practitioner.

While the concept of an outline format was well received by the authors and publisher, the difficulties inherent in working with this style were not initially apparent. That the series has been published and received enthusiastically is a tribute to the authors who worked long and diligently to produce books that are stylistically consistent and comprehensive in content.

The task of producing the *National Medical Series* required more than the efforts of the authors, however, and the missing elements have been supplied by highly competent and dedicated developmental editors and support staff. Editors, compositors, proofreaders, and layout and design staff have all polished the outline to a fine form. It is with deep appreciation that I thank all who have participated, in particular, the staff at Harwal—Debra L. Dreger, Jane Edwards, Gloria Hamilton, Jeanine Kosteski, Wieslawa B. Langenfeld, Keith LaSala, June A. Sangiorgio, Mary Ann C. Sheldon, and Jane Velker.

The Publisher

Introduction

Pharmacology is one of seven basic science review books in a series entitled *The National Medical Series for Independent Study*. This series has been designed to provide students and house officers, as well as physicians, with a concise but comprehensive instrument for self-evaluation and review within the basic sciences. Although *Pharmacology* would be most useful for students preparing for the National Board of Medical Examiners examinations (Part I, FLEX, and FMGEMS), it should also be useful for students studying for course examinations. These books are not intended to replace the standard basic science texts but, rather, to complement them.

The books in this series present the core content of each basic science area, using an outline format and featuring a total of 300 study questions. The questions are distributed throughout the book at the end of each chapter and in a pretest and posttest. In addition, each question is accompanied by the correct answer, a paragraph-length explanation of the correct answer, and specific reference to the outline points under which the information necessary to answer the question can be found.

We have chosen an outline format to allow maximal ease in retrieving information, assuming that the time available to the reader is limited. Considerable editorial time has been spent to ensure that the information required by all medical school curricula has been included and that each question parallels the format of the questions on the National Board examinations. We feel that the combination of the outline format and board-type study questions provides a unique teaching device.

We hope you will find this series interesting, relevant, and challenging. The authors, as well as the John Wiley and Harwal staffs, welcome your comments and suggestions.

Pretest

QUESTIONS

Directions: Each question below contains five suggested answers. Choose the **one best** response to each question.

1. A postmenopausal woman presents with a breast carcinoma that is rich in estrogen receptors. The drug most likely to be administered is

(A) bleomycin
(B) vinblastine
(C) mitomycin
(D) dacarbazine
(E) tamoxifen

2. Scopolamine most closely resembles which of the following agents in its pharmacologic actions?

(A) Hexamethonium
(B) Atropine
(C) Succinylcholine
(D) Acetylcholine
(E) Curare

3. Physiologic doses of glucocorticoids can result in all of the following changes EXCEPT

(A) decreased liver glycogen stores
(B) increased gluconeogenesis
(C) increased lipolysis
(D) increased hemoglobin synthesis
(E) decreased cardiovascular function

4. Basic considerations for the treatment of hypertension should include all of the following EXCEPT

(A) initial drug therapy for mild hypertension could include minoxidil
(B) a combination of a diuretic and a β-adrenergic blocking agent can be used if either drug is ineffective alone
(C) when arteriolar vasodilators are used, appropriate sympathetic blockers are administered to prevent a reflex sympathetic response
(D) hypertensive emergencies are best treated with parenteral therapy
(E) diuretic agents are effective for patients requiring long-term treatment of hypertension

5. Which of the following statements concerning physiologic or pharmacologic antagonism is correct?

(A) In physiologic antagonism, the agonist has no intrinsic activity
(B) In physiologic antagonism, the antagonist has no intrinsic activity
(C) In physiologic antagonism, the antagonist and the agonist act on the same receptor
(D) In pharmacologic antagonism, the agonist has intrinsic activity
(E) In pharmacologic antagonism, the agonist has no intrinsic activity

Questions 6 and 7

A 10-year-old boy is admitted to the hospital with an initial diagnosis of acute lymphoblastic leukemia. His liver, spleen, and lymph nodes are extensively infiltrated.

6. Which of the following drug combinations would be most appropriate for inducing remission?

(A) Prednisone and vincristine
(B) Cyclophosphamide and methotrexate
(C) Cyclophosphamide and vinblastine
(D) 6-Mercaptopurine and methotrexate
(E) Cytarabine and 5-fluorouracil

7. The patient is given allopurinol to reduce the complications of his cancer chemotherapy. The rationale underlying the allopurinol therapy is that

(A) allopurinol increases the renal clearance of uric acid
(B) the most effective therapeutic regimens interfere with purine biosynthesis
(C) rapid lympholysis produces large quantities of uric acid
(D) lower doses of the remission-inducing drugs can be given
(E) allopurinol inhibits the metabolism of pyrimidine analogs

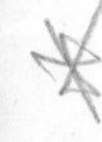

8. Mercury is toxic because it

(A) complexes with hemoglobin to form methemoglobin
(B) inhibits hemoglobin synthesis, producing anemia
(C) binds to ferric ions of the cytochrome a–a_3 complex
(D) inhibits anaerobic glycolysis
(E) binds to sulfhydryl groups

9. The diuretic of choice for a patient receiving the nephrotoxic antitumor agent cisplatin is

(A) ethacrynic acid
(B) mercaptomerin
(C) acetazolamide
(D) chlorothiazide
(E) mannitol

10. During a regular prenatal checkup, Mrs. Jones is found to have a normochromic, megaloblastic anemia. The most likely cause is a deficiency of

(A) iron
(B) vitamin B_{12}
(C) vitamin K
(D) folic acid
(E) intrinsic factor

11. Untoward effects seen with nitrites include all of the following EXCEPT

(A) headache
(B) increased intracerebral pressure
(C) methemoglobinemia due to oxidation of hemoglobin by the nitrite ion
(D) postural hypotension
(E) impotence

12. Exacerbation of petit mal seizures, gastrointestinal irritation, gingival hyperplasia, and facial hirsutism are all possible side effects of which one of the following anticonvulsant drugs?

(A) Phenobarbital
(B) Carbamazepine
(C) Acetazolamide
(D) Phenytoin
(E) Valproic acid

13. Furosemide is useful for the treatment of all of the following conditions EXCEPT

(A) congestive heart failure
(B) acute pulmonary edema
(C) hypocalcemia
(D) edema resulting from hepatic or renal disease
(E) hypertensive crisis

14. All of the following statements about untoward effects of cardiac glycosides are true EXCEPT that

(A) they have a high margin of safety
(B) intoxication is often precipitated by the depletion of potassium
(C) decreased renal function can predispose to toxicity
(D) the glycosides can cause vision changes
(E) the glycosides can cause ventricular tachycardia

15. The first-pass effect occurs most often after

(A) oral administration of a drug
(B) sublingual administration of a drug
(C) intravenous administration of a drug
(D) subcutaneous administration of a drug
(E) intramuscular administration of a drug

16. Atropine is useful in treating poisoning produced by organophosphate insecticides because it

(A) reactivates inhibited acetylcholinesterase
(B) stimulates α receptors directly
(C) stimulates β receptors directly
(D) inhibits normal ganglionic transmission
(E) blocks the action of acetylcholine at both central and peripheral sites

17. A patient with a history of glaucoma, epilepsy, and edema would be a candidate for treatment with which of the following diuretics?

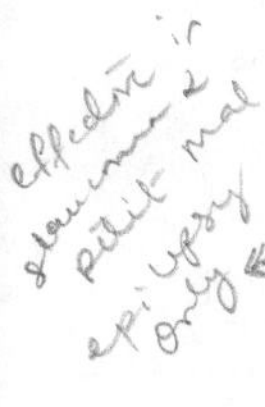

(A) Ethacrynic acid
(B) Chlorothiazide
(C) Furosemide
(D) Acetazolamide
(E) Spironolactone

18. Characteristics of the partial agonist–antagonist opioid agents (e.g., pentazocine) include

(A) severe nausea as a side effect
(B) a lack of correlation, at all therapeutic doses, between analgesic potency and depressant potency
(C) an increase in peripheral resistance and pulmonary vascular resistance, resulting in increased cardiac work
(D) a lack of constipating effects
(E) absence of tolerance to the analgesic effect

19. The potential for digitalis-induced cardiac arrhythmias is increased by each of the following diuretics EXCEPT

(A) ethacrynic acid
(B) chlorothiazide
(C) spironolactone
(D) furosemide
(E) mercaptomerin

20. Which of the following statements best characterizes morphine?

(A) It has a more rapid onset of action than heroin
(B) It has low addiction capabilities compared with heroin
(C) It can increase biliary tract pressure
(D) It always produces euphoria
(E) It blocks the chemoreceptor trigger zone

Directions: Each question below contains four suggested answers of which **one or more** is correct. Choose the answer

A if **1, 2, and 3** are correct
B if **1 and 3** are correct
C if **2 and 4** are correct
D if **4** is correct
E if **1, 2, 3, and 4** are correct

21. Ascariasis can be effectively treated by

(1) piperazine
(2) metronidazole
(3) pyrantel pamoate
(4) suramin

22. A patient with arthritis presents with a sore throat, fever, and dependent edema. The patient had been in good health previously. A complete blood count reveals a white count of 500 (normal, 5,000–8,000). Drugs capable of causing this effect include

(1) aspirin
(2) indomethacin
(3) sulindac
(4) phenylbutazone

SUMMARY OF DIRECTIONS

A	B	C	D	E
1, 2, 3 only	1, 3 only	2, 4 only	4 only	All are correct

23. Which of the following statements would be true of H_1 receptor blockers?

(1) They are substituted imidazoles
(2) They increase the heart rate
(3) They decrease gastric secretion
(4) They cause sedation

Questions 24 and 25

A 70-year-old woman with a history of congestive heart failure, for which she takes digoxin and a diuretic agent, is seen because of an arrhythmia. Electrolyte determination reveals a serum K^+ of 2.8 mEq/L.

24. Diuretics capable of producing this patient's hypokalemia include

(1) furosemide
(2) ammonium chloride
(3) hydrochlorothiazide
(4) aminophylline

25. Immediate therapy for this patient should include

(1) high doses of spironolactone
(2) insulin and glucose administration
(3) high doses of triamterene
(4) potassium supplementation

26. Correct statements concerning procaine include which of the following?

(1) It has an ester linkage
(2) It interferes with sodium influx during depolarization
(3) It is relatively short-acting
(4) It produces a lupus-like syndrome

27. A 67-year-old male presents with acute pulmonary coccidioidomycosis. Proper therapy would include

(1) high doses of penicillin G
(2) griseofulvin
(3) flucytosine
(4) amphotericin B

28. The concomitant administration of antacids with tetracycline will reduce the effectiveness of the antibiotic because

(1) antacids inhibit the absorption of tetracycline
(2) antacids stimulate the drug microsomal metabolizing system, so that the tetracycline is metabolized more rapidly
(3) ions in antacids chelate the tetracycline
(4) antacids enhance the renal excretion of tetracycline

29. Drug metabolism can be influenced by which of the following factors?

(1) Age
(2) Hepatic disease
(3) Concomitant drug therapy
(4) Apparent volume of distribution

30. Oral contraceptives containing norethindrone act basically by which of the following mechanisms?

(1) Speeding up the growth of ovarian follicles
(2) Increasing the secretion of follicle-stimulating hormone (FSH)
(3) Hastening the release of luteinizing hormone (LH)
(4) Suppressing ovulation

31. An 18-year-old woman presents with urgency, frequency, and burning urination. She is afebrile. Urinalysis reveals the presence of red blood cells. Appropriate therapy after urine culture could include which of the following?

(1) Trimethoprim-sulfamethoxazole
(2) Carbenicillin
(3) Sulfisoxazole
(4) Gentamicin

32. Characteristics of ergot alkaloids include which of the following?

(1) They are useful in treating migraine headaches
(2) They show CNS stimulating effects
(3) They can produce vasoconstriction
(4) They can be blocked by propranolol

33. Untoward effects of corticosteroids include

(1) suppression of the pituitary–adrenal axis
(2) increased susceptibility to infection
(3) behavioral disturbances
(4) muscle hypertrophy

34. Lidocaine, when used intravenously, will

(1) suppress premature ventricular contractions
(2) reverse atrial arrhythmias
(3) decrease sodium conductance in automatic cells
(4) decrease potassium conductance in automatic cells

35. True statements about the purine analog 6-mercaptopurine include which of the following?

(1) It is a structural analog of hypoxanthine
(2) It decreases the synthesis of 5-phosphoribosylamine
(3) It interferes with the formation of adenosine monophosphate
(4) Its metabolism is stimulated by allopurinol

36. Which of the following agents should not be administered to a patient whose renal function is severely compromised?

(1) Tobramycin
(2) Erythromycin
(3) Penicillin
(4) Doxycycline

37. Which of the following drugs and descriptions are correctly matched?

(1) Lidocaine—an ester but metabolized in the liver
(2) Mepivacaine—an amide metabolized in the liver
(3) Procaine—rapidly inactivated by acetylcholinesterase
(4) Tetracaine—a good spinal anesthetic

Questions 38 and 39

A patient presents with a 5-day history of a nonproductive cough, a fever of 101°F, and malaise. The chest x-ray is consistent with a diagnosis of *Mycoplasma pneumoniae* pneumonia.

38. Proper therapy could include which of the following?

(1) Doxycycline
(2) Chlortetracycline
(3) Erythromycin
(4) Streptomycin

39. Two days later the patient is re-diagnosed as having Legionnaires' disease. Correct therapy would include

(1) streptomycin
(2) doxycycline
(3) chloramphenicol
(4) erythromycin

40. Aspirin is characterized by which of the following?

(1) Its analgesic, antipyretic, and anti-inflammatory actions are due to inhibition of prostaglandin synthesis
(2) Toxic doses are capable of producing a respiratory and metabolic acidosis
(3) It can increase mean bleeding time
(4) Excretion can be increased by acidifying the urine

41. Which of the autacoids listed below will cause vasoconstriction in the microcirculation of humans?

(1) Bradykinin
(2) Angiotensin II
(3) Prostaglandin F
(4) Serotonin

42. Characteristics of carbachol (carbamylcholine) include which of the following?

(1) It is a parasympathetic agent
(2) It is purely muscarinic in action
(3) It is resistant to acetylcholinesterase
(4) It is purely nicotinic in action

43. Characteristics of antineoplastic agents include which of the following?

(1) They frequently are self-limiting in their killing of cancer cells
(2) They kill a constant fraction of the tumor cells
(3) They are preferentially toxic to nonproliferating cells
(4) They are usually used in combination with each other

44. Side effects most frequently seen with benzodiazepines include

(1) drowsiness
(2) ataxia
(3) lethargy
(4) seizures

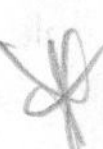

SUMMARY OF DIRECTIONS

A	B	C	D	E
1, 2, 3 only	1, 3 only	2, 4 only	4 only	All are correct

45. Adrenocortical drugs that are anti-inflammatory in pharmacologic doses include which of the following?

(1) Desoxycorticosterone
(2) Corticotropin (ACTH)
(3) Aldosterone
(4) Cortisol (hydrocortisone)

46. Quinidine administration can produce which of the following actions on the heart?

(1) A reduction in the maximal rate of rise ($\dot{V}_{max}$) of depolarization
(2) An increase in the effective refractory period (ERP)
(3) A decrease in automaticity
(4) An increase in inotropic action

47. The properties of carrier-mediated facilitated diffusion include which of the following?

(1) The process is not saturable
(2) It is specific for the chemical structure of the drug
(3) It requires energy
(4) It cannot move against a concentration gradient

48. Which of the following are true statements concerning the autacoids?

(1) Autacoids are circulating or locally active hormones from diffuse tissues
(2) All autacoids are believed to be involved with local circulatory adjustments and/or inflammation
(3) Kinins, like histamine, are associated with a "triple response"
(4) Stimulation of histamine receptors has been linked to calcium influx

49. Bleomycin is an antitumor agent that has which of the following characteristics?

(1) It intercalates with DNA
(2) It causes both single- and double-strand breaks in DNA
(3) It requires ferrous ion for its action
(4) It kills cells in G_2 and M phase

50. A patient presents with respiratory failure, pinpoint pupils, and cardiovascular collapse. The drugs which might reverse these symptoms include which of the following?

(1) Digoxin
(2) Nalorphine
(3) Epinephrine
(4) Naloxone

51. A poorly controlled diabetic patient is complaining of hunger, diaphoresis, and palpitations. Examination also reveals a "thready" pulse. Which of the following can be deduced from her symptoms?

(1) The patient is approaching a diabetic coma
(2) Her insulin dose is probably too high
(3) She is probably "spilling" sugar in her urine
(4) Her symptoms are premonitory of insulin shock

52. Diisopropyl fluorophosphate (DFP) increases which of the following effects?

(1) Lacrimation
(2) Salivation
(3) Muscle twitching
(4) Bronchodilation

Directions: The groups of questions below consist of lettered choices followed by several numbered items. For each numbered item select the **one** lettered choice with which it is **most** closely associated. Each lettered choice may be used once, more than once, or not at all.

Questions 53–56

For each description that follows, select the drug most likely to be associated with it.

(A) Halothane
(B) Diethyl ether
(C) Nitrous oxide
(D) Isoflurane
(E) Thiopental

53. Given intravenously and not adequate for prolonged surgery

54. Has the highest minimum alveolar concentration (MAC) value

55. Highly explosive agent

56. Widely used inhalation agent that can cause liver necrosis

Questions 57–60

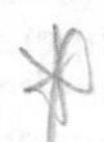

For each of the following diuretic agents, choose the anatomic site in the renal nephron where the principal action of the agent occurs.

(A) Glomerulus
(B) Proximal tubule
(C) Ascending limb of the loop of Henle
(D) Distal tubule
(E) Collecting duct

57. Acetazolamide

58. Spironolactone

59. Furosemide

60. Chlorothiazide

ANSWERS AND EXPLANATIONS

1. The answer is E. *(Chapter 11, II E 5; III D 5; IV E, F 5; V B 2, 4)* Tamoxifen is a nonsteroidal antiestrogen which competes with estrogen for the cytoplasmic estrogen receptor. Tumors with many estrogen receptors are frequently dependent on estrogen for cell proliferation. Thus, tamoxifen blocks the growth of such tumors. Bleomycin, mitomycin, and vinblastine are natural products that have little activity against breast carcinomas. Dacarbazine (DTIC) is a triazene alkylating agent which is effective against melanomas but is not effective against breast carcinomas.

2. The answer is B. *(Chapter 2, VI B)* Scopolamine is a competitive muscarinic blocker and therefore most closely resembles atropine in its mechanism of action. It is more potent than atropine in decreasing bronchial, salivary, and sweat gland secretions, in its sedative effect, and in producing mydriasis and cycloplegia. It is less potent than atropine in its effects on the heart, bronchial muscle, and intestines.

3. The answer is E. *(Chapter 10, I C 3 a)* Cardiovascular function is usually maintained when physiologic doses of glucocorticoids are given. This is probably so because glucocorticoids have the ability to potentiate norepinephrine. Physiologic doses of glucocorticoids can result in all of the other changes listed in the question.

4. The answer is A. *(Chapter 5, V A 3, B, C 2 b, 3 c)* Minoxidil is reserved for the treatment of moderate to severe hypertension. It is used in combination with a β-adrenergic blocking agent and a diuretic to minimize the dosage requirement. All of the other statements in the question are correct basic considerations for the treatment of hypertension.

5. The answer is D. *(Chapter 1, VIII E)* In physiologic antagonism, both agonists may have intrinsic activity; the agonist and the antagonist, however, act upon different receptors. In pharmacologic antagonism, the agonist has intrinsic activity but the antagonist has little or no intrinsic activity. Partial antagonists, such as nalorphine, possess some intrinsic activity.

6. The answer is A. *(Chapter 11, IV F 5 b (5))* Vincristine is far superior to vinblastine in the treatment of lymphocytic leukemia. When combined with prednisone, it is the treatment of choice for inducing remission in acute lymphoblastic leukemia in children.

7. The answer is C. *(Chapter 9, X A 3 a)* Rapid lympholysis produces large quantities of uric acid via nucleic acid release and catabolism. Therefore, the xanthine oxidase inhibitor allopurinol is given because it inhibits uric acid formation and thus is effective in preventing acute gouty arthritis attacks during antineoplastic therapy. Because allopurinol is an inhibitor of xanthine oxidase, it increases the renal excretion of xanthine and hypoxanthine. Since allopurinol is an analog of hypoxanthine it inhibits the metabolism of purines, not pyrimidines.

8. The answer is E. *(Chapter 13, III B 1, 4)* Mercury, like arsenic, binds to sulfhydryl groups on proteins, frequently inactivating those proteins that are enzymes, or producing structural damage. Interactions with the ferric ions of the cytochrome oxidase system is the principal mechanism of cyanide damage. Hemoglobin synthesis is disrupted by lead, which causes a microcytic hypochromic anemia. A number of substances can cause methemoglobinemia (nitrites, nitrates, chlorates, quinones), but mercury is not one of them.

9. The answer is E. *(Chapter 6, VIII B 4; Chapter 11, VI D 6; Chapter 13, II F 3)* The antitumor agent cisplatin causes severe nephrotoxicity if it is given without concomitant hydration or a diuretic. The osmotic diuretic mannitol is most commonly employed to reduce this side effect. Mannitol is also useful prophylactically to reduce the risk of acute renal failure in conditions such as cardiovascular operations and severe trauma. The other listed diuretics are not as effective as mannitol in these situations.

10. The answer is D. *(Chapter 7, II B 5)* Although iron-deficiency anemia is common during pregnancy, it is a hypochromic, microcytic anemia. A deficiency of vitamin B_{12} or intrinsic factor (or both) causes megaloblastic anemia, but is not especially likely to occur during pregnancy. Vitamin K deficiency can affect blood clotting, but does not cause an anemia. Because folic acid requirements increase during pregnancy, the most likely cause of Mrs. Jones's anemia is a folic acid deficiency.

11. The answer is E. *(Chapter 5, IV A 3 a, 8)* All of the listed untoward effects are seen except impotence. Headache usually decreases after the first few days of treatment. Dilation of cerebral vessels can result in increased intracerebral pressure. Dizziness and cerebral ischemia can be associated with postural hypotension. When present in large amounts, nitrite ions can oxidize hemoglobin to methemoglobin.

12. The answer is D. *(Chapter 3, III C 3 e, g)* Phenytoin can exacerbate petit mal seizures. Other untoward effects include gastrointestinal irritation, ataxia and diplopia, gingival hyperplasia, hypersensitivity reactions, hirsutism, hepatitis, and drug interactions.

13. The answer is C. *(Chapter 6, VII B)* The therapeutic uses of furosemide are many, but hypocalcemia is not one of these. To the contrary, furosemide is useful for the treatment of *hyper*calcemia because it increases the renal excretion of calcium. Other clinical uses include the treatment of both acute and chronic edema from such conditions as cirrhosis, renal disease, acute pulmonary edema, and congestive heart failure.

14. The answer is A. *(Chapter 5, II H)* Digitalis glycosides have a low margin of safety. In most patients the lethal dose is likely to be only 5 to 10 times the minimal effective dose. Intoxication can be precipitated by hypokalemia, a condition that is often the result of diuretic therapy but can also be the result of protracted vomiting or diarrhea. Other signs of toxicity include abnormal color perception and, more importantly, ventricular tachycardia.

15. The answer is A. *(Chapter 1, II B 1 c (4))* After oral administration, a drug is absorbed in the intestine and then passes through the liver. Some drugs (e.g., propranolol) can undergo extensive hepatic metabolism before reaching the site of action. With most other routes of administration, this first-pass effect does not occur because extensive hepatic passage immediately after drug absorption is avoided.

16. The answer is E. *(Chapter 2, VI A 1, 4 f)* Atropine is both a central and a peripheral muscarinic blocker. Atropine competes reversibly with acetylcholine at muscarinic receptors, antagonizes the action of acetylcholine in the central nervous system, and, at high levels, blocks acetylcholine action at ganglionic synapses and motor nerve endings.

17. The answer is D. *(Chapter 6, IV B, C)* The carbonic anhydrase inhibitor acetazolamide, although a weak diuretic, is useful in the treatment of glaucoma and petit mal epilepsy. The high-ceiling diuretics, namely ethacrynic acid and furosemide, the thiazide diuretic chlorothiazide, and the postassium-sparing diuretic spironolactone are not effective agents in the treatment of glaucoma or epilepsy, although they are more effective as diuretics.

18. The answer is C. *(Chapter 3, IX F)* Pentazocine produces less nausea than other opioids, and shows a correlation between dose, analgesic potency, and depressant potency. It can cause constipation like other narcotics, and tolerance to the analgesic effect can occur. Pentazocine can cause an increase in cardiac work by increasing pulmonary and peripheral vascular resistance.

19. The answer is C. *(Chapter 5, II H 3; Chapter 6, IX B; Chapter 13, III D)* Reduction in serum potassium levels (hypokalemia) is an extremely common untoward effect of most diuretics. Hypokalemia greatly increases the potential for digitalis-induced cardiac arrhythmias. The potassium-sparing diuretics, such as spironolactone, do not produce hypokalemia and thus do not add to the toxic potential of digitalis.

20. The answer is C. *(Chapter 3, IX C 1, 4)* Heroin has a more rapid onset of action than morphine. Tolerance and dependence occur frequently with both opioids. Morphine increases biliary tract pressure by causing constriction at the sphincter of Oddi. When administered to a pain-free person morphine can produce dysphoria. It has a stimulatory effect on the chemoreceptor trigger zone, producing nausea or vomiting.

21. The answer is B (1, 3). *(Chapter 12, XI G, H; XII A, C)* Both piperazine and pyrantel pamoate are effective in the treatment of ascariasis. Metronidazole is useful in the treatment of protozoal and anaerobic bacterial infections, while suramin is useful in the treatment of trypanosomiasis and onchoceriasis.

22. The answer is D (4). *(Chapter 9, II B 6; IV B 1, 3; V B 3; VI B)* Phenylbutazone, by directly affecting the renal tubules, can cause significant salt and water retention, leading to edema. Phenylbutazone can cause agranulocytosis or aplastic anemia. Although indomethacin also can cause blood dyscrasias, its salt-retaining properties are much less significant than with phenylbutazone. The properties of sulindac are similar to those of indomethacin.

23. The answer is D (4). *(Chapter 8, III A 1)* Most H_2 receptor blockers are substituted imidazoles; H_1 receptor blockers are substituted ethylamines. H_1 blockers have minimal cardiac effects. As a class the

H_1 blockers do not alter gastric secretion, since this is primarily mediated by H_2 receptors. H_1 blockers are, however, capable of producing unpleasant sedation.

24. The answer is B (1, 3). *(Chapter 6, VI D 1; VII D 1)* Hypokalemia is a potential complication of both furosemide and hydrochlorothiazide therapy. If a patient is concurrently receiving digoxin therapy, aggravated toxicity of this cardiac glycoside can become a major therapeutic problem. Correcting the hypokalemia is essential.

25. The answer is D (4). *(Chapter 6, VI D 1; IX A 2, B 2 a)* Both spironolactone and triamterene are used as adjunct diuretics for preventing hypokalemia, but they are not used for the treatment of hypokalemia once it occurs. Insulin and glucose are used for the treatment of hyperkalemia. Immediate potassium supplementation with oral preparations is indicated.

26. The answer is A (1, 2, 3). *(Chapter 4, II A 3, C 2)* Procaine is a diethylaminoethanol ester and para-aminobenzoic acid. It does interfere with sodium influx during depolarization. It has a short duration of action and is metabolized by pseudocholinesterase. Unlike procainamide, procaine does not cause a lupus-like syndrome.

27. The answer is D (4). *(Chapter 12, IX B 5)* Amphotericin B is effective in the treatment of acute pulmonary coccidioidomycosis. The other agents listed would be ineffective. Griseofulvin is used for mycotic diseases of the skin, hair, and nails. Flucytosine is used for systemic infections caused by *Candida albicans* or *Cryptococcus meningitidis.* Penicillin G has no antifungal activity.

28. The answer is B (1, 3). *(Chapter 13, II C 2 b)* Antacids inhibit the absorption of tetracycline because ions such as aluminum in antacids can chelate the tetracycline. Antacids do not stimulate or inhibit the drug microsomal metabolizing system, nor do they enhance the renal excretion of tetracycline.

29. The answer is A (1, 2, 3). *(Chapter 1, VI C)* Factors known to affect drug metabolism in humans include the chemical properties of the drug; the dose; the route of administration; concomitant drug therapy; the patient's genetic makeup, age, gender, and diet; circadian rhythms; and the presence of significant disease. No direct relationship between the apparent volume of distribution and drug metabolism has been established.

30. The answer is D (4). *(Chapter 10, II A, B)* Oral contraceptives interfere with pituitary function by blocking the surge of luteinizing hormone (LH) and follicle-stimulating hormone (FSH) that normally occurs in the middle of the menstrual cycle. In this way, they suppress ovulation and ovarian follicle growth.

31. The answer is B (1, 3). *(Chapter 12, II E 1)* The major indication for the use of sulfa drugs is in the treatment of acute uncomplicated urinary tract infections. Carbenicillin and gentamicin represent very broad-spectrum therapy, which is unnecessary for the treatment of an uncomplicated cystitis.

32. The answer is A (1, 2, 3). *(Chapter 2, III A 4)* Ergot alkaloids, by directly stimulating vascular smooth muscle, are useful in treating migraine headaches. Their chemical structure resembles LSD and thus CNS stimulation can occur. Ergot alkaloids are weak α-blockers and therefore would not be blocked by propranolol.

33. The answer is A (1, 2, 3). *(Chapter 10, I C 9)* Corticosteroids, especially when used for long periods, can result in all of the untoward effects listed in the question except for muscle hypertrophy. Rather, a myopathy can occur which is characterized by proximal arm and leg weakness.

34. The answer is B (1, 3). *(Chapter 4, II A 1–3, C 4 d; Chapter 5, III E 3)* Lidocaine is an effective antiarrhythmic agent and is the drug of choice for premature ventricular contractions, although it is ineffective in atrial arrhythmias. It decreases sodium but not potassium conductance in automatic cells.

35. The answer is A (1, 2, 3). *(Chapter 11, III C 1)* Allopurinol blocks rather than stimulates the metabolism of 6-mercaptopurine. In addition, allopurinol blocks the formation of uric acid from hypoxanthine and xanthine. All of the other statements about 6-mercaptopurine in the question are correct.

36. The answer is B (1, 3). *(Chapter 12, III E 2, H 2 b; V C 2 b, VI F 1 g (2); VIII D 1 d)* In a patient with renal disease, any antibiotic which is renally excreted should be administered with caution. Penicillin and tobramycin are two such antibiotics. Both erythromycin and doxycycline (in contrast to other tetracyclines) are excreted in the bile and feces; thus, they are useful in the treatment of infections in renally compromised patients.

37. The answer is C (2, 4). *(Chapter 4, II B 2, C 2 c, 3 c (1), 4 a, c, 8 a)* Lidocaine is an amide and, like mepivacaine, is metabolized in the liver. Procaine is metabolized by pseudocholinesterase. Tetracaine is the most frequently used spinal anesthetic agent.

38. The answer is A (1, 2, 3). *(Chapter 12, V E 1; VI C 2, E 2 c; VIII E 1 b)* Both the tetracyclines and erythromycin are effective in the treatment of primary atypical pneumonias. Streptomycin is most often used in combination with other drugs for the treatment of tuberculosis.

39. The answer is D (4). *(Chapter 12, VIII E 1)* Erythromycin is effective for the treatment of Legionnaires' disease. It is initially difficult to differentiate this disease from mycoplasmal pneumonia.

40. The answer is A (1, 2, 3). *(Chapter 9, I B; II B 1 b, 2 d, 3 c, 6 b, D 4 c)* Aspirin has analgesic, antipyretic, and anti-inflammatory activity, all of which are mediated by an inhibition of prostaglandin synthesis. Aspirin can increase mean bleeding time, while toxic doses can produce respiratory and metabolic acidosis. Excretion is increased by alkalinizing, not acidifying, the urine.

41. The answer is C (2, 4). *(Chapter 8, II B 3, C 2 a (2), D 2 a, G 2 c (3))* Bradykinin and prostaglandin F are vasodilators in the human microcirculation. Serotonin is capable of constricting arteries and veins, especially in the renal vasculature. Angiotensin II is one of the most potent vasoconstrictors known, causing a pronounced increase in blood pressure.

42. The answer is B (1, 3). *(Chapter 2, IV C)* Carbachol (carbamylcholine) is a parasympathetic agent which is resistant to cholinesterase because of its carbamic acid–ester link. It exerts both muscarinic and nicotinic effects.

43. The answer is C (2, 4). *(Chapter 11, I C, D)* Each dose of an antineoplastic agent kills a constant fraction of the tumor cells rather than a fixed number of cells. Many of the commonly used antineoplastic agents have been found to be much more effective when administered in combination with other antitumor drugs; the MOPP regimen, which combines mechlorethamine, vincristine (Oncovin), procarbazine, and prednisone, is an example. One reason why combinations are effective is that the individual drugs may kill different tumor cell populations; moreover, because their toxic effects on the patient do not overlap, dose reductions of the individual drugs are not necessary. Although some drugs, such as methotrexate, are self-limiting, most agents are not. Only a few of the antitumor agents, for example vincristine, act on cells in mitosis; most drugs that are phase-specific affect cells in other phases of the cell cycle.

44. The answer is A (1, 2, 3). *(Chapter 3, VI C 7)* All of the listed untoward effects can be seen with benzodiazepine administration except seizures. Drugs of this class possess significant anticonvulsant activity.

45. The answer is C (2, 4). *(Chapter 10, I A 6, 7, B 3, C 3 b; Table 10-1)* Both desoxycorticosterone and aldosterone are mineralocorticoids and thus have no anti-inflammatory effects. Corticotropin (ACTH) and cortisol (hydrocortisone) possess anti-inflammatory properties, ACTH because it stimulates glucocorticoid synthesis, and cortisol because it is a glucocorticoid.

46. The answer is A (1, 2, 3). *(Chapter 5, III B 3, 8 a)* Quinidine reduces the maximal rate of rise ($\dot{V}_{max}$) of depolarization during phase O. It increases the effective refractory period (ERP) but decreases automaticity in ventricular tissue. Quinidine depresses myocardial contractility, and caution must therefore be used if quinidine is administered to patients with any degree of congestive heart failure.

47. The answer is C (2, 4). *(Chapter 1, III E 2)* Carrier-mediated facilitated diffusion is a saturable process and does not require energy. It is specific for the chemical structure of the drug. Since it is a diffusion process it cannot move against a concentration gradient.

48. The answer is E (all). *(Chapter 8, I A 1, B 1; II A 3, D 2 a)* All of the statements in the question are true statements about autacoids. Autacoids are a heterogeneous collection of substances that originate in diffuse tissues and act locally or on distant organs after transport in the circulation. The primary function of autacoids is currently believed to be in modulating inflammation or local circulation. Both histamine and kinins are potent vasodilators and cause the "triple response" of reddening, flare, and halo. Histamine is believed to act either by altering cell permeability to calcium ions or by elevating cyclic AMP.

49. The answer is E (all). *(Chapter 11, IV D)* Bleomycin is a natural product that intercalates with DNA and causes both single- and double-strand scissions in DNA. It requires ferrous ion and molecular oxygen to produce the superoxide and hydroxyl free radicals necessary for the DNA strand breaks. The most sensitive cells are cells in G_2 and M phase of the cell cycle.

50. The answer is C (2, 4). *(Chapter 3, IX C, F)* This patient appears to have taken an overdose of a narcotic. Both naloxone and nalorphine are opioid antagonists and would be capable of reversing these symptoms. The latter, however, is a partial antagonist, while the former is a pure antagonist.

51. The answer is C (2, 4). *(Chapter 10, IV K 1 b)* This patient is rapidly approaching insulin shock. Her insulin dose is probably too high. Because of her low glucose level she would not be "spilling" sugar into her urine.

52. The answer is A (1, 2, 3). *(Chapter 2, V D 1)* Diisopropyl fluorophosphate (DFP) is an irreversible cholinesterase inhibitor which increases acetylcholine levels. Increased lacrimation, salivation, and increased muscle twitching are cholinergic (cholinomimetic) effects; increased bronchodilation is not.

53–56. The answers are: 53-E, 54-C, 55-B, 56-A. *(Chapter 4, III A 2, 4–6, B 3)* Thiopental is administered intravenously for induction of anesthesia but is not adequate alone except for short procedures. Nitrous oxide has a minimum alveolar concentration (MAC) of 105.2 percent, making it the least potent inhalation anesthetic agent used. Diethyl ether is a highly explosive anesthetic agent and thus has limited usefulness. Halothane is the most widely used anesthetic agent in the United States and has been associated with hepatitis and liver necrosis which may be due to toxic or immunogenic products.

57–60. The answers are: 57-B, 58-D, 59-C, 60-C. *(Chapter 6, I F; IV A 1; VI A 2; VII A 1; IX B 1 b)* Although acetazolamide acts on both the proximal and distal convoluted tubules, its effects on the proximal tubules are quantitatively most important for its diuretic actions. Spironolactone, a potassium-sparing diuretic, acts as a competitive antagonist of aldosterone. The receptor for aldosterone is located in the distal convoluted tubule, and thus this is the site of action for spironolactone. Furosemide is a high-ceiling diuretic and, like ethacrynic acid, it inhibits Cl^- reabsorption in the ascending limb of the loop of Henle. Chlorothiazide is one of a variety of thiazide diuretics. The thiazides, like the high-ceiling diuretics, act primarily on the ascending limb of the loop of Henle. Cl^- reabsorption is inhibited and there is an increased renal excretion of Na^+, Cl^-, HCO_3^-, and K^+.

1
General Pharmacologic Principles

I. SOME BASIC DEFINITIONS

A. PHARMACOLOGY: The study of the biochemical and physiologic aspects of drug effects, including absorption, distribution, metabolism, elimination, toxicity, and specific mechanisms of drug action.

B. PHARMACOKINETICS: The quantitative aspects of drug absorption, distribution, and excretion. Once the pharmacokinetics of a drug is determined, rational dosage regimens can be instituted.

C. RECEPTOR: A specific drug-binding site in a cell or on its surface which mediates the action of the drug. Some drugs (e.g., mannitol) are believed not to have specific receptors.

II. FACTORS AFFECTING DRUG ABSORPTION

A. DOSAGE is an important determinant of the drug's concentration at its site of action and, thus, greatly influences the biological response to the drug. The larger the dose the greater will be the effect, until a maximum effect is achieved. This is called the **dose–response relationship**.

B. ROUTE OF ADMINISTRATION is an important determinant of the rate and efficiency of absorption.

1. **Alimentary routes** are the most common routes of administration.
   - **a.** Examples of alimentary routes:
     - **(1)** Oral.
     - **(2)** Rectal.
     - **(3)** Sublingual.
   - **b. Advantages of alimentary administration**
     - **(1)** An alimentary route is generally the safest route of administration. The delivery of the drug into the circulation is slow after oral administration, so that rapid, high blood levels and untoward effects are avoided.
     - **(2)** Alimentary routes allow for convenient dosage forms that do not require sterile technique.
   - **c. Disadvantages of alimentary administration**
     - **(1)** The rate of absorption is variable. This becomes a problem if only a small range in blood levels separates a drug's desired therapeutic effect from its toxic effects.
     - **(2)** Irritation of mucosal surfaces can occur.
     - **(3)** The compliance of the patient is not ensured.
     - **(4)** With oral administration of some drugs, extensive hepatic metabolism (**"first-pass effect"**) may occur before the drug reaches its site of action. Passage through the liver, and, thus, extensive initial hepatic metabolism, is avoided by the sublingual route.
2. **Parenteral routes** bypass the alimentary canal and result in direct drug absorption.
   - **a.** Examples of parenteral routes:
     - **(1)** Intravenous (IV).
     - **(2)** Intramuscular (IM).
     - **(3)** Subcutaneous (SC).
     - **(4)** Intraperitoneal (IP).
     - **(5)** Intra-arterial (IA).

(6) Intrathecal (IT).
(7) Transdermal.

b. **Advantages of parenteral administration**
   (1) There is a rapid response, which may be required in an emergency.
   (2) The dose is accurate because of complete absorption.
   (3) Parenteral administration provides an alternative when the alimentary route is not feasible; for example, when the patient is unconscious.

c. **Disadvantages of parenteral administration**
   (1) The more rapid absorption can lead to an increase in untoward effects.
   (2) Both a sterile formulation and the use of aseptic technique are required.
   (3) Local irritation may occur at the site of injection.

3. **Miscellaneous routes**
   a. **Topical administration** is useful in the treatment of local conditions; there is little systemic absorption.
   b. **Inhalation** provides a rapid route of administration; it is used for volatile anesthetics and many bronchodilators.

III. DRUG TRANSPORT

A. **BIOAVAILABILITY** is the relative rate at which an administered drug reaches the general circulation, and is important when a drug is administered orally. Factors which influence bioavailability are:

1. Solubility of the drug in the contents of the stomach.
2. Dietary patterns.
3. Tablet size.
4. Quality control in manufacturing and formulation.

B. The absorption of a drug through the mucosal lining of the gastrointestinal tract or through capillary walls depends on the physical and chemical properties of the drug.

C. Drugs can cross cellular membranes by passive diffusion, carrier-mediated diffusion, active transport, or endocytosis. The cell membrane, being a bimolecular lipid layer, can act as a barrier to some drugs.

D. **PASSIVE DIFFUSION.** Most foreign compounds penetrate cells by diffusing as the **un-ionized moiety** through the lipid membrane. Factors affecting the passage of a molecule through a membrane are the molecule's size and charge, the lipid–water partition coefficient, and the concentration gradient. The two types of passive drug transport are **simple diffusion** and **filtration.**

1. **Simple diffusion**
   a. Simple diffusion is based on **Fick's law**:

$$dQ/dt = (-D)(A)(dc/dx)$$

where dQ/dt is the rate of drug flux (i.e., the change in concentration of a drug within a given time); D is a temperature-dependent diffusion constant of the molecule; A is the area of the absorbing surface; and dc/dx is the concentration gradient.

   (1) The greater the concentration gradient, the greater the rate of absorption.
   (2) The larger the absorbing surface, the greater the drug flux.
   (3) The diffusion constant, D, is directly proportional to the temperature and is inversely related to the molecular size.
   (4) The greater the lipid–water partition coefficient, the greater the drug flux.

   b. In simple diffusion, molecules cross the lipid membrane in an **uncharged form**. The distribution of the uncharged form is a function of the pK_a of the compound and the pH of the medium, and is expressed by the **Henderson-Hasselbalch equation**:
   (1) If the drug is a weak acid:

$$pK_a = pH + \log \frac{\text{concentration of un-ionized acid}}{\text{concentration of ionized acid}}$$

(2) If the drug is a weak base:

$$pK_a = pH + \log \frac{\text{concentration of ionized base}}{\text{concentration of un-ionized base}}$$

c. The pH of the medium therefore affects the absorption and excretion of a passively diffused drug.

(1) Aspirin and other weak acids are best absorbed in the stomach because of its acidic environment.

(2) Basic drugs are best absorbed in the small intestine, which has a higher pH.

(3) Since the pH of urine is acidic, a weakly acidic drug can be extensively reabsorbed into the body from the urine. If the pH of the urine is increased, excretion of the drug can be increased.

2. Filtration

a. Water, ions, and some polar and nonpolar molecules of low molecular weight can diffuse through membranes, suggesting that "pores" or "channels" may exist.

b. The capillaries of some vascular beds (e.g., in the kidney) have larger pores which permit the passage of molecules as large as proteins.

E. CARRIER-MEDIATED FACILITATED DIFFUSION

1. In this type of transport, movement across the membrane is facilitated by a macromolecule.

2. The properties of carrier-mediated diffusion are as follows:

a. It is a saturable process; that is, external concentrations can be achieved in which increasing the external/internal concentration gradient will not increase the rate of influx.

b. It is specific for the chemical structure of a drug.

c. It requires no energy.

d. It cannot move against a concentration gradient and, therefore, is still a diffusion process.

F. ACTIVE TRANSPORT

1. Active transport is similar to carrier-mediated diffusion in several ways:

a. Movement across the membrane is mediated by a macromolecule.

b. It is a saturable process.

c. It is specific for chemical structure.

2. Several important features, however, distinguish active transport from diffusion processes:

a. Active transport requires metabolic energy; this is often generated by the enzyme known as Na^+-K^+-ATPase.

b. It transports molecules against a concentration gradient.

G. ENDOCYTOSIS is a minor method by which some drugs are transported into cells.

1. A vacuolar apparatus in some cells is responsible for this process.

2. There exist both **fluid-phase endocytosis** for substances such as sucrose and **adsorptive-phase endocytosis** for substances such as insulin.

IV. DRUG DISTRIBUTION

A. Once in the circulatory system, some drugs can bind nonspecifically and reversibly to various plasma proteins; that is, to albumin or globulins.

1. In this case, an equilibrium is produced between bound and free drug.

2. Only the **free drug** exerts a biologic effect; bound drug can not leave the vascular space, and is not metabolized or eliminated.

B. In general, the distribution of a drug to a particular region of the body depends on the blood flow to that region and on the physical and chemical properties of the drug; an example is the distribution of barbiturates to the central nervous system (see Chapter 3, II A).

C. Some areas of the body are not readily accessible to drugs due to anatomic barriers; examples are the brain and the fetus.

D. Some drugs may be sequestered in storage depots; for example, lipid-soluble drugs in fatty tissue. These depots are in equilibrium with free circulating drug.

E. Eventually the drug achieves a free state and is excreted either directly or after it has been metabolized.

V. EXCRETION

A. THE KIDNEY is the most important excretory organ for drugs. Excretion of drugs and their metabolites into the urine involves three processes:

1. Glomerular filtration.
2. Active tubular secretion.
3. Passive tubular reabsorption.

B. THE BILIARY TRACT AND THE FECES are important in the excretion of some drugs that are metabolized in the liver. In general, the minimum molecular weight of substances eliminated in the bile is probably 300 to 600 daltons.

C. OTHER ROUTES. Drugs and their metabolites can also be eliminated in expired air, in sweat, saliva, and tears, and in breast milk.

VI. DRUG METABOLISM

A. PRINCIPLES

1. The liver is the major site of metabolism for many drugs, but many nonhepatic organs, such as the lungs, kidneys, and adrenal glands, can also metabolize drugs.
2. Many lipid-soluble, weak organic acids or bases are not readily eliminated from the body and must be metabolized to compounds that are more polar and less lipid-soluble.
3. Metabolism often but not always results in **inactivation** of the compound.
4. Some drugs (often called **prodrugs**) are **activated** by metabolism.

B. BIOCHEMICAL REACTIONS INVOLVED IN DRUG METABOLISM

1. **Oxidation.** The most common type of metabolic reaction, oxidation involves the addition of oxygen or the removal of hydrogen from the drug.
   a. **Microsomal oxidation**
      (1) A collection of membrane-associated enzymes are located in the smooth endoplasmic reticulum (ER) of cells in many organs, especially the liver, and are responsible for drug oxidation.
      (2) The subcellular components of the ER, called **microsomes**, can be isolated by centrifugation of organ homogenates.
      (3) Primary components of this enzyme system are cytochrome P-450 reductase and cytochrome P-450.
      (4) This enzyme system has been termed a **mixed-function oxygenase** because one oxygen atom in molecular oxygen is incorporated into a drug in the form of a hydroxyl (–OH) moiety and the other is incorporated into water. Reduced nicotinamide adenine dinucleotide phosphate (NADPH) provides the reducing equivalents.
      (5) Types of microsomal oxidation reactions are:
         (a) Carbon oxidation–hydroxylation of aliphatic or aromatic groups.
         (b) *N*- or *O*-dealkylation.
         (c) *N*-oxidation or *N*-hydroxylation.
         (d) Sulfoxide formation.
         (e) Deamination.
         (f) Desulfuration.
      (6) The microsomal oxidative system also metabolizes endogenous fatty acids and steroids.
      (7) A number of drugs and environmental substances can induce (increase) or inhibit the microsomal enzyme system (see Chapter 13, II E 5).
   b. **Nonmicrosomal oxidation**
      (1) Soluble enzymes found in the cytosol or mitochondria of cells are responsible for the metabolism of a relatively few compounds. These enzyme activities are, however, important.

(2) Examples include:

(a) Alcohol dehydrogenase and aldehyde dehydrogenase, which oxidize ethanol to acetaldehyde and then to acetate, respectively, in reactions requiring oxidized nicotinamide adenine dinucleotide (NAD^+).

(b) Xanthine oxidase, which converts hypoxanthine to xanthine, and xanthine to uric acid.

(c) Tyrosine hydroxylase, which is important in the synthesis of adrenergic neurotransmitters because it hydroxylates tyrosine to dopa (L-β-3,4-dihydroxyphenylalanine).

(d) Monoamine oxidase, which is important in the metabolism of catecholamines and serotonin.

2. **Reduction**. Reduction occurs in both the microsomal and nonmicrosomal metabolizing systems; it is less common than oxidation. Examples are the reduction of nitro and azide groups.

3. **Hydrolysis**. Nonmicrosomal hydrolases exist in a wide variety of body systems, including the plasma. Microsomal hydrolases have also been identified. Examples of nonmicrosomal hydrolases are:

a. Nonspecific esterases for drugs such as acetylcholine, succinylcholine, and procaine.

b. Peptidases.

c. Phosphatases.

d. Amidases for drugs such as procainamide and nicotinamide.

4. **Conjugation** involves the coupling of a drug or its metabolite with an endogenous substrate, usually inorganic sulfate, a methyl group, acetic acid, an amino acid, or a carbohydrate.

a. **Glucuronide conjugation** is the most common conjugation reaction. It occurs frequently with phenols, alcohols, and carboxylic acids.

(1) "Activated" glucuronic acid (uridine diphosphoglucuronic acid; UDP-glucuronide) is formed from glucose 1-phosphate, which then reacts as follows:

$$\text{UDP-glucuronide} + \text{ROH} \rightarrow \text{RO-glucuronide} + \text{UDP}$$

where ROH is the drug or its metabolite.

(2) Glucuronides are generally inactive and are rapidly excreted in urine or bile by anionic transport systems.

(3) Glucuronides eliminated in the bile can be hydrolyzed by intestinal or bacterial β-glucuronidases, and free drug can be reabsorbed. This **enterohepatic recirculation** can greatly extend the action of a drug.

b. **Other conjugation reactions**. All conjugations except glucuronide formation are catalyzed by nonmicrosomal enzymes. These reactions include:

(1) Sulfate formation, in which phenols, alcohols, and aromatic amines are converted to sulfates and sulfanilates; 3′-phosphoadenosine 5′-phosphosulfate (PAPS) is the sulfate donor.

(2) *O*-, *S*-, and *N*-methylation; *S*-adenosylmethionine is the methyl donor.

(3) *N*-acetylation; acetyl coenzyme A is the acetyl donor.

(4) Glycine and glutamine conjugation with acids (e.g., salicylic acid).

(5) Glutathione conjugation.

C. FACTORS AFFECTING DRUG METABOLISM

1. The **chemical properties** of the drug.

2. The **route of administration**. The oral route, for example, can result in extensive hepatic metabolism of some drugs (the **"first-pass" effect**).

2. **Genetics**.The acetylation of isoniazid and related drugs is under genetic control.

4. **Diet**. Starvation can deplete glycine stores and alter glycine conjugation.

5. **Dosage**. Toxic doses can deplete enzymes needed for detoxification reactions.

6. **Age**. The liver can not detoxify drugs such as chloramphenicol as well in neonates as it can in adults.

7. **Gender**. Young males are more prone to sedation from barbiturates than females are.

8. **Disease**. Liver disease decreases the ability of an individual to metabolize drugs, while kidney disease hampers the excretion of drugs.

9. **Species differences.** Experimental findings in animals do not necessarily translate to humans.

10. **Circadian rhythm.** In rats and mice the rate of hepatic metabolism of some drugs follows a diurnal rhythm. This may be true in humans as well.

VII. PHARMACOKINETICS

A. ABSORPTION

1. After any route of administration except IV, the absorption of most drugs follows **first-order (exponential) kinetics**; thus, a constant *fraction* of drug is absorbed.

2. After IV administration, the absorption of a drug follows **zero-order kinetics**; thus, a constant *amount* (i.e., 100 percent) of drug is absorbed.

B. ELIMINATION

1. For most drugs, elimination from the blood follows exponential (first-order) kinetics.

2. Saturation of the elimination process can occur after high doses of some drugs, and zero-order kinetics will follow. Ethanol is a prototypic example.

3. For drugs that are eliminated by first-order kinetics, the fractional change in the amount of drug in the plasma or blood per unit of time is expressed by the **half-time ($t_{1/2}$)**; that is, the time it takes for one-half of the drug to be eliminated, or by the **rate constant** (k), which is equal to $0.693/t_{1/2}$.

C. DISTRIBUTION

1. **One-compartment model.** This is the simplest and most commonly used pharmacokinetic model system.
   a. Distribution of the drug within the compartment is assumed to be **uniform**, and is assumed to occur **rapidly** in comparison to absorption and elimination.
   b. The **apparent volume of distribution** (V_d) is a quantitative estimate of the tissue localization of a drug and can be determined by measuring the plasma level of the drug:

$$V_d = \frac{\text{total amount of drug in body}}{\text{concentration of drug in plasma}}$$

   c. The **total body clearance** is the product of the volume of distribution times the elimination rate constant:

$$\text{Total body clearance} = (V_d)(k)$$

2. **Two-compartment model**
   a. This model is generally more useful for drugs that are not given IV because it can better describe both distribution and elimination.
   b. The distribution rate constant in this model is known as the **alpha half-time**, or $t_{1/2\alpha}$.
   c. The elimination rate constant in this model, known as the **beta half-time**, or $t_{1/2\beta}$, is therapeutically more important than the $t_{1/2\alpha}$.

3. The **multicompartment model** is necessary for a number of drugs that are stored in body depots, and for drugs with extensive metabolism or elimination mechanisms.

D. EFFECT OF REPEATED DOSES

1. A drug accumulates in the body if the time interval between doses is less than four half-times, in which case the total body stores of the drug increase exponentially to a plateau.

2. The **average total body store** of a drug at the plateau is a function of the dose, the interval between doses, and the elimination half-time of the drug; when the drug is administered at the half-time of elimination, the average total body store of the drug is approximately equal to **1.5 times** the amount administered.

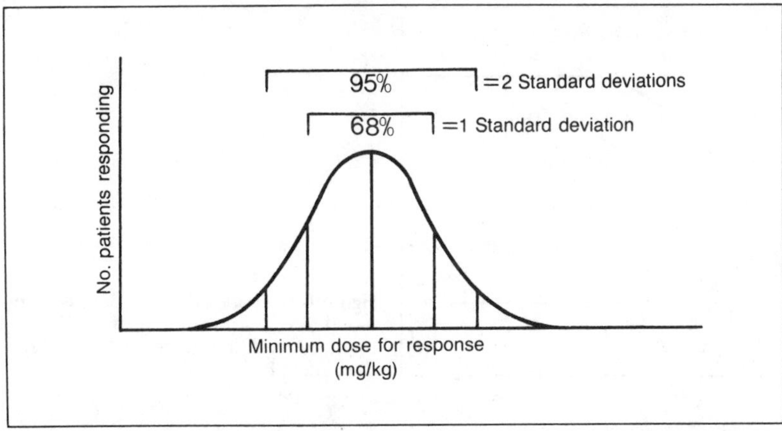

Figure 1-1. Frequency distribution curve, plotting the number of patients showing a quantal response to a drug against the minimum dose needed to produce the response.

VIII. DOSE–RESPONSE RELATIONSHIPS

A. QUANTAL DOSE–RESPONSE CURVE

1. A **quantal response** is an all-or-none response to a drug, and relates to the frequency with which a specified dose of a drug produces a specified response (e.g., death; or a 50 percent increase in blood pressure) in a population.
2. The smallest amount of a drug that will produce a quantal response is not the same for all the members of a population. If the frequency of response is plotted against the minimum dose necessary to produce the response, the result is often a gaussian distribution. A graphic representation of this gaussian **frequency distribution curve** is shown in Figure 1-1.
3. The **quantal dose–response curve** is a cumulative graph of the frequency distribution curve (Fig. 1-2).

B. GRADED DOSE–RESPONSE CURVE (Fig. 1-3)

1. As the dose administered to a single subject or isolated tissue is increased, the pharmacologic effect will also increase (the **graded dose–response**).
2. At a certain dose, the effect will reach a maximum level (the **ceiling effect**).
3. **Efficacy versus potency**
   a. The maximum effect of a drug, E_{max} (see Fig. 1-3), is a measure of drug **efficacy**.
   b. Efficacy is independent of the slope or position of the dose–response curve. In Figure 1-3, drugs A and B have equal efficacies (namely, E_{max}).
   c. Drugs such as aspirin and morphine produce the same pharmacologic effect (analgesia) but have very different levels of efficacy.

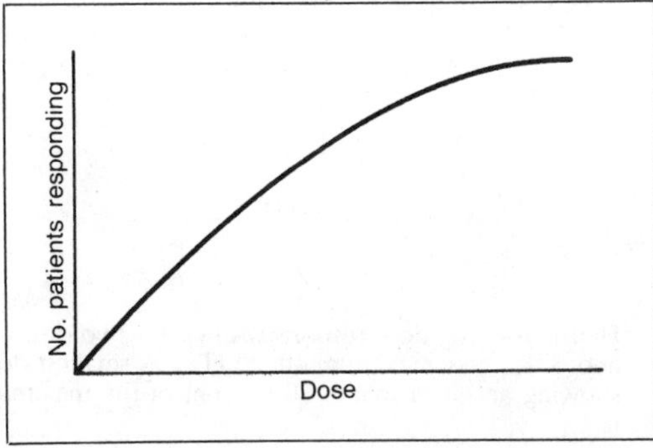

Figure 1-2. Quantal dose–response curve, cumulating the data used in plotting Figure 1-1.

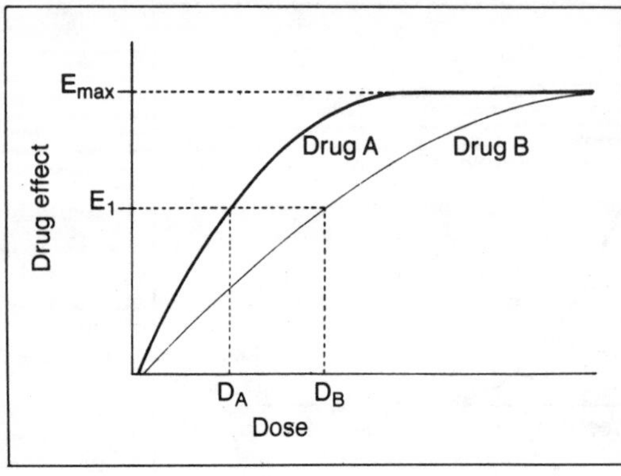

Figure 1-3. Graded dose–response curves for two drugs, A and B. E_{max} = maximum effect; D_A and D_B = amount of drug A and drug B, respectively, needed to produce drug effect E_1.

d. **Potency**, a comparative measure, refers to the different doses of two drugs that are needed to produce the same effect. In Figure 1-3, drug A is more potent than drug B, since the dose of drug B (D_B) must be larger than the dose of drug A (D_A) to produce a given effect (E_1).

e. Meaningful comparisons of potency can be made only when the drugs being compared have log dose–response curves (see VIII C, below) of the same slope.

f. Potency is independent of efficacy, and efficacy is usually more important than potency in selecting drugs for use in a clinical situation.

C. LOG DOSE–RESPONSE CURVE

1. To construct the log dose–response curve, the log of the dose is plotted on the abscissa and the drug effect on the ordinate. This causes the hyperbolic graded dose–response curve to become sigmoidal. Log dose–response curves for two drugs, A and B, are shown in Figure 1-4.
   a. The ED_{50}, the smallest dose showing an effect that is 50 percent of the maximum, is a measure of drug potency: the smaller the ED_{50}, the greater the potency. Thus, in Figure 1-4, drug A is more potent than drug B.
   b. Efficacy is indicated by the height of the log dose–response curve. Drug B in Figure 1-4 is less efficacious than drug A; the E_{max} of the two drugs is, therefore, different.

2. One advantage of plotting on a logarithmic scale is that drugs with the same action at a receptor, but with different potencies, will usually show dose–response curves that are parallel.

D. DRUG–RECEPTOR INTERACTIONS

1. It is currently believed that, for most drugs, the drug (D) combines reversibly with a receptor

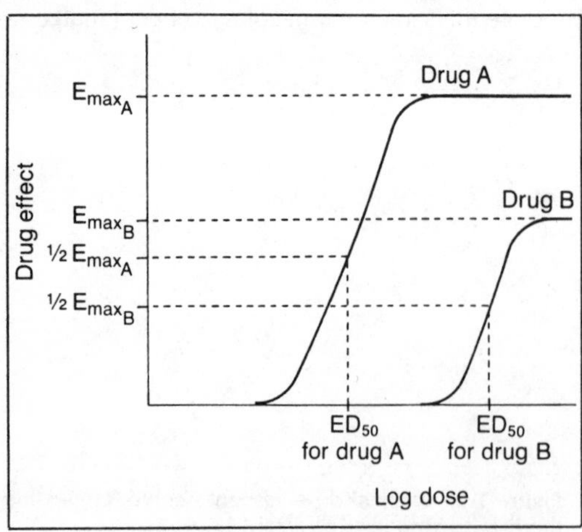

Figure 1-4. Log dose-response curves for two drugs, A and B. E_{max} = maximum effect; ED_{50} = smallest dose showing an effect that is 50 percent of the maximum (E_{max}).

site (R) within a cell or on its surface to form a drug–receptor complex (DR).

$$D + R \rightleftharpoons DR$$

2. A sequence of events then takes place, often intracellularly, by which the drug–receptor complex produces an effect (E)—for example, a decrease in blood pressure.

$$DR \xrightarrow{\text{via sequence}} \dashrightarrow \dashrightarrow \xrightarrow[\text{of events}]{} E$$

3. In general, E is a function of the quantity of the drug–receptor complex, and can be expressed as

$$E = \alpha[DR]$$

   a. The magnitude of E depends on the amount of DR, which in turn depends on the amount of drug given. Once all receptors are saturated, the maximum effect is achieved.
   b. Alpha (α) is a constant for a given drug, and is a partial determinant of whether an effect occurs.
   c. Alpha (α) is determined experimentally, and is considered to be a measure of a drug's **intrinsic activity**; that is, its inherent ability to produce an effect. If α is zero, the drug has no intrinsic pharmacologic activity and, therefore, if the drug binds to the receptor, it must be an effective antagonist.

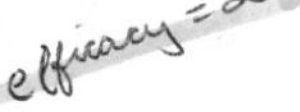

E. ANTAGONISMS BETWEEN DRUGS

1. **Agonists versus antagonists**
   a. An **agonist** is a drug that produces a pharmacologic effect (E) when it combines with a receptor.
   b. An **antagonist** is a drug which reduces or abolishes the effect of an agonist.
      (1) Examples of pure antagonists are atropine and curare, which inhibit the effect of acetylcholine.
      (2) The agonist, acetylcholine, possesses intrinsic activity, while both atropine and curare have zero intrinsic activity. They occupy cholinergic receptor sites (curare in nicotinic skeletal muscle, atropine in muscarinic smooth muscle; see Chapter 2, I D), preventing the further binding of acetylcholine to these receptors.
   c. Some drugs, for example nalorphine, are **partial antagonists**; that is, they possess some intrinsic activity. (same as partial agonist?)

2. **Pharmacologic antagonism** occurs when an antagonist prevents an agonist from acting upon its receptors to produce an effect. This type of antagonism can be either competitive or noncompetitive.
   a. **Competitive antagonism**
      (1) Competitive antagonists compete with agonists in a reversible fashion for the same receptor site.
      (2) When the antagonist is present, the log dose–response curve is shifted to the right, indicating that a higher concentration of agonist is necessary to achieve the same response as when the antagonist is absent.
      (3) In the presence of the antagonist, if enough agonist is given, the E_{max} can be achieved, indicating that the action of the antagonist has been overcome. This results in a parallel shift of the dose–response curve, as shown in Figure 1-5.

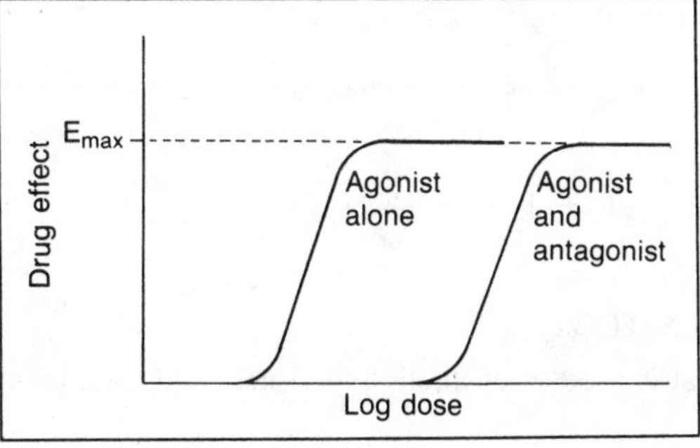

Figure 1-5. Shift in the log dose–response curve that occurs when an agonist is administered in the presence of a competitive antagonist.

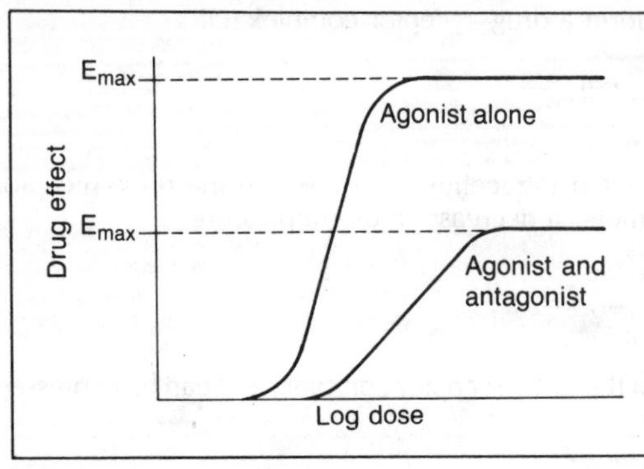

Figure 1-6. Shift in the log dose–response curve and lowering of the E_{max} that occurs when an agonist is given in the presence of a noncompetitive antagonist.

b. Noncompetitive antagonism

(1) The noncompetitive antagonist binds irreversibly to the receptor site or to another site that inhibits the response to the agonist.

(2) No matter how much agonist is given, the action of the antagonist can not be overcome.

(3) This results in a nonparallel shift of the log dose–response curve, with a lower E_{max} (Fig. 1-6).

3. **Physiologic antagonism**. With pharmacologic antagonism, the agonist and antagonist compete for the *same* receptor site. In contrast, with physiologic antagonism, the drugs act independently on two *different* receptors.
   - **a.** An example of physiologic antagonism is provided by drugs which act on the sympathetic and the parasympathetic nervous systems, which are antagonistic to one another.
   - **b.** The drug acting on the sympathetic nervous system increases the heart rate and causes vasoconstriction, whereas the parasympathetic drug decreases the heart rate and causes vasodilation.
4. **Antagonism by neutralization** occurs when two drugs combine with one another to form an inactive compound. For example, drugs containing sulfhydryl (–SH) groups, when combined with mercury or arsenic, no longer show agonistic actions.

F. ENHANCEMENT OF DRUG EFFECTS

1. **Additive drug effects** occur if two drugs with the same effect, when given together, produce an effect that is **equal in magnitude** to the sum of the effects when the drugs are given individually:

$$E_{AB} = E_A + E_B \qquad 1 + 1 = 2$$

2. **Synergism** occurs if two drugs with the same effect, when given together, produce an effect that is **greater in magnitude** than the sum of the effects when the drugs are given individually:

$$E_{AB} > E_A + E_B \qquad 1 + 1 > 2$$

3. **Potentiation** occurs if a drug lacking an effect of its own increases the effect of a second, active drug.

$$E_{AB} > E_A + E_B \qquad 0 + 1 > 1$$

G. THERAPEUTIC INDEX AND MARGIN OF SAFETY

1. The **therapeutic index** is a measure that is used in evaluating the safety and usefulness of a drug.

2. The formula for the therapeutic index is

$$TI = \frac{LD_{50}}{ED_{50}}$$

where LD_{50} is the minimum dose that is *lethal* for 50 percent of the population, and ED_{50} is the minimum dose that is *effective* for 50 percent of the population.*

3. Ideally, the LD_{50} should be a much higher dose than the ED_{50}, so that the TI would be large.

4. A more useful expression is the **margin of safety** of a drug, which is the ratio

$$\frac{LD_{0.1}}{ED_{99.9}}$$

where $LD_{0.1}$ is the minimum lethal dose for 0.1 percent of the population, and $ED_{99.9}$ is the minimum effective dose for 99.9 percent of the population.

---

*Note that the definition for ED_{50} here is for a population rather than a single individual or tissue and thus differs from that in VIII C 1 a.

STUDY QUESTIONS

Directions: Each question below contains five suggested answers. Choose the **one best** response to each question.

1. All of the following factors might be considered advantages of oral administration EXCEPT

(A) it is relatively safe and convenient
(B) the patient can administer the agent easily
(C) oral administration allows for slow absorption
(D) oral administration avoids extensive hepatic metabolism
(E) oral administration allows the medication to be administered in a nonsterile fashion

2. The maximum effect (E_{max}) achieved by a drug is a measure of

(A) potency
(B) efficacy
(C) the quantal response
(D) antagonist magnitude
(E) the therapeutic index

3. All of the following statements about the therapeutic index (TI) are true EXCEPT

(A) a high TI means that the drug is safe to use
(B) a low TI means that the drug is dangerous to use therapeutically
(C) a high TI indicates that the ED_{50} far exceeds the LD_{50}
(D) aspirin has a high TI
(E) the TI is a less useful expression than the margin of safety

4. Which of the following statements best characterizes potentiation?

(A) Potentiation occurs if a drug lacking an effect of its own increases the effect of a second, active drug
(B) Potentiation occurs if two drugs with the same effect, when given together, produce an effect that is equal in magnitude to the sum of the effects when the drugs are given individually
(C) Potentiation occurs if two drugs with the same effect, when given together, produce an effect that is greater in magnitude than the sum of the effects when the drugs are given individually
(D) Potentiation occurs if two drugs with the same effect, when given together, produce an effect that is equal in magnitude to the effect of only one of the drugs given individually
(E) None of the above statements correctly characterizes potentiation

5. Which of the following statements concerning drug receptors is true?

(A) Gamma globulin can bind to a drug and serve as a drug receptor
(B) A drug cannot act unless it is first bound to a receptor
(C) A drug cannot act unless it is first released from a drug receptor
(D) Drug receptors play a role in the bioavailability of a drug
(E) A drug can act as an antagonist even if it is bound to a drug receptor

Directions: Each question below contains four suggested answers of which **one or more** is correct. Choose the answer

A if **1, 2, and 3** are correct
B if **1 and 3** are correct
C if **2 and 4** are correct
D if **4** is correct
E if **1, 2, 3, and 4** are correct

6. Absorption of a drug from the gastrointestinal tract is influenced by

(1) the patient's dietary patterns
(2) the plasma half-time of the drug
(3) the pH of the stomach
(4) stress

7. Correct statements about drug transport include which of the following?

(1) Little, if any, of an ionized drug passively diffuses into cells
(2) "Bioavailability" refers to the percentage of drug which is not bound to plasma protein
(3) Simple diffusion depends upon the area of the absorbing surface
(4) Diffusion is a saturable process

8. Correct statements concerning drug metabolism, distribution, and elimination include which of the following?

(1) A lipid-soluble drug metabolite will not be sequestered in fatty tissue
(2) For a weakly acidic drug ($pK_a = 3$) at equilibrium, the ratio $(HA)/(A^-)$ equals 1 when the pH of the medium equals 3
(3) Glucuronide conjugates are readily excreted through the lungs
(4) Acidification of the urine favors excretion of basic drugs

9. Correct statements concerning the hepatic microsomal metabolizing enzyme system include which of the following?

(1) It requires reduced nicotinamide adenine dinucleotide phosphate (NADPH) and molecular oxygen
(2) It is concerned only with exogenous substances
(3) Its oxidation reactions include hydrocarbon chain hydroxylations and *N*- and *O*-dealkylations
(4) It includes alcohol dehydrogenase activity

10. A weak acid drug (A), with $pK_a = 6$, is given orally. Assuming that the pH of the stomach equals 3 and the pH of the blood equals 7, which of the following expressions are true? [Recall that $pK_a = pH + \log (HA/A^-)$.]

(1) At steady state, there is roughly 1000 times more undissociated drug than dissociated drug in the stomach
(2) At steady state, the ratio of dissociated to undissociated drug in the blood is approximately 10
(3) Drug will accumulate on the blood side of the stomach barrier
(4) Drug will be absorbed more readily in the stomach than in the small intestine

11. Propranolol is a competitive antagonist of norepinephrine. If one compares the log dose–response curve seen with both norepinephrine and propranolol to that seen with norepinephrine alone, the norepinephrine-propranolol curve would

(1) have a greater E_{max}
(2) be shifted to the right of the norepinephrine curve
(3) have a lower E_{max}
(4) have the same E_{max}

12. True statements about potency and efficacy include which of the following?

(1) The slope of the dose–response curve gives a good idea of a drug's efficacy
(2) Potency refers to the different amounts of two or more drugs that are needed to produce the same effect
(3) The log dose–response curve allows comparison of the relative potency of two drugs, but not a comparison of their efficacy
(4) Potency and efficacy are unrelated properties

ANSWERS AND EXPLANATIONS

1. The answer is D. *(II B 1)* Orally administered drugs are usually safe and convenient, and need not be sterile. Rapid absorption occurs after sublingual administration, but often not after oral administration. In addition, the rate of absorption is frequently variable, after oral administration, and extensive hepatic metabolism (''first-pass effect'') may occur with some drugs. Although the oral route is safe, convenient, and easy, one additional problem is that patient compliance is not ensured.

2. The answer is B. *(VIII B 3)* E_{max} reflects the efficacy of a drug and is indicated by the height of the dose–response curve. Potency refers to the different doses of two drugs that are needed to produce the same effect. Potency is independent of efficacy, and efficacy is more important than potency in selecting drugs for a particular clinical situation. The quantal response of a drug relates to the all-or-none relationship seen in a population with a given dose of a drug. The therapeutic index is defined as the LD_{50}/ED_{50} and is independent of the E_{max}.

3. The answer is C. *(VIII G)* The therapeutic index is a measure that is used in evaluating the safety and usefulness of a drug. The formula for the therapeutic index is

$$TI = \frac{LD_{50}}{ED_{50}}$$

where LD_{50} is the minimum dose that is *lethal* for 50 percent of the population, and ED_{50} is the minimum dose that is *effective* for 50 percent of the population. Thus, choice C is untrue. Therapeutically, the margin of safety has been considered more useful because the numerator is more restrictive

4. The answer is A. *(VIII F)* Potentiation occurs if a drug lacking an effect of its own increases the effect of a second, active drug. If two drugs with the same effect, when given together, produce an effect that is equal in magnitude to the sum of the effects when the drugs are given individually, then the effects of the two drugs are additive. If two drugs with the same effect, when given together, produce an effect that is greater in magnitude than the sum of the effects when the drugs are given individually, then synergism has occurred. If two drugs with the same effect, when given together, produce an effect that is less than the combined effect of the two drugs individually, then antagonism has occurred.

5. The answer is E. *(I C; III A; IV A; VIII D 2, 3 c)* A drug receptor is a specific drug-binding site in a cell or on its surface which mediates the action of the drug. Some drugs bind to various plasma proteins, such as gamma globulin, but these molecules do not serve as drug receptors. Most drugs combine reversibly with their receptors to form a drug–receptor complex, and it is this complex that exerts a biologic effect—for example, a decrease in blood pressure. However, some drugs are believed not to have specific receptors, and act by some other mechanism. If a drug has no inherent pharmacologic activity but binds to a receptor, it acts as an antagonist.

6. The answers is B (1, 3). *(III A, D 1 c)* Tablet size, solubility of the drug in the contents of the stomach, quality control of the manufacturer, the patient's dietary patterns, and the pH of the surrounding environment influence the absorption of a drug from the gastrointestinal tract. In general, the plasma half-time of a drug is independent of the absorption process, and stress has not been shown to be an important factor.

7. The answer is B (1, 3). *(III A, D)* Ionized drugs will not passively diffuse across cell membranes. Simple diffusion is not saturable, requires no energy, and is governed by Fick's law; thus, it is a function of the area of the absorbing surface, the diffusion constant of the drug, and the concentration gradient. Bioavailability is a measure of the relative rate at which an administered drug reaches the general circulation.

8. The answer is C (2, 4). *(III D 1 b, c; IV C; VI B 4)* A lipid-soluble drug metabolite would be readily sequestered in fatty tissue, and these deposits are in equilibrium with the circulating drug. For a weak acid, $3 = 3 + \log (HA)/(A^-) = 1$, according to the Henderson-Hasselbalch equation. Glucuronide conjugates are not excreted through the lungs but, rather, through the liver. Acidification of the urine favors ionization of the basic drug, which would generally favor urinary excretion.

9. The answer is B (1, 3). *(VI B 1 a)* In the hepatic microsomal enzyme metabolizing system, molecular oxygen is incorporated into the substrate, and reduced nicotinamide adenine dinucleotide phosphate (NADPH) is required as a reducing equivalent to reduce oxygen. It involves both exogenous and endogenous substrates. Oxidation reactions include hydrocarbon chain hydroxylations as well as *N*- and *O*-dealkylations. Alcohol dehydrogenase activity is a nonmicrosomal or soluble oxidation reaction.

10. The answer is E (all). *(III D 1 b)* If $pK_a = pH + \log(HA/A^-)$, then

$$\begin{aligned} 6 &= 3 + \log(HA/A^-) \\ 3 &= \log(HA/A^-) \\ 1000 &= HA/A^- \\ 6 &= 7 + \log(HA/A^-) \\ {}^-1 &= \log(HA/A^-) \\ 1/10 &= HA/A^- \end{aligned}$$

Therefore all statements are true.

11. The answer is C (2, 4). *(VIII E 2)* With competitive antagonism, the log dose–response curve will be shifted to the right and will have the same E_{max}. With noncompetitive antagonism there is a nonparallel shift of the log dose–response curve, with a lower E_{max}.

12. The answer is C (2, 4). *(VIII B 3, C)* The maximum effect of a drug, E_{max}, is a measure of the drug's efficacy. Potency is a comparative measure that refers to the different doses of two or more drugs that are needed to produce the same effect. The log dose–response curve allows both the efficacy and the potency of two or more drugs to be compared. The height (not the slope) of the log dose–response curve indicates a drug's efficacy, while drugs with the same action but with different potencies will usually have parallel curves. Potency is independent of efficacy, and efficacy is usually more important than potency in selecting drugs for use in a clinical situation.

2
Drugs Affecting Peripheral Neurohumoral Transmission

I. INTRODUCTION: THE PERIPHERAL EFFERENT NERVOUS SYSTEM

A. THE PERIPHERAL EFFERENT NERVOUS SYSTEM consists of the somatic and the autonomic nervous systems.

1. **The somatic nervous system** innervates and controls the motor functions of the body. Axons from the spinal cord innervate skeletal muscle; the neurotransmitter (see I C) is acetylcholine.

2. **The autonomic nervous system**
   - **a.** Axons from preganglionic neurons within the spinal cord connect to neurons in ganglia outside the spinal cord.
   - **b.** Postganglionic axons from the ganglia innervate smooth and cardiac muscle and exocrine glands.
   - **c.** The autonomic nervous system has two parts: the parasympathetic and sympathetic nervous systems. These two divisions control homeostatic functions that are primarily involuntary.

B. THE PARASYMPATHETIC AND SYMPATHETIC NERVOUS SYSTEMS

1. **Anatomic differences**
   - **a. Location of preganglionic neurons**
     - **(1)** In the parasympathetic (craniosacral) nervous system, preganglionic neurons are located in cranial and sacral portions of the spinal cord.
     - **(2)** In the sympathetic (thoracolumbar) nervous system, the neurons are located in lumbar and thoracic portions of the spinal cord.
   - **b. Location of ganglia**
     - **(1)** In the parasympathetic nervous system, the ganglia are close to the innervated organ, so that the preganglionic axons are long and the postganglionic axons are short.
     - **(2)** In the sympathetic nervous system, the ganglia are close to the spinal cord, so that the preganglionic axons are short and the postganglionic axons are long.

2. **Innervation of organs**
   - **a.** Both sympathetic and parasympathetic nervous systems innervate the heart, bronchial smooth muscle, iris, salivary glands, and urinary bladder.
   - **b.** The sympathetic system also innervates most vascular smooth muscle, the spleen, and the sweat glands. The adrenal medulla is considered to be a part of the sympathetic nervous system, replacing the ganglionic neuron.
   - **c.** Under normal conditions, the heart, eye, gastrointestinal tract, urinary bladder, bronchi, and salivary glands are under parasympathetic control, while blood vessels are controlled by the sympathetic division.

C. NEUROTRANSMITTERS. These are chemical mediators which transmit nerve impulses across junctions such as synapses.

1. In both the sympathetic and the parasympathetic nervous systems, the neurotransmitter at the ganglionic synapse is acetylcholine (see IV A, below).

2. At the postganglionic synapse, the two systems differ.
   - **a.** The parasympathetic neurotransmitter is acetylcholine.
   - **b.** The sympathetic transmitter is usually norepinephrine (see II A), but at sweat glands and at some blood vessels, it is acetylcholine.

D. RECEPTORS OF THE NERVOUS SYSTEM. More than one type of receptor exists for each neurotransmitter. The receptors are distinguished on the basis of their affinity for various agonists and antagonists.

1. **Cholinergic receptors** (for acetylcholine). There are several types of cholinergic receptors:
   a. **Muscarinic receptors**. Muscarine is an agonist and atropine is an antagonist. Muscarinic receptors are found on the innervated organ.
   b. **Nicotinic receptors.** Nicotine is an agonist. Nicotinic receptors are of two types:
      (1) **Skeletal muscle nicotinic receptors** are found at skeletal neuromuscular junctions; antagonists are decamethonium and *d*-tubocurarine.
      (2) **Ganglionic nicotinic receptors** are found on neurons in autonomic ganglia; hexamethonium is an antagonist.

2. **Adrenergic receptors** (for norepinephrine and epinephrine) are also of several types, and these are subdivided on the basis of the relative response to agonists and antagonists.
   a. **α-Adrenergic receptors**. Agonists for α receptors, in decreasing order of potency, are epinephrine, norepinephrine, and isoproterenol. Antagonists are phentolamine and phenoxybenzamine.
      (1) **α_1-Adrenergic receptors** are found on blood vessels, on the radial muscle of the eye, in the gastrointestinal tract, and on the splenic capsule; these are postsynaptic sites. The relative potency of agonists is epinephrine $\geq$ norepinephrine $\gg$ isoproterenol.
      (2) **α_2-Adrenergic receptors** are found on dendrites at some presynaptic sympathetic sites and at postsynaptic sites in the adrenal medulla and brain. Presynaptic α_2 receptors, when activated, inhibit the release of further neurotransmitter. Isoproterenol is ineffective on α_2 receptors.
   b. **β-Adrenergic receptors.** Agonists for β receptors, in decreasing order of potency, are isoproterenol, epinephrine, and norepinephrine. Propranolol is an antagonist. The β receptors are also subdivided on the basis of their relative response to agonists and antagonists:
      (1) **β_1-Adrenergic receptors** are found predominantly on cells in the heart and intestine. The relative potency of agonists is isoproterenol $>$ epinephrine $=$ norepinephrine.
      (2) **β_2-Adrenergic receptors** are found on bronchial and vascular smooth muscle. The relative potency of agonists is isoproterenol $\geq$ epinephrine $\gg$ norepinephrine.

E. DIRECT EFFECTS OF PARASYMPATHETIC AND SYMPATHETIC STIMULATION ON VARIOUS ORGANS. A direct effect occurs when the nerve innervating an organ is stimulated. (Indirect responses are mediated by changes caused in other organs.)

1. **Heart**
   a. **Sympathetic stimulation** increases the heart rate **(chronotropic effect)** and the contractile force **(inotropic effect)**.
   b. **Parasympathetic stimulation** decreases the heart rate but has little effect on contractile force because there is no parasympathetic innervation of the ventricles.

2. **Blood vessels**
   a. **Sympathetic stimulation**
      (1) Stimulation of α receptors causes constriction of arteries, arterioles, and veins.
      (2) Stimulation of β receptors causes dilation of skeletal muscle arteries.
   b. **Parasympathetic stimulation** has no effect on blood vessels because most have no parasympathetic innervation.

3. **Gastrointestinal tract. Sympathetic stimulation** decreases the activity of the gastrointestinal tract, while **parasympathetic stimulation** increases it.

4. **Eye**
   a. **Sympathetic stimulation** contracts the radial muscle, causing dilation of the pupil.
   b. **Parasympathetic stimulation** produces contraction of the circular and ciliary muscles, causing pupillary constriction and changes in accommodation.

5. **Bronchial smooth muscle** is relaxed by sympathetic stimulation and contracted by parasympathetic stimulation.

6. **Glycogenolysis** is increased in liver and muscle by sympathetic stimulation.

F. Drugs can affect neurohumoral transmission at various steps. They can affect:

1. The synthesis, storage, or release of a neurotransmitter.

2. The interaction between transmitter and receptor.
3. The enzymatic destruction of a neurotransmitter.
4. The transport of a transmitter into cells.
5. The recovery of a cell membrane after the transmitter–receptor interaction.

II. SYMPATHOMIMETIC (ADRENERGIC) AGENTS.
These are drugs which mimic the actions of the sympathetic nervous system.

A. CATECHOLAMINES: NOREPINEPHRINE AND EPINEPHRINE

1. Structure

HO, HO, H, C–CH_2–NH_2, OH

Norepinephrine

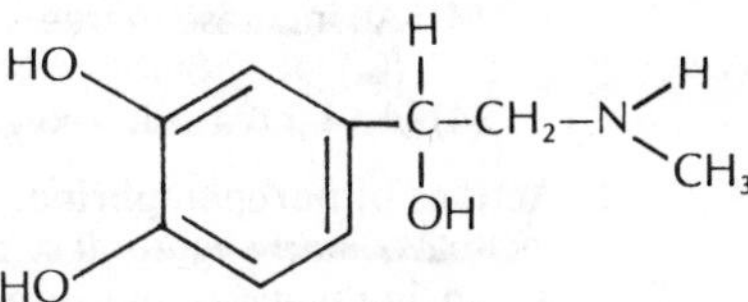

Epinephrine

2. Biosynthesis

a. Tyrosine is hydroxylated on the aromatic ring by tyrosine hydroxylase, yielding **dopa** (dihydroxyphenylalanine); this step is the rate-limiting step in the biosynthesis of adrenergic transmitters.
b. Dopa is decarboxylated to give **dopamine**.
c. Dopamine is hydroxylated on the β-carbon to give **norepinephrine**.
d. **Epinephrine** is formed in the adrenal medulla by the methylation of norepinephrine. The medulla releases 85 percent epinephrine and 15 percent norepinephrine.

3. Actions of epinephrine. Epinephrine interacts strongly with both β and α receptors. Its effects on some body systems depend on the concentration of epinephrine present as well as the type of receptor. At low concentrations, β effects predominate, and at high concentrations, α effects predominate.

a. **Effects on blood pressure**
   (1) A large dose of epinephrine, administered intravenously, causes an increase in blood pressure, the systolic pressure increasing more than the diastolic. Subsequently, the mean pressure falls below normal before returning to the control value. The rise in pressure is due to:
      (a) Vasoconstriction through activation of α receptors.
      (b) Increased ventricular contraction through activation of β receptors.
      (c) An initial increase in heart rate which, at the height of the vasopressor response, will be slowed by a compensatory vagal discharge.
   (2) Low doses cause a fall in blood pressure because the β_2 (vasodilator) receptors are more sensitive to epinephrine than are the α (vasoconstrictor) receptors.

b. **Vascular effects**. Epinephrine exerts its action on small arterioles and precapillary sphincters. Its vascular effects include:
   (1) Decreased cutaneous blood flow.
   (2) Increased blood flow to skeletal muscle at low concentrations, and decreased flow at higher concentrations.
   (3) Increased hepatic blood flow, with decreased splanchnic vascular resistance.
   (4) Increased renal vascular resistance, producing decreased renal blood flow.
   (5) Increased arterial and venous pulmonary pressure.
   (6) Increased coronary blood flow, caused indirectly by an increase in the work of the heart, and mediated by local effectors.

c. **Effects on the heart** produced by epinephrine include:
   (1) A direct effect on β_1 receptors, producing a slight initial increase in heart rate which is slowed by a compensatory vagal discharge.
   (2) Increased stroke volume.
   (3) Increased cardiac output.
   (4) A propensity toward arrhythmias.

d. **Effects on smooth muscle** depend on the predominant type of adrenergic receptor in the muscle:
   (1) Epinephrine relaxes gastrointestinal smooth muscle (α_2 and β receptor stimulation), while it usually increases sphincter contraction (α stimulation).
   (2) Uterine contractions are inhibited in the nonpregnant individual (β), while in the pregnant woman contractions occur (α).
   (3) In the bladder, the detrusor muscle relaxes (β), while the trigone and sphincter contract (α).
   (4) Bronchiolar smooth muscle relaxes (β_2).

e. **Metabolic effects** of epinephrine also depend on the type of adrenergic receptor. These effects include:
   (1) An increase in glucose and lactate production via liver and muscle glycogenolysis (β_2).
   (2) Inhibition of insulin secretion (α).
   (3) An increase in free fatty acids, mediated by cyclic adenosine monophosphate (cAMP) (β_1).
   (4) An increase in oxygen consumption.

4. **Actions of norepinephrine**. Norepinephrine is equipotent to epinephrine in its action on β_1 receptors, and slightly less potent on α receptors. It has very little effect on β_2 receptors.
   a. An intravenous infusion raises both systolic and diastolic pressure by constriction of vascular smooth muscle (α receptors).
   b. The increased peripheral vascular resistance produces a compensatory vagal reflex that slows the heart rate. Cardiac output may actually decrease although coronary blood flow is increased.

5. **Termination of action**
   a. **Transport**, or **uptake into the cells**, is an important mechanism for terminating the action of many neurotransmitters. There are two active **amine transport systems:**
      (1) A system in the plasma membrane transports amines from the extracellular fluid to the cytosol.
      (2) A system in the secretory granular membrane transports amines into granules.
   b. **Deactivation** by **conversion to inactive metabolites** is also a way of terminating action. Two enzymes are involved:
      (1) Catechol-O-methyltransferase (COMT) adds a methyl group to the hydroxyl of the catechol ring.
      (2) Monoamine oxidase (MAO) removes the amine group. When metabolic breakdown or transport is prevented (in patients taking MAO inhibitors or tricyclic antidepressants), then the dosage of sympathomimetic agents must be reduced.

6. **Pharmacokinetics of epinephrine and norepinephrine**
   a. Absorption is poor with oral administration because the drugs are rapidly conjugated and oxidized.
   b. Absorption is slow with subcutaneous administration because the drugs cause local vasoconstriction.
   c. Nebulized and inhaled solutions are usually used for their actions on the respiratory tract.
   d. The drugs can be given intravenously, but this route must be used with caution so that the heart does not fibrillate.
   e. The liver is important in the degradation of epinephrine and norepinephrine. The majority of the dose is metabolized by COMT and MAO, and the metabolites are excreted in the urine.

7. **Therapeutic uses**
   a. Epinephrine is used:
      (1) To treat bronchospasm.
      (2) For relief of hypersensitivity reactions; it is the primary treatment for anaphylactic shock.
      (3) To prolong the duration of infiltrative anesthesia.
      (4) To restore cardiac activity in cardiac arrest.
   b. Norepinephrine is used for treating hypotension during anesthesia when tissue perfusion is good.

8. **Untoward effects**. Both epinephrine and norepinephrine can cause:
   a. Anxiety.
   b. Headache.
   c. Cerebral hemorrhage, from the vasopressor effects.

d. Cardiac arrhythmias, especially in the presence of digitalis and certain anesthetic agents.
e. Pulmonary edema, from pulmonary hypertension.

B. ISOPROTERENOL

1. **Actions**
   a. Isoproterenol has an *N*-alkyl substitution, which makes it act almost entirely on β receptors and have very little effect on α receptors.
   b. Intravenous infusion produces a reduction of peripheral vascular resistance in skeletal muscles and in renal and mesenteric vascular beds.
   c. Diastolic blood pressure falls but, owing to increased venous return and positive inotropic and chronotropic effects, cardiac output is increased.
   d. Systolic blood pressure may increase, but mean pressure decreases.
   e. Renal blood flow decreases in normotensive individuals, but increases in patients with nonhemorrhagic shock.
   f. Relaxation of both bronchial and gastrointestinal smooth muscle occurs.
   g. A release of free fatty acids occurs; hyperglycemia is less than with epinephrine.
   h. Pancreatic islet cells are activated, stimulating insulin secretion.

2. **Pharmacokinetics**
   a. Absorption of orally administered isoproterenol is unreliable.
   b. It is readily absorbed when given parenterally or as an inhaled aerosol.
   c. It is principally metabolized by COMT; MAO plays a much smaller role than in epinephrine or norepinephrine metabolism.

3. **Therapeutic uses**. Isoproterenol is used as a bronchodilator and as a cardiac stimulant.

4. **Untoward effects**
   a. These are similar to the untoward effects of epinephrine.
   b. Overdosage by inhalation can induce fatal ventricular arrhythmias.
   c. Tolerance to the desired effects occurs with overuse in the asthmatic.

C. DOPAMINE

1. **Biosynthesis**. Dopamine is an intermediate in the synthesis of norepinephrine (see II A 2).

2. **Actions**
   a. Dopamine is an important neurotransmitter in the central nervous system. It is a direct agonist, acting on β_1 receptors, and also releases norepinephrine from nerve terminals. The result is a positive inotropic effect on the myocardium.
   b. Low or intermediate doses of dopamine reduce arterial resistance in the mesentery and kidney, an effect mediated by a receptor for dopamine.
   c. Dopamine increases systolic pressure but has little effect on diastolic pressure.
   d. At higher doses it acts on α receptors and causes vasoconstriction, with a consequent reduction in renal function.

3. **Pharmacokinetics**. Dopamine resembles epinephrine and norepinephrine in its pharmacokinetics.

4. **Therapeutic uses**. Dopamine is used in the treatment of cardiogenic and septic shock, and in chronic refractory congestive heart failure.

5. **Untoward effects**
   a. Overdosage results in excessive sympathomimetic activity.
   b. Anginal pain, arrhythmias, nausea, and hypertension can occur, but these effects are short-lived because of dopamine's rapid metabolism.

D. DOBUTAMINE

1. **Actions**
   a. Though dobutamine resembles dopamine chemically, it is a direct β_1 receptor agonist. It has a greater inotropic than chronotropic effect.
   b. Dobutamine does not act on dopaminergic receptors.

2. **Pharmacokinetics**
   a. Dobutamine is not absorbed when given orally.
   b. It has a half-life of 2 minutes when given by intravenous injection.

3. **Therapeutic uses**. Dobutamine is used to improve myocardial function in congestive heart

failure. Oxygen demands are less than with other sympathetic agonists because dobutamine causes minimal changes in heart rate and systolic pressure.

4. **Untoward effects and precautions**
   a. Dobutamine increases atrioventricular conduction and must therefore be used with caution in atrial fibrillation.
   b. Other adverse effects are similar to those of other catecholamines.

E. PHENYLEPHRINE

1. **Actions**
   a. Phenylephrine is a direct-acting sympathomimetic agent. Its effects are similar to those of norepinephrine, but it is less potent and has a longer duration of action.
   b. Vasoconstriction, increased arterial pressure, and reflex bradycardia occur with parenteral administration.
2. **Therapeutic uses**. Phenylephrine is used:
   a. As a nasal decongestant.
   b. As a pressor agent.
   c. To provide local vasoconstriction for use with local anesthetics.
   d. For relief of paroxysmal atrial tachycardia.
3. **Untoward effects**
   a. Large doses cause cardiac irregularities.
   b. Rebound nasal congestion occasionally occurs with chronic use as a nasal decongestant.

F. EPHEDRINE

1. **Actions**
   a. Ephedrine is a mixed-acting sympathomimetic agent; that is, it has both direct and indirect actions.
      (1) Its primary action is indirect: it causes the release of norepinephrine from storage in nerve terminals, apparently by competing with norepinephrine for transport into the granules.
      (2) It also produces direct stimulation of adrenergic receptors.
   b. When administered intravenously its action is similar to that of epinephrine. However,
      (1) Its pressor response occurs more slowly and lasts ten times longer.
      (2) Its potency is 1/250 that of epinephrine in producing an equivalent pressor response.
   c. Ephedrine increases arterial pressure by causing peripheral vasoconstriction and cardiac stimulation.
   d. Its effects on the bronchi and other smooth muscle are qualitatively similar to those of epinephrine.
   e. It causes CNS stimulation, which can result in effects such as insomnia, nervousness, nausea, and agitation.
   f. Tachyphylaxis occurs with repeated administration.
2. **Pharmacokinetics**
   a. Ephedrine is absorbed when taken orally.
   b. It is resistant to COMT and MAO, so that its action is prolonged.
3. **Therapeutic uses**. Ephedrine is used:
   a. In the treatment of bronchial asthma.
   b. As a nasal decongestant.
   c. As a pressor agent in spinal anesthesia.
   d. As a mydriatic.
4. **Untoward effects and precautions**
   a. These are similar to the untoward effects seen with epinephrine.
   b. In addition, CNS effects may occur.
   c. Ephedrine must be used with caution in patients with cardiovascular disease or hyperthyroidism because it is a powerful heart stimulator.

G. AMPHETAMINE

1. **Actions**
   a. Amphetamine acts indirectly by releasing norepinephrine.
   b. Amphetamine is a CNS stimulant (see Chapter 3, VIII A).
   c. The dextrorotatory (*d*-) form is more active in the CNS than the levorotatory (*l*-) form.
   d. Amphetamine depresses the appetite, decreasing food intake, by affecting the feeding

center in the lateral hypothalamus.

e. It increases metabolism to a small extent.

2. **Therapeutic uses**
   a. Amphetamine is used in the treatment of narcolepsy and the hyperkinetic syndrome in children (see Chapter 3, VIII A 3).
   b. The control of obesity is not a recommended use because abuse of amphetamine is not rare and because tolerance to the anorexic effects develops within a few weeks.

3. **Untoward effects and precautions**
   a. Tolerance to amphetamine can occur within several weeks.
   b. Psychic and physical dependence can occur.
   c. Toxic psychosis can result from large doses.
   d. Prolonged use can lead to mental depression and fatigue.
   e. Reactions attributable to CNS stimulation occur, such as restlessness or insomnia.
   f. Cardiovascular stimulation can result in tachycardia and hypertension.
   g. Mydriasis and dry mouth can occur.
   h. Amphetamine is contraindicated in patients with cardiovascular disease, because it stimulates the heart, and also in those receiving MAO inhibitors or guanethidine, since these compounds increase norepinephrine concentrations outside the cells, as amphetamine does.
   i. Treatment of acute intoxication should include:
      (1) Acidification of the urine by ammonium chloride administration.
      (2) Administering chlorpromazine, which is effective for treating both the CNS symptoms and the elevated blood pressure because of its α-blocking activity.

H. METHAMPHETAMINE

1. Methamphetamine is related chemically to both amphetamine and ephedrine. A mixed-acting sympathomimetic agent, it is equal to amphetamine in central stimulant activity and is more potent than ephedrine in pressor activity.

2. Therapeutic indications are limited to those which make use of its CNS effects, such as narcolepsy.

I. MEPHENTERMINE

1. Mephentermine is a mixed-acting sympathomimetic. Its peripheral vasopressor actions are similar to those of methamphetamine; it lacks significant central actions.

2. Its major therapeutic use is in the treatment of hypotension.

J. METHOXAMINE

1. Methoxamine is a direct-acting stimulator of α-adrenergic receptors with pharmacologic properties similar to those of phenylephrine. → N-Epi

2. It produces little CNS stimulation.

3. Its large pressor effect is due to an increase in total peripheral resistance.

4. It causes a reflex bradycardia.

5. Methoxamine is used therapeutically in hypotensive states and to end attacks of paroxysmal atrial tachycardia.

K. METARAMINOL

1. Metaraminol is a mixed-acting sympathomimetic that is similar to norepinephrine in its actions, although it is less potent.

2. Metaraminol increases systolic and diastolic blood pressure via vasoconstriction, and produces a marked reflex bradycardia.

3. It has little stimulant effect on the CNS.

4. Its major therapeutic use is in the treatment of hypotensive states.

L. METAPROTERENOL

1. Metaproterenol is primarily a β_2 agonist, relaxing bronchial muscle. It has little effect on cardiac β_1 receptors.

2. It is used therapeutically for the treatment of bronchial asthma or bronchospasm, where its lack of cardiac stimulation is a decided advantage.

3. Untoward effects are those seen with the sympathomimetic drugs listed above. Even though metaproterenol is primarily a β_2 agonist, it should be used with caution in patients with cardiovascular disease or hyperthyroidism because it can still stimulate (though minimally) β_1 receptors of the heart. In diabetics it can mask the symptoms of lack of insulin.

M. TERBUTALINE

1. Terbutaline is a β_2 agonist that is similar to metaproterenol in its pharmacologic actions.

2. Its major therapeutic use is as a bronchodilator.

3. Its untoward effects are similar to those produced by other sympathomimetic agents.

III. SYMPATHETIC ANTAGONISTS

A. α-ADRENERGIC BLOCKING AGENTS (α-BLOCKERS)

1. Phenoxybenzamine and dibenamine

a. Mechanism of action

(1) These agents are haloalkylamines and are closely related to nitrogen mustards.
(2) They covalently bind to the α receptor, producing an irreversible blockade.
(3) Phenoxybenzamine is somewhat more potent in blocking α_1 (postsynaptic) receptors than in blocking α_2 (presynaptic) receptors.

b. Actions. The drugs antagonize sympathetic responses mediated by α-adrenergic receptors.

(1) **Cardiovascular effects**. Both agents induce postural hypotension due to a lack of compensatory sympathetic vasoconstriction. In addition, phenoxybenzamine increases cardiac output and decreases total peripheral resistance.
(2) Most **metabolic effects** produced by catecholamines are the result of their effects on β receptors, and thus α-adrenergic blocking agents do not have significant metabolic actions.
(3) Phenoxybenzamine and dibenamine stimulate the CNS, producing nausea, hyperventilation, and loss of time perception.

c. Therapeutic uses. These agents are used:

(1) For acute hypertensive episodes due to sympathomimetics, MAO inhibitors, or pheochromocytomas.
(2) To reverse vasoconstriction in shock. If use is attempted in shock, the patient must have an elevated central venous pressure.
(3) To relieve vasospasm in Raynaud's syndrome.
(4) For control of autonomic hyperreflexia due to spinal cord transection.

d. Untoward effects

(1) Postural hypotension and reflex tachycardia may occur, especially in patients who are hypovolemic.
(2) Ejaculation may be inhibited.
(3) Miosis and nasal stuffiness may occur.
(4) Nausea and vomiting may occur with oral administration.
(5) Both agents are usually given intravenously because of their irritant properties.

2. Phentolamine and tolazoline act by a reversible α-adrenergic blockade.

a. Actions

(1) These agents produce vasodilation and reflex cardiac stimulation.
(2) They decrease peripheral resistance and increase venous capacity.
(3) Both stimulate salivary, lacrimal, pancreatic, and respiratory tract secretions.
(4) They cause a gastric secretion that resembles the effect of histamine.
(5) Phentolamine is more potent than tolazoline.
(6) Tolazoline is absorbed when given orally and is rapidly excreted by the kidneys; phentolamine is excreted more slowly. Both can be given parenterally.

b. Therapeutic uses

(1) Phentolamine has been used to control acute hypertensive episodes due to sympathomimetics.
(2) In the past, phentolamine was used as a diagnostic test for pheochromocytoma, but has been replaced by assays for urinary catecholamines.
(3) Tolazoline can be used to relieve vasospasm and in the treatment of Raynaud's syndrome.

c. **Untoward effects and precautions**
   (1) Both drugs can cause cardiac stimulation, leading to arrhythmias and anginal pain, especially after parenteral administration; they must be used with caution in patients with coronary artery disease.
   (2) Tolazoline can produce a paradoxical hypertension.
   (3) Because they induce gastrointestinal stimulation, both drugs must be used with caution in patients with peptic ulcer disease.

3. **Prazosin** is a selective blocker of postsynaptic α_1 receptors, producing vasodilation.
   a. **Actions**
      (1) Prazosin reduces vascular tone in both resistance and capacitance vessels.
      (2) Because prazosin has no effect on α_2 receptors, neurotransmitter feedback inhibition is maintained, so that prazosin causes only a small degree of tachycardia.
      (3) It decreases arterial pressure with little change in cardiac output, heart rate, and right atrial pressure.
   b. Further information about prazosin can be found in Chapter 5, V D 2.

4. **Ergot alkaloids**
   a. **Mechanism of action**
      (1) These agents are weak α-adrenergic blockers as well as being serotonin antagonists.
      (2) They are also partial agonists at α-adrenergic receptors, and agonists at receptors for tryptamine and dopamine.
   b. **Actions**
      (1) Ergot alkaloids are CNS stimulants, and therefore may cause effects such as confusion, irregular respiration, and anxiety.
      (2) They directly stimulate smooth muscle.
      (3) They cause a significant elevation of blood pressure via peripheral vasoconstriction.
   c. **Therapeutic uses**
      (1) Ergotamine tartrate, by virtue of its vasoconstricting effects, is used in the treatment of migraine.
      (2) Ergonovine maleate is a powerful oxytocic but lacks the adrenergic blocking activity of ergotamine. It causes direct contraction of uterine smooth muscle, and is used to decrease postpartum bleeding.
   d. **Untoward effects**
      (1) Ergot preparations often cause nausea and vomiting.
      (2) Their vasoconstricting effects can cause vascular insufficiency, leading to gangrene.

B. β-ADRENERGIC BLOCKING AGENTS (β-BLOCKERS)

1. **Propranolol** is a nonselective β antagonist: it competes for both β_1 and β_2 receptors.
   a. **Actions**
      (1) Propranolol decreases the heart rate and cardiac output, and prolongs systole.
      (2) It decreases total coronary blood flow and oxygen consumption.
      (3) It reduces blood flow to most tissues except the brain.
      (4) Its antihypertensive effect is slow to develop, and the mechanisms that cause the effect are not clear. However, propranolol inhibits the renal secretion of renin, which may play a part.
      (5) Propranolol depresses sodium excretion because it alters renal hemodynamics, an effect that is secondary to the decrease in cardiac output.
      (6) Propranolol increases airway resistance by β_2 blockade.
      (7) Since most of the effects of catecholamines on carbohydrate and fat metabolism are mediated by β receptors, propranolol will interfere with these events.
   b. **Pharmacokinetics**
      (1) Although propranolol is completely absorbed from the gastrointestinal tract, a large portion of the drug is extracted by the liver before it enters the systemic circulation.
      (2) Wide variation in the hepatic metabolism of the drug among individuals causes significant differences in the plasma concentrations attained.
      (3) Propranolol is approximately 90 percent bound to plasma proteins.
      (4) The elimination half-time is approximately 3 hours for a small dose, but it is prolonged with larger doses and is significantly prolonged in the presence of cirrhosis.
      (5) A metabolic product, 4-hydroxypropranolol, is active but has a short half- life.
   c. **Therapeutic uses**. Propranolol is used for:
      (1) Treatment of hypertension, often in combination with a diuretic.
      (2) Prophylaxis of angina pectoris (see Chapter 5, IV B).
      (3) Prophylaxis of supraventricular and ventricular arrhythmias (see Chapter 5, III G).

(4) Management of hypertrophic obstructive cardiomyopathies, to reduce the force of myocardial contractions.
(5) Management of hyperthyroidism and anxiety states, to decrease the heart rate.
(6) Prophylaxis of migraine headaches.

d. Untoward effects and precautions
(1) Propranolol can induce heart failure, especially in patients with compromised myocardial function.
(2) Rapid withdrawal can lead to "supersensitivity" of β-adrenergic receptors, which can provoke anginal attacks, arrhythmias, or myocardial infarction.
(3) Because propranolol increases airway resistance, it must be used with caution in asthmatics.
(4) Because of its effects on carbohydrate metabolism, the hypoglycemic action of insulin may be augmented. Therefore, diabetics being treated with insulin and persons prone to hypoglycemia must use propranolol with caution.
(5) Rash, fever, and purpura are characteristic of an allergic response and require discontinuation of the drug.

2. **Timolol** is a nonselective β-adrenergic antagonist that is 5 to 10 times more potent than propranolol.
   a. Timolol lowers intraocular pressure by reducing the production of aqueous humor; the mechanism is not clear.
   b. It does not change the size of the pupil, and vision is not affected.
   c. Timolol, in the form of eyedrops, is therefore useful in the treatment of glaucoma.
   d. It is now also used as propranolol is.
   e. Systemic absorption can occur with ocular use, but the amount absorbed is usually not enough to affect patients with asthma or heart failure.

3. **Nadolol** is a nonselective β-adrenergic blocking agent that is not metabolized and is excreted unchanged in the urine. Its effects and adverse reactions are similar to those of propranolol.

4. **Metoprolol** is a selective β_1-adrenergic antagonist.
   a. Actions
   (1) Metoprolol inhibits the inotropic and chronotropic cardiac responses to isoproterenol.
   (2) It is 1/50 as potent as propranolol in inhibiting the vasodilator response to isoproterenol; however, it is long-acting.
   (3) It is absorbed well when given orally.
   b. The major **therapeutic use** of metoprolol is in the treatment of hypertension.
   c. Untoward effects
   (1) Metoprolol produces fewer deleterious effects in asthmatic patients because of its selective β_1-adrenergic antagonism, but its use in asthmatics still requires caution.
   (2) Other adverse effects are similar to those of propranolol.

5. **Atenolol** is a selective β_1-adrenergic antagonist, which is administered once a day.

C. AGENTS THAT INHIBIT THE ACTION OF ADRENERGIC NERVES

1. Reserpine
   a. **Mechanism of action**. Reserpine, a rauwolfia alkaloid, acts via catecholamine depletion. It inhibits the uptake of norepinephrine into vesicles, and intraneuronal degradation of norepinephrine by MAO then occurs. This action takes place both centrally and peripherally.
   b. Actions
   (1) Large doses given parenterally may cause a transient sympathomimetic effect as stored catecholamines are released from the cell, because uptake into vesicles is inhibited.
   (2) Blood pressure decreases, which usually triggers reflex tachycardia in normal people through sympathetic stimulation. However, because sympathetic stores are depleted, bradycardia may ensue in people taking reserpine.
   (3) Sedation often results, owing to the depleted stores of catecholamines and 5-hydroxytryptamine (5-HT) in the brain.
   c. The major **therapeutic use** of reserpine is in the treatment of hypertension (see Chapter 5, V F 1).
   d. **Untoward effects** include:
   (1) Sedation.
   (2) Psychic depression that may result in suicide.

(3) Abdominal cramps and diarrhea.
(4) Gastrointestinal ulceration.
(5) Possible increased incidence of breast carcinoma.

2. **Guanethidine**
   a. **Mechanism of action**
      (1) Guanethidine acts presynaptically. It impairs the response to sympathetic stimulation by inhibiting the release of neurotransmitters from peripheral adrenergic neurons.
      (2) Guanethidine is taken up by adrenergic nerves and displaces norepinephrine from intraneuronal storage granules. This action does not inhibit the release of granule contents; that occurs through another, unknown, mechanism.
      (3) Much of the norepinephrine released from the adrenergic nerve terminals is deaminated by intraneuronal MAO. Some norepinephrine will still leak from the cell.
   b. **Actions**
      (1) A large intravenous dose causes a rapid fall in blood pressure due to the direct action of guanethidine on resistance vessels.
      (2) This is followed by a fall in systemic and pulmonary arterial pressures that is much more intense in the erect than in the supine individual.
      (3) Other effects include increased gastrointestinal motility and retention of fluid.
   c. **Pharmacokinetics**
      (1) Oral absorption varies.
      (2) With oral administration, the onset of action is slow.
      (3) The drug is rapidly cleared by the kidney.
   d. **Therapeutic uses.** The major therapeutic indication is as a potent, long-acting antihypertensive agent (see Chapter 5, V F 2).
   e. **Untoward effects** include:
      (1) Postural hypotension.
      (2) Syncope, especially with strenuous exercise.
      (3) Diarrhea.
      (4) Edema.

3. **Bretylium**
   a. **Actions**
      (1) Bretylium is taken up by adrenergic nerve terminals and produces a block in the release of norepinephrine.
      (2) It also inhibits the re-uptake of norepinephrine into nerve terminals.
      (3) Initially, bretylium produces a sympathomimetic effect, before it blocks the action of the nerves.
   b. **Therapeutic uses**. Bretylium is no longer used for hypertension but is used mainly as an antiarrhythmic agent (see Chapter 5, III H). It is poorly absorbed when given orally.
   c. **Untoward effects** include cardiac stimulation due to the sympathomimetic effects of bretylium, and strong hypotension.

IV. PARASYMPATHETIC (CHOLINERGIC) AGONISTS

A. ACETYLCHOLINE

1. Acetylcholine is a quaternary ammonium ester that is rapidly hydrolyzed by acetylcholinesterase and plasma cholinesterase.

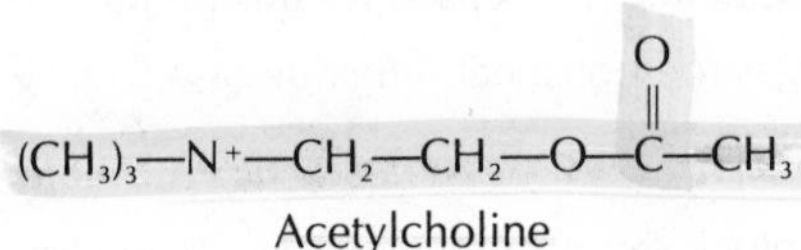

Acetylcholine

2. **Actions**
   a. **Cardiovascular system**
      (1) Acetylcholine produces:
         (a) A negative inotropic effect.
         (b) A negative chronotropic effect.
         (c) Vasodilation.
      (2) Its actions on the heart are the same as the effects of vagal stimulation.
      (3) Large intravenous doses cause an increase in blood pressure, owing to the release of catecholamines from the adrenal medulla and activation of sympathetic ganglia.

b. Other systems

(1) Acetylcholine increases gastrointestinal motility and secretory activity.

(2) It contracts smooth muscle in the uterus, ureters, bladder, and bronchioles, and the constrictor muscles of the iris.

(3) It stimulates the salivary, sweat, and lacrimal glands.

3. **Therapeutic uses**. Acetylcholine has no therapeutic application.

B. METHACHOLINE (ACETYL-β-METHYLCHOLINE)

1. Methacholine differs chemically from acetylcholine by the addition of a methyl group to the β position of choline. As a result,
   - **a.** Methacholine is hydrolyzed only by acetylcholinesterase, and therefore has a longer duration of action than acetylcholine.
   - **b.** It becomes virtually a pure muscarinic-acting agent.
2. **Actions and therapeutic uses**
   - **a.** The effects of methacholine on the cardiovascular system and other systems are similar to those of acetylcholine.
   - **b.** Methacholine is sometimes used clinically in combination with neostigmine for the emergency treatment of narrow-angle glaucoma.

C. CARBACHOL (CARBAMYLCHOLINE)

1. Carbachol has a carbamic acid–ester link which is not readily susceptible to hydrolysis by cholinesterases.

2. **Actions**. Carbachol has all the pharmacologic properties of acetylcholine. It exerts both nicotinic and muscarinic effects.

3. **Therapeutic uses**. Carbachol is used ophthalmically as a miotic agent.

D. BETHANECHOL

1. Chemically, bethanechol has the structural features of both methacholine and carbachol. It is resistant to hydrolysis by cholinesterases, and is mainly muscarinic in action.

2. It is used therapeutically to stimulate the smooth muscle of the gastrointestinal tract and urinary bladder.

E. PILOCARPINE

1. Pilocarpine is a tertiary amine alkaloid.

2. Its actions are similar to those of methacholine. When applied locally to the eye it causes miosis and an eventual fall in intraocular pressure.

3. Its major therapeutic indication is in the treatment of glaucoma.

F. METOCLOPRAMIDE

1. Metoclopramide possesses cholinergic effects.

2. It stimulates the gastrointestinal tract.

3. It is an effective antiemetic, and is used for this purpose during cancer chemotherapy.

4. It may be useful in gastroesophageal reflux disease.

G. UNTOWARD EFFECTS AND PRECAUTIONS FOR PARASYMPATHETIC AGONISTS

1. Atropine will often block serious untoward effects, such as the increase in gastrointestinal motility, muscle paralysis, and stimulation of glandular secretion, that can occur with these drugs.

2. Use of these drugs is contraindicated in patients with coronary insufficiency, hyperthyroidism, peptic ulcer, or asthma.

V. ANTICHOLINESTERASE AGENTS

A. PHYSOSTIGMINE

1. **Mechanism of action**. This alkaloid forms a reversible complex at the site of acetylcholinesterase where acetylcholine is broken down.

2. **Actions**. The pharmacologic properties of physostigmine mimic those of acetylcholine.
   a. It produces miosis and thus can antagonize the mydriasis induced by atropine.
   b. When given in large doses it causes fasciculation, then paralysis, of skeletal muscle because of the accumulation of acetylcholine at the neuromuscular junction that results when acetylcholine is not broken down.

3. **Pharmacokinetics**
   a. Physostigmine is well absorbed from the gastrointestinal tract, subcutaneous tissues, and mucous membranes.
   b. Its metabolism is at the ester linkage by hydrolytic cleavage.

4. **Therapeutic uses** include:
   a. Treatment of atropine, phenothiazine, and tricyclic antidepressant intoxication.
   b. Treatment of glaucoma, especially simple and secondary glaucoma.

B. NEOSTIGMINE

1. Neostigmine is a synthetic reversible anticholinesterase that contains a quaternary nitrogen.

2. **Actions**
   a. The pharmacologic properties of neostigmine mimic those of acetylcholine.
   b. It also has a direct action on nicotinic receptors, in addition to blocking acetylcholinesterase.
   c. It reverses the neuromuscular blockade produced by curare and its derivatives; the mechanism of action involves the release of increased amounts of acetylcholine from nerve endings, cholinesterase inhibition, and a direct action on the skeletal muscle cholinergic receptor.

3. **Pharmacokinetics**
   a. Neostigmine is not well absorbed orally.
   b. It does not penetrate the blood–brain barrier, which minimizes the toxicity due to inhibition of acetylcholinesterase that is in the brain.
   c. It is destroyed by plasma esterases and is excreted in the urine.

4. **Therapeutic uses**
   a. Neostigmine is used to reverse the effects of competitive neuromuscular blocking agents (see VIII).
   b. It is used in the management of paralytic ileus and atony of the urinary bladder.
   c. It is also used in the symptomatic treatment of myasthenia gravis.

C. EDROPHONIUM

1. **Actions**. In its actions, edrophonium is similar to neostigmine, except that with high doses it can stimulate the neuromuscular junction without affecting muscarinic effector organs.

2. **Pharmacokinetics**. Edrophonium is more rapidly absorbed and has a shorter duration of action than neostigmine. It is administered parenterally.

3. Its major **therapeutic uses** include:
   a. Diagnosis of myasthenia gravis.
   b. Antagonism of curare-like agents.

Irreversible →

D. ORGANOPHOSPHATE CHOLINESTERASE INHIBITORS

1. **Diisopropyl fluorophosphate (DFP)**
   a. **Mechanism of action**. DFP is an organophosphate compound which forms a covalent bond between its phosphorus atom and the esteratic site of cholinesterase. The enzyme–inhibitor complex thus formed is irreversible.
   b. **Therapeutic use** is limited to the treatment of certain types of glaucoma.
   c. **Untoward effects** of DFP and other organophosphate cholinesterase inhibitors include:
      (1) Miosis.
      (2) Increased bronchial secretions, profuse sweating, and increased lacrimation.
      (3) Anorexia, vomiting, and involuntary diarrhea.
      (4) Bradycardia.
      (5) Weakness of all skeletal muscles, but especially those of respiration, after twitching and fasciculations.
      (6) Anxiety, confusion, and convulsions, followed by vasomotor depression.

2. **Echothiophate** is a long-acting organophosphate cholinesterase inhibitor with pharmacologic properties similar to those of DFP. Spontaneous regeneration of the phosphorylated enzyme can occur. Its major use is in the treatment of glaucoma.

3. **Parathion** is an organophosphate anticholinesterase agent used as an insecticide. Its active form is **paraoxon**, a metabolite. Pharmacologic and untoward effects are similar to those of DFP.

4. **Reversal of cholinesterase inhibition**. Pyridine-2-aldoxime methyl chloride (PAM, pralidoxime) reverses the effects of the organophosphate anticholinesterase agents.
   a. It combines with and splits off the phosphorus from the esteratic site on cholinesterase in such a way that the enzyme is restored.
   b. With reactivation of the enzyme the effects of acetylcholine begin to disappear.
   c. Treatment must be within hours, for the phosphorylated enzyme slowly changes to a form that cannot be reversed.

VI. PARASYMPATHETIC ANTAGONISTS

A. **ATROPINE.** Atropine is an alkaloid derived from the plant *Atropa belladonna* (deadly nightshade). The active component is the racemic mixture *dl*-hyoscyamine, an ester composed of tropic acid and the organic base tropine.

1. **Mechanism of action**
   a. Atropine competes reversibly with acetylcholine at muscarinic receptors.
   b. At very high concentrations it blocks acetylcholine at ganglionic synapses and motor nerve endings.
   c. Atropine antagonizes the action of acetylcholine in the CNS.

2. **Actions**
   a. **Heart**
      (1) The heart rate slows initially, owing to medullary stimulation of the cardioinhibitory center.
      (2) Tachycardia then follows, with increased cardiac output and shortening of the P–R interval. Higher doses cause only tachycardia.
   b. **Blood pressure**
      (1) Oral or intramuscular doses have little effect on blood pressure.
      (2) With intravenous injection, total peripheral resistance increases.
      (3) Owing to the rise in heart rate and cardiac output, arterial pressure increases.
      (4) Atropine has a direct vasodilating effect on small blood vessels.
   c. **Central nervous system**
      (1) Large doses can produce hallucinations and, ultimately, coma, but therapeutic doses exert little effect.
      (2) Atropine possesses antitremor activity via a central antimuscarinic mechanism.
   d. **Involuntary muscles**
      (1) Atropine decreases the amplitude and frequency of peristaltic contractions and reduces the tone of the stomach, small intestine, and colon.
      (2) It also relaxes the smooth muscle of the biliary tract.
      (3) Bladder and ureter tone are decreased, while vesical sphincter tone is increased.
   e. **Eye**. Atropine blocks the acetylcholine response of the ciliary muscle of the lens and of the circular smooth muscles of the iris, producing cycloplegia and mydriasis.
   f. **Secretions**
      (1) Sweat gland secretions are greatly reduced.
      (2) Bronchial and salivary secretions are decreased.
      (3) There is a reduction in gastric secretion during both the psychic and gastric phases, and a reduction in total acid content, especially at doses greater than 1 mg.
   g. **Bronchi**. Atropine produces slight bronchodilation.

3. **Pharmacokinetics**
   a. Atropine is rapidly but poorly absorbed when given orally.
   b. It disappears rapidly from the blood and is excreted in the urine.

4. **Therapeutic uses**
   a. Ophthalmic administration is used for producing cycloplegia and mydriasis.
   b. Its ability to reduce secretions in the upper and lower respiratory tract makes it useful as a preanesthetic agent.
   c. It is used in myocardial infarction to treat sinus node bradycardia or a high-grade A–V block.
   d. It is effective for prophylaxis of motion sickness.
   e. Combined with an opioid, it is used for the treatment of renal and biliary colic.
   f. It may be used in large doses for the treatment of poisoning by anticholinesterase agents and for the rapid type of mushroom poisoning, because it antagonizes the actions of acetylcholine.

5. **Untoward effects** include:
   a. Rapid pulse.
   b. Dilated pupils, resulting in photophobia.
   c. Dry mouth.
   d. Flushed skin.
   e. A rise in body temperature, especially in children.
   f. Restlessness, confusion, and disorientation.

6. The antidote in atropine poisoning is physostigmine.

B. **SCOPOLAMINE (HYOSCINE),** like atropine, is an alkaloid and is an ester of tropic acid, but with the organic base scopine.

1. **Actions**. Like atropine, scopolamine has antimuscarinic actions.
   a. It is more potent than atropine in producing mydriasis and cycloplegia, in decreasing bronchial, salivary, and sweat gland secretions, and in its sedative effect.
   b. It is less potent than atropine in its effects on the heart, bronchial muscle, and intestines.
   c. Atropine has a longer duration of action and in therapeutic doses does not depress the CNS.

2. **Therapeutic uses** and **untoward effects** are generally similar to those of atropine. Scopolamine is excellent for motion sickness.

C. **PROPANTHELINE** is a synthetic antimuscarinic agent. High doses produce skeletal neuromuscular blockade. It is useful in the treatment of bladder spasm and enuresis. PROBANTHINE

D. **DICYCLOMINE** is another synthetic antimuscarinic drug.

1. At normal therapeutic doses it decreases spasm in most smooth muscles without producing atropine-like effects on the heart, eye, or salivary and sweat glands.

2. It is thought to act by direct relaxation of muscle rather than by competitive antagonism of acetylcholine at muscarinic receptors.

E. TROPICAMIDE - MYDRIACYL (R)   F. METHSCOPOLAMINE - PAMINE (R)

VII. GANGLIONIC STIMULATORS AND BLOCKERS

A. NICOTINE

1. **Mechanism of action**
   a. Nicotine interacts with the acetylcholine receptor on the postsynaptic membrane of autonomic ganglia.
   b. It causes an initial stimulation of the ganglion similar to the effect of acetylcholine.
   c. Larger amounts produce a prolonged blockade following the initial stimulation.
   d. In small doses it causes the release of catecholamines from the adrenal medulla, while larger doses prevent their release.
   e. Nicotine affects chemoreceptors in the carotid and aortic bodies and centers in the medulla oblongata.

2. **Pharmacologic actions**
   a. Nicotine is a CNS stimulant.
      (1) Via motor cortex excitation it produces tremors which, with larger doses, can be followed by convulsions.
      (2) Small doses stimulate respiration while toxic doses depress it.
      (3) Nicotine stimulates the release of antidiuretic hormone.
   b. Tachycardia, increased blood pressure, and increased total peripheral resistance result from stimulation of sympathetic ganglia and the adrenal medulla.
   c. Increased bowel motility results predominantly from parasympathetic ganglionic stimulation.
   d. Salivary and bronchial secretions are first stimulated, then blocked.

3. **Pharmacokinetics**
   a. Nicotine is readily absorbed through the skin, respiratory tract, and buccal membranes.
   b. It is metabolized in the liver, kidney, and lung, and is eliminated via the kidney.
   c. It is excreted in the breast milk of lactating women who are heavy smokers.

4. No therapeutic uses for nicotine exist. Its inherent toxicity has been applied in the control of insects. Its presence in tobacco is, of course, of major medical importance.

B. HEXAMETHONIUM

1. **Structure**. Hexamethonium $[(CH_3)_3—N^+—(CH_2)_6—^+N—(CH_3)_3]$ has a bridge of six methylene groups between two quaternary nitrogen atoms. The addition of more intervening carbon groups decreases the activity at the ganglionic receptor and increases activity at the skeletal muscle receptor. Ten carbons (as in decamethonium) will produce maximal activity at the skeletal muscle receptor.

2. **Mechanism of action**. Hexamethonium produces competitive ganglionic blockade by occupying ganglionic cholinergic receptors.

3. **Actions**
   - **a.** Hexamethonium reduces systemic vascular resistance, venous return, and cardiac output.
   - **b.** Gastric secretions are reduced in volume and acidity, and gastric motility is reduced.
   - **c.** Salivary secretions are decreased, and some bronchodilation occurs.
   - **d.** The glomerular filtration rate is decreased and renal vascular resistance is increased.
   - **e.** Urinary excretion may be impaired because of reduced bladder contractions.
   - **f.** Partial mydriasis and loss of accommodation may occur.
   - **g.** Dryness of the skin and flushing occur.

4. Hexamethonium is not used therapeutically.

C. TRIMETHAPHAN is a sulfonium ganglionic blocking agent with a very short duration of action. It is used therapeutically in treating hypertensive crises, in the management of autonomic hyperreflexia, and to provide controlled hypotension in order to reduce bleeding in the operative field during surgery.

VIII. NEUROMUSCULAR BLOCKING AGENTS.

These agents, which act by blocking transmission at the neuromuscular junction, can be divided into two classes on the basis of their mechanism of action: **depolarizing agents** (succinylcholine, decamethonium) and **competitive**, or **stabilizing, blocking agents** (tubocurarine, gallamine, pancuronium).

A. MECHANISM OF ACTION

1. **Depolarizing agents** (succinylcholine, decamethonium)
   - **a.** Like acetylcholine, depolarizing agents react with receptors at the muscle end-plate, leading to depolarization of the excitable membrane. This so-called **phase I block** is seen clinically as fasciculation.
   - **b.** With prolonged exposure, a reduction in receptor sensitivity occurs, leading to a **phase II**, or **desensitization, block** manifested by flaccid paralysis. This phase II block is not competitive in nature.

2. **Competitive blocking agents** (tubocurarine, gallamine, pancuronium)
   - **a.** Competitive blocking agents combine with acetylcholine receptors at the muscle end-plate but do not activate them.
   - **b.** By decreasing the number of available acetylcholine receptors, these agents reduce the height of the end-plate potential; thus, the threshold for excitation is not reached.

B. PHARMACOKINETICS

1. After injection of a neuromuscular blocking agent, it is found in high concentration in venous blood flowing to the heart, and ultimately in the extracellular space around the muscle end-plate.

2. Succinylcholine has a rapid onset of action, which facilitates rapid endotracheal intubation.

3. **Metabolism**
   - **a.** Metabolism of gallamine, tubocurarine, and decamethonium is negligible.
   - **b.** Pancuronium is deacetylated, and its metabolites show some activity.
   - **c.** Succinylcholine is rapidly metabolized to succinylmonocholine and choline, which accounts for its brief duration of action.

C. THERAPEUTIC USES.

Neuromuscular blocking agents are used:

1. As surgical adjuvants to anesthesia
   - **a.** For promoting skeletal muscle relaxation.
   - **b.** For facilitating endotracheal intubation.

2. With electroconvulsant shock therapy, to prevent trauma.

3. In the diagnosis of myasthenia gravis (tubocurarine), although provocative tests of this sort are potentially hazardous procedures.

D. UNTOWARD EFFECTS

1. **Neuromuscular blocking agents** do not affect the sensorium, so that despite the paralysis, individuals remain conscious and are able to feel pain.

2. **Depolarizing agents**
   a. The fasciculations can cause muscle pain, which occurs most frequently in young patients.
   b. Fasciculation of the abdominal muscles can result in increased intragastric pressure. This is of importance in patients at risk of aspirating gastric contents.
   c. Contraction of extraocular muscles can lead to an increase in intraocular pressure.
   d. The muscle fasciculations and the increased intraocular and intragastric pressure may be diminished by the prior administration of a small dose of a competitive blocking agent.
   e. Succinylcholine may exert some action at other acetylcholine receptors, such as stimulation of autonomic ganglia and muscarinic receptors.
   f. The resulting effects, such as bradycardia and increased bronchial secretions, are seen more commonly with repeated intravenous administration in children; cardiac arrest has occurred.
   g. In some genetically predisposed individuals, the combination of succinylcholine and halothane results in a rapid and potentially fatal rise in temperature (malignant hyperthermia).

3. **Tubocurarine**
   a. A dose-related fall in arterial pressure, the most common side effect, is the result of both ganglionic blockade and histamine release.
   b. Histamine release can also result in bronchospasm.

4. **Gallamine** causes tachycardia and increased arterial pressure, the results of both vagolytic and tyramine-like effects.

5. **Pancuronium** also causes an increase in the heart rate and in arterial pressure, but to a lesser extent than gallamine does; the mechanism is not understood.

E. FACTORS INFLUENCING THE ACTION OF NEUROMUSCULAR BLOCKING AGENTS

1. Serum cholinesterase is determined genetically; the normally transient effects of succinylcholine will be greatly prolonged in an individual with deficient serum cholinesterase.

2. Because serum cholinesterase is synthesized in the liver, hepatic disease can double the duration of action of succinylcholine.

3. Echothiophate, an irreversible cholinesterase inhibitor used in the treatment of glaucoma, can significantly decrease cholinesterase activity and thereby increase the duration of action of succinylcholine.

4. Patients with myasthenia gravis are highly sensitive to competitive neuromuscular blocking agents, and phase II block occurs sooner than in normal individuals when depolarizing blockers are given.

5. Patients with Eaton-Lambert syndrome (small-cell, or oat-cell, carcinoma of the lung) have increased sensitivity to both competitive and depolarizing neuromuscular blockers.

6. Depolarizing neuromuscular blockers increase serum potassium; this is exacerbated in conditions that are associated with hyperkalemia, such as burns.

7. Aminoglycoside antibiotics and lincomycin exert a synergistic neuromuscular blockade when given with either competitive or depolarizing neuromuscular blocking agents; the mechanism is presynaptic.

8. All inhalation anesthetics increase the effects of neuromuscular blocking agents.

F. REVERSAL OF NEUROMUSCULAR BLOCKADE

1. Competitive neuromuscular blockers can be antagonized by cholinesterase inhibitors such as edrophonium, neostigmine, or pyridostigmine.

2. No antagonists currently exist for depolarizing blockers.
   a. Controlled ventilation is used until spontaneous recovery occurs.
   b. If an anticholinesterase is given, phase I block increases, but an anticholinesterase may reverse phase II block.

STUDY QUESTIONS

Directions: Each question below contains five suggested answers. Choose the **one best** response to each question.

1. Atropine and its analogs produce which of the following effects?

(A) Pupillary constriction
(B) Increased gastric secretion
(C) Decreased secretion in the respiratory tract
(D) Increased peristalsis
(E) Micturition

2. Agents that produce neuromuscular blockade act by inhibiting which of the following events?

(A) Synthesis of acetylcholine from acetyl coenzyme A and choline
(B) Release of acetylcholine from the prejunctional membrane
(C) Packaging of acetylcholine into synaptic vesicles
(D) Interaction of acetylcholine with cholinergic receptors
(E) Re-uptake of acetylcholine into the nerve ending

3. A patient who is using a sympathomimetic agent that is direct-acting, is not a monoamine oxidase inhibitor, and is used clinically as a decongestant is most likely to be taking

(A) ephedrine
(B) amphetamine
(C) phenylephrine
(D) metaraminol
(E) mephentermine

4. A cholinesterase-inhibiting agent that also has a direct nicotinic effect is

(A) physostigmine
(B) diisopropyl fluorophosphate (DFP)
(C) neostigmine
(D) scopolamine
(E) none of the above

5. Which of the following agents is capable of inhibiting insulin secretion, increasing glucose blood levels via liver glycogenolysis, and increasing free fatty acids?

(A) Epinephrine
(B) Phentolamine
(C) Phenoxybenzamine
(D) Atropine
(E) Propranolol

6. A patient is taking a mixed-acting sympathomimetic as a nasal decongestant. This agent, which exhibits tachyphylaxis and qualitatively resembles epinephrine in its cardiovascular effects, most likely is

(A) ephedrine
(B) phenylephrine
(C) metaproterenol
(D) terbutaline
(E) amphetamine

Directions: Each question below contains four suggested answers of which **one or more** is correct. Choose the answer

A if **1, 2, and 3** are correct
B if **1 and 3** are correct
C if **2 and 4** are correct
D if **4** is correct
E if **1, 2, 3, and 4** are correct

7. Correct statements about agents that affect adrenergic receptors include which of the following?

(1) Phentolamine is a reversible β-blocker
(2) Propranolol causes bronchiolar constriction
(3) Phenoxybenzamine is an α-agonist
(4) Ergotamine is a weak α-blocker

8. Acetylcholine can stimulate

(1) ganglionic (nicotinic) receptors
(2) muscarinic receptors
(3) the release of epinephrine
(4) the release of norepinephrine

SUMMARY OF DIRECTIONS

A	B	C	D	E
1, 2, 3 only	1, 3 only	2, 4 only	4 only	All are correct

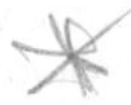

9. Characteristics of pilocarpine include which of the following?

(1) It is a quaternary compound
(2) It possesses mainly muscarinic activity
(3) It can be blocked by neostigmine
(4) It can be blocked by atropine

10. Characteristics of adrenergic receptors include which of the following?

(1) β_1-Adrenergic receptors predominate in cardiac tissue
(2) β_2-Adrenergic receptors are found in smooth muscle
(3) α_2-Adrenergic receptors mediate presynaptic feedback inhibition
(4) α_1-Adrenergic receptors are found at postsynaptic effector sites

11. Characteristics of pancuronium include which of the following?

(1) Its effects on the heart are similar to the effects of succinylcholine
(2) It can cause apnea
(3) It produces analgesia
(4) It causes less histamine release than *d*-tubocurarine

12. A patient comes into the emergency room with a pulse of 140 and a blood pressure of 190/120; he is nervous, restless, and complaining of insomnia. Which of the following drugs could have caused these symptoms?

(1) Metaraminol
(2) Ephedrine
(3) Phenylephrine
(4) Amphetamine

Directions: The group of questions below consists of lettered choices followed by several numbered items. For each numbered item select the **one** lettered choice with which it is **most** closely associated. Each lettered choice may be used once, more than once, or not at all.

Questions 13–16

For each of the following descriptions of drug actions, select the agent with which it is most likely to be associated.

(A) Phenylephrine
(B) Amphetamine
(C) Diisopropyl fluorophosphate (DFP)
(D) Neostigmine
(E) Methacholine (acetyl β-methylcholine)

13. Purely muscarinic in its action
14. Irreversible cholinesterase inhibitor
15. Closely resembles norepinephrine in its cardiovascular actions
16. Enzyme inhibitor as well as receptor agonist

ANSWERS AND EXPLANATIONS

1. The answer is C. *(VI A 2)* The muscarinic blocker atropine will produce pupillary dilation, decreased gastric acid secretion, reflex tachycardia, and difficulty with micturition. Its ability to decrease bronchial secretions makes it clinically useful as a preanesthetic agent.

2. The answer is D. *(VIII A)* Both competitive and noncompetitive neuromuscular blocking agents interact with cholinergic receptors to produce neuromuscular blockade. Competitive agents such as α-tubocurarine act at the skeletal muscle cholinergic receptor in a reversible fashion. Succinylcholine, however, acts at this site in a more complex manner, and metabolism is required for the termination of its action.

3. The answer is C. *(II E–G, I, K)* All of the substances listed in the question are sympathomimetic agents. Ephedrine, amphetamine, mephentermine, and metaraminol are all mixed-acting agents. Phenylephrine is direct-acting and is used clinically as a decongestant.

4. The answer is C. *(V B; VI B)* Scopolamine is a muscarinic blocker. All of the other agents listed are cholinesterase inhibitors but only neostigmine has, in addition, a direct nicotinic stimulating effect.

5. The answer is A. *(II A 3 e)* The adrenal medullary substance epinephrine is the only agent listed in the question which is capable of producing all of the effects noted. Because epinephrine interacts with both α- and β-adrenergic receptors, its effects on some body systems depend on the concentration as well as the receptor.

6. The answer is A. *(II E, F, G, L, M)* Phenylephrine, metaproterenol, and terbutaline are all direct-acting sympathomimetic agents, while amphetamine is indirect-acting. Ephedrine is mixed-acting and is used as a nasal decongestant. While its primary action is indirect, causing release of norepinephrine from storage in nerve terminals, it also directly stimulates sympathetic receptors.

7. The answer is C (2, 4). *(III A 1, 2, 4, B 1)* Phentolamine is a reversible α-blocker, while phenoxybenzamine is an irreversible α-antagonist. Propranolol by reversible β blockade can cause bronchiolar constriction, and ergotamine is a weak α-blocker

8. The answer is E (all). *(I D 1; IV A 2)* Acetylcholine can stimulate the release of epinephrine from the adrenal medulla. In addition, by stimulating postganglionic adrenergic nerves, it will cause the release of norepinephrine.

9. The answer is C (2, 4). *(IV E)* Pilocarpine is a tertiary amine which possesses mainly muscarinic activity. It is not blocked by the acetylcholinesterase inhibitor neostigmine but can be blocked by the muscarinic blocker atropine.

10. The answer is E (all). *(I D 2)* All of the statements regarding receptors are true. Those drugs that act principally on β_1 receptors will produce cardiac effects, while those acting on β_2 receptors produce minimal cardiac effects but possess significant smooth muscle (e.g., bronchiolar) relaxant activity. α_1 Receptors are found at postsynaptic effector sites, while α_2 receptors mediate presynaptic feedback inhibition.

11. The answer is C (2, 4). *(VIII)* Pancuronium is a competitive neuromuscular blocker which can cause apnea and, unlike tubocurarine, causes minimal histamine release. Unlike succinylcholine, it can increase the heart rate. None of the neuromuscular blocking agents affect sensory awareness.

12. The answer is D (4). *(II E–G, K)* The only agent listed that is capable of producing the significant peripheral and central adrenergic symptoms described is amphetamine.

13–16. The answers are 13-E, 14-C, 15-A, 16-D. *(II E 1, G 1; IV B; V B 2, D1)* Methacholine, because of the addition of the β-methyl group, is purely muscarinic in action. DFP is an irreversible organophosphate cholinesterase inhibitor. Neostigmine is a reversible cholinesterase inhibitor. Phenylephrine, though less potent, resembles norepinephrine in its cardiovascular effects. Neostigmine, besides being a reversible cholinesterase inhibitor, also stimulates nicotinic receptors.

3
Agents Acting on the Central Nervous System

I. INTRODUCTION

A. TRANSMISSION OF NERVE IMPULSES

1. The brain and spinal cord are involved in information transfer via electrical signals passing along axons **(action potentials)**.
2. The locus of communication between neurons is the **synapse**.
   a. In general, a chemical **neurotransmitter** is released from a presynaptic neuron, diffuses across the synaptic cleft, and interacts with a specific cell-surface receptor located on a second, postsynaptic, neuron.
   b. The neurotransmitter–receptor complex initiates a sequence of events (e.g., the opening of channels for particular ions) which can either excite, inhibit, or otherwise modulate the electrical activity of the postsynaptic neuron.
3. Although the basic mechanisms underlying many of the agents affecting the central nervous system (CNS) are only incompletely understood, most are believed to alter either the basic cellular functioning of neurons or the communication between neurons.
   a. Any agent that slows or blocks the axonal electrical conduction (e.g., a local anesthetic) will have an effect on behavior.
   b. However, at therapeutic doses, most of the pharmacologically useful agents that affect the CNS are believed to act at various specific synaptic sites.
4. Synaptic transmission between neurons can be affected by altering the levels of neurotransmitter in the presynaptic neuron. This can be accomplished by various agents which:
   a. Block or enhance the biosynthesis of the neurotransmitter.
   b. Block or enhance the metabolic degradation of the neurotransmitter.
   c. Alter the re-uptake and re-utilization of the neurotransmitter in presynaptic terminals.
5. In some cases it is possible to alter the amount of neurotransmitter that is released, by activating **presynaptic receptors (autoreceptors)** which are located at some synapses.
6. Many drugs are believed to bind to receptors, and, bypassing the normal neurotransmitter, to either activate or block the response of the postsynaptic neuron, serving respectively as agonists or antagonists.
7. Some drugs may act directly on ion channels, bypassing the neurotransmitter–receptor interaction entirely.

B. THE BLOOD–BRAIN BARRIER. The ability of an agent to affect CNS function is also dependent on its ability to cross the so-called **blood–brain barrier**.

1. Agents that are lipid-soluble, are un-ionized at physiologic pH, and bind poorly to plasma proteins are better able to diffuse across the blood–brain barrier.
2. Some metabolically important compounds (e.g., nutrients) apparently are actively transported across this barrier.
3. The morphologic basis for the blood–brain barrier appears to be the structure of the endothelial cell layer lining the brain capillaries. The capillaries in the brain, unlike those in other tissues, have few pinocytotic vesicles or fenestrations.

II. SEDATIVE–HYPNOTICS

A. BARBITURATES

1. Chemistry

a. The parent compound, barbituric acid (Fig. 3-1), is derived from a dehydration of urea and malonic acid. Barbituric acid itself has no depressant effect on the CNS.

b. The common barbiturates are listed in Table 3-1; the radicals given in the table are those shown in Figure 3-1 (R_1 and R_2).

c. Changes in structure that favor increased lipid solubility will speed up the onset of action, shorten the duration of action, and increase the hypnotic potency.

d. When the oxygen at C-2 of oxybarbiturates is replaced with a sulfur it becomes a thiobarbiturate, a compound with enhanced lipid solubility.

2. Classification. Barbiturates are classified on the basis of their onset and duration of action.

a. **Ultra-short-acting** barbiturates (e.g., **thiopental**) act within seconds, and their duration of action is 30 minutes. Their principal use is as intravenous adjuvants to anesthesia.

b. **Short-acting** barbiturates (e.g., **pentobarbital**) have a duration of action of about 2 hours; their principal use is as sleep-inducing hypnotics.

c. **Intermediate-acting** barbiturates (e.g., **amobarbital**) have an effect lasting 3 to 5 hours. Their principal use is as hypnotics; however, they have a "hangover" liability, the result of residual depression of the CNS.

d. **Long-acting** barbiturates (e.g., **phenobarbital**) have a duration of action greater than 6 hours. They are effective hypnotics and sedatives, and at low doses are useful as antiepileptic agents, but they are likely to cause "hangover."

3. Mechanism of action

a. At low doses, barbiturates either have a GABA-like action or enhance the effects of GABA (γ-aminobutyric acid).

b. The mechanism of their GABA-like action is unclear. Barbiturates may inhibit a neuronal uptake system for GABA or may stimulate the release of GABA.

c. Barbiturates are less selective than benzodiazepines, which also have GABA-like actions, because elevating the dose of barbiturates produces a generalized CNS depression in addition to selective depression at synaptic sites.

4. Pharmacologic actions

a. Barbiturates depress the CNS at all levels in a dose-dependent fashion.

b. As hypnotics, they decrease the amount of time spent in REM sleep.

c. Barbiturates are not analgesic and at low doses are thought to be hyperalgesic.

d. All barbiturates will suppress convulsant activity if given in sufficient doses.

e. Respiration is depressed at multiple levels. As CNS depression develops and the neurogenic respiratory drive is eliminated, the respiratory drive shifts to the carotid and aortic bodies. The hypoxic drive is affected at lower doses than the chemoreceptor drive, but it persists beyond complete blockade of the response to CO_2. Eventually, at high doses, the hypoxic drive also fails.

f. At sedative doses barbiturates have little effect on the cardiovascular system.

- **(1)** As the dose of barbiturate is increased, depressed ganglionic transmission results in decreased blood pressure and heart rate.
- **(2)** Toxic dose levels can cause circulatory collapse which is due, in part, to medullary vasomotor depression.

g. Most barbiturates, but especially phenobarbital, are capable of inducing the hepatic microsomal drug-metabolizing enzyme system.

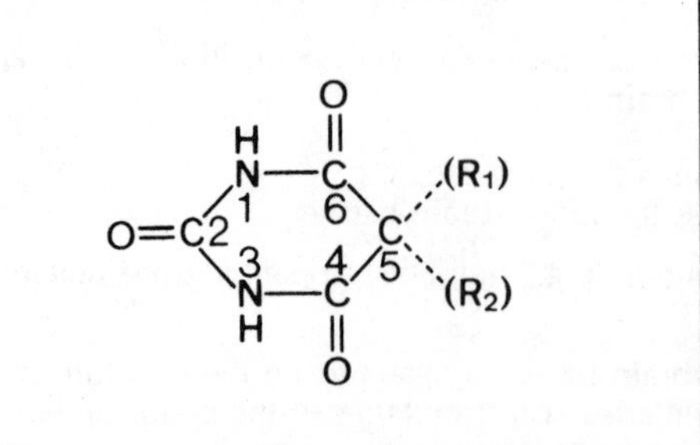

Figure 3-1. Structure of barbituric acid. The radicals (R_1 and R_2) of the common barbiturates are given in Table 3-1.

Table 3-1. Common Barbiturates: Radicals and Duration of Action

Drug	Radical 1 (R_1)*	Radical 2 (R_2)*	Duration of Action
Thiopental	Ethyl	1-Methylbutyl	Ultra-short
Hexobarbital	Methyl	1-Cyclohexen-1-yl	Short
Pentobarbital	Ethyl	1-Methylbutyl	Short
Secobarbital	Allyl	1-Methylbutyl	Short
Amobarbital	Ethyl	Isopentyl	Intermediate
Butabarbital	Ethyl	*sec*-Butyl	Intermediate
Barbital	Ethyl	Ethyl	Long
Phenobarbital	Ethyl	Phenyl	Long

*See Figure 3-1.

(1) This results in increased degradation of the barbiturate, ultimately leading to barbiturate tolerance.
(2) It also causes increased inactivation of other compounds, such as the anticoagulants, phenytoin, digitoxin, and glucocorticoids, leading to potentially serious problems with drug interactions.

h. Anesthetic doses of barbiturates may suppress renal tubular transport.
i. Barbiturate-induced porphyria can occur.

5. Pharmacokinetics

a. The duration of action of a barbiturate depends on
   (1) Its rate of metabolic (hepatic) degradation.
   (2) Its degree of lipid solubility.
   (3) The extent to which it binds to serum proteins, which reduces renal excretion.
b. Long-acting barbiturates are metabolized principally in the liver, by a slow oxidation of the radicals at C-5, which produces more polar derivatives with low lipid solubility.
c. Ultra-short-acting barbiturates are highly lipid-soluble and thus have a short onset and duration of action. High lipid solubility allows rapid transport across the blood–brain barrier.
d. Removal of the ultra-short-acting barbiturates from the brain occurs via redistribution to other tissues (e.g., muscle).
e. Barbiturates are absorbed from the stomach, small intestine, rectum, and intramuscular sites.
f. They readily cross the placental barrier, and concentrations in the fetal blood approach those in maternal blood.
g. Barbiturates and their metabolites are principally excreted via the renal route.
   (1) If renal function is impaired, barbiturates can cause severe CNS and cardiovascular depression.
   (2) Alkalinization of the urine profoundly expedites the excretion of barbiturates with lower lipid solubility such as phenobarbital. These drugs are only partially bound to plasma protein and are weak organic acids.

6. Therapeutic indications

a. Although still used as sedatives and hypnotic agents, barbiturates are being replaced for this purpose by benzodiazepines (see VI C).
b. Due to their rapid onset of action, barbiturates (phenobarbital, pentobarbital, amobarbital, and thiopental) are used in the emergency treatment of convulsions, as in status epilepticus, but the benzodiazepines are again the drugs of choice. (See also III A, below.)
c. The ultra-short-acting thiobarbiturates are useful as intravenous adjuncts to surgical anesthetics.
d. Barbiturates, especially in anesthetic doses, significantly decrease oxygen utilization by the brain. This may be of value in lessening cerebral edema caused by surgery or trauma and in protecting against cerebral infarction during cerebral ischemia.
e. The ability of barbiturates to stimulate liver glucuronyl transferase has been applied successfully in the treatment of hyperbilirubinemia and kernicterus in the neonate.

7. Barbiturate dependence and intoxication

a. Physiologic as well as psychological dependence can occur.
b. Withdrawal of a barbiturate may result in grand mal seizures, severe tremors, vivid hallucinations, and psychoses. Abrupt withdrawal should therefore be avoided.
c. Acute barbiturate overdoses can result in coma; diminished reflexes (although deep tendon reflexes are usually intact); severe respiratory depression; hypotension, leading to cardiovascular collapse; and renal failure.

d. Treatment of acute barbiturate overdosage
   (1) Primary treatment consists of supporting respiration and circulation.
   (2) Excretion of the drug is fostered by alkalinizing the urine and promoting diuresis. These measures are most effective with the longer-acting barbiturates.
   (3) Hemodialysis or peritoneal dialysis is useful and often needed.

B. NONBARBITURATE SEDATIVE–HYPNOTICS

1. Chloral hydrate

a. Chloral hydrate is a relatively safe hypnotic drug, inducing sleep in half an hour and lasting about 6 hours.
b. It causes a relatively small reduction in REM sleep.
c. Chloral hydrate is quite bad-tasting and is irritating to the gastrointestinal tract.
d. It is metabolized in the liver by alcohol dehydrogenase to trichloroethanol, which is thought to be the active metabolite producing the CNS effects. In addition, chloral hydrate enhances the ability of hepatic microsomes to metabolize drugs.
e. Trichloroethanol, and, to a smaller extent, chloral hydrate, are oxidized to trichloroacetic acid, which is excreted in the kidney as the glucuronide conjugate.
f. In patients with significant liver or kidney disease chloral hydrate should not be used.
g. The CNS depressant effects are potentiated by alcohol (the combination being dubbed a "Mickey Finn").
h. Addiction can occur, and when it does the patient often presents with chronic gastritis and skin eruptions. Dependent individuals may lose the mechanisms that detoxify the drug.

2. Paraldehyde

a. Paraldehyde is a trimer of acetaldehyde; its structure is shown in Figure 3-2.
b. Paraldehyde produces hypnosis in about 15 minutes and lasts 4 to 8 hours.
c. Its CNS depressant activity resembles that of alcohol, chloral hydrate, and the barbiturates.
d. Besides its use as a hypnotic, it is also used in the treatment of delirium tremens and for obstetrical anesthesia.
e. Paraldehyde can be administered orally, parenterally, or rectally. When used rectally it is combined with two volumes of olive oil.
f. About 70 percent is detoxified in the liver and the remainder is expired through the lungs.
g. Both addiction and untoward effects are rare. However,
   (1) Its strong odor and disagreeable taste limit its use mainly to hospitals.
   (2) It is a gastrointestinal irritant.
   (3) Pulmonary disease, peptic ulcer disease, and hepatic insufficiency are relative contraindications to paraldehyde administration.
   (4) It should not be used with disulfiram.

3. Glutethimide. The use of glutethimide as a therapeutic agent is hard to justify.

a. Its clinical use is now limited by its high addiction liability, the severity of withdrawal symptoms, and the problems caused by acute intoxication.
b. Glutethimide is erratically absorbed from the gastrointestinal tract and most is metabolized in the liver. After metabolism most is excreted by the kidney.
c. Chronic abuse of glutethimide can lead to toxic psychoses, convulsions, and hyperpyrexia.
d. Acute intoxication produces symptoms similar to those of barbiturate poisoning. In addition, atropine-like effects are observed and convulsions can occur. The plasma half-life during acute intoxication can be as long as 4 days, but can be reduced to ½ day by hemodialysis. Although the plasma levels decline after dialysis, a secondary rise in plasma levels is then observed. This is thought to result from additional intestinal absorption of glutethimide.

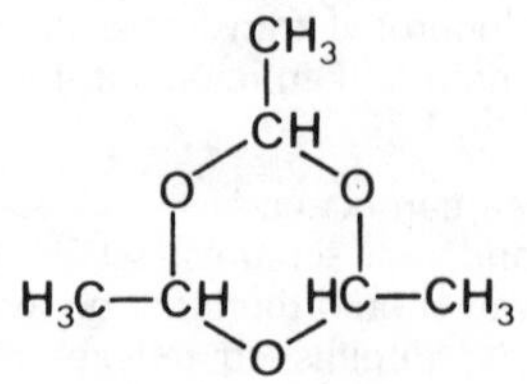

Figure 3-2. Paraldehyde.

4. **Methyprylon**
   a. Methyprylon closely resembles secobarbital in its onset and duration of action. It is absorbed from the gastrointestinal tract and is used as an oral hypnotic.
   b. It significantly suppresses REM sleep.
   c. Untoward effects include a hangover-like effect, skin rashes, and addiction liabilities.
   d. Acute intoxication resembles that of barbiturates; treatment is supportive.

5. **Ethchlorvynol**
   a. Ethchlorvynol is classified as a tertiary alcohol which, in addition to its sedative–hypnotic properties, possesses muscle-relaxant and anticonvulsant properties.
   b. It is absorbed from the gastrointestinal tract and shows an onset of action in 30 minutes and a 5-hour duration of action.
   c. Untoward effects include suppression of REM sleep, ataxia, hypotension, and facial numbness.
   d. Physical dependence can occur. An acute overdose is treated as for barbiturate poisoning.

6. **Methaqualone**
   a. Methaqualone (Quaalude) is highly abused because it is said to cause a heroin-like "high." It is also believed to have aphrodisiac properties.
   b. Large doses exert a selective depressant effect on polysynaptic spinal reflexes.
   c. It possesses local anesthetic, anticholinergic, antihistaminic, and anticonvulsant properties.
   d. It enhances the analgesic effect of codeine.
   e. Methaqualone is well absorbed from the gastrointestinal tract and is metabolized by the hepatic microsomal metabolizing system. The majority of the metabolites are excreted in the urine.
   f. Untoward effects include pulmonary and cutaneous edema, and at large doses tonic convulsions can occur.
   g. Paresthesias may precede the onset of sleep, and a hangover effect is common.
   h. An overdose resulting in death most often occurs with the concomitant ingestion of alcohol.
   i. Physical dependence and tolerance occur with methaqualone abuse.

7. **Flurazepam**
   a. Flurazepam, a benzodiazepine derivative (see VI C), produces hypnotic effects that begin in 20 to 40 minutes after an oral dose and last for 6 to 8 hours.
   b. In contrast to the various other hypnotic sedatives, the benzodiazepines are not general neuronal depressants.
   c. Flurazepam offers diminished suppression of REM sleep.
   d. Overdosage can occur and is treated as for other benzodiazepines.
   e. At moderate dosage, addiction liability is low, as is withdrawal insomnia, which is often seen with many of the other hypnotics.
   f. As mentioned earlier, the benzodiazepines are now generally considered to be the preferred drug for hypnosis–sedation. Whether the antianxiety features of the benzodiazepines are distinct from the hypnotic–sedative effects is presently unclear. A full description of the benzodiazepines is given below (see VI C).

III. ANTISEIZURE AGENTS

A. BARBITURATES (see II A, above)

1. The prototype agent is **phenobarbital**, which is most frequently used in doses far below the sedative–hypnotic range.
2. It is effective in controlling generalized seizure states (generalized tonic–clonic seizures, simple and complex partial seizures). It can be used alone or in combination with other antiseizure agents.
3. Sedation is the most frequent untoward effect, while drug allergy occurs in about 1 percent of patients treated.
4. If barbiturate therapy is withdrawn it should be done gradually in order to prevent the occurrence of status epilepticus.

B. DEOXYBARBITURATES

1. The prototype agent of this class is primidone, which is useful for the same types of seizures as phenobarbital.

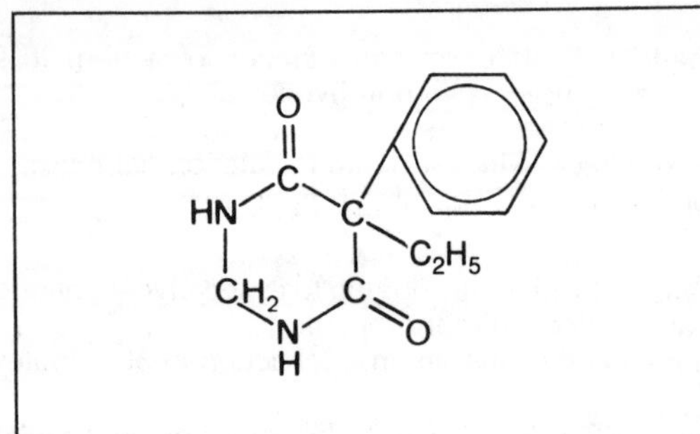

Figure 3-3. Primidone.

2. Primidone does not have a true barbituric acid ring structure but bears a close resemblance to the barbiturates (Fig. 3-3).
3. It is well absorbed from the gastrointestinal tract. Two major metabolites are seen, one of which is phenobarbital.
4. It may initially produce sedation but this decreases with continued use.
5. Primidone may exacerbate petit mal epilepsy.
6. Other serious untoward reactions include
   a. Skin rashes which are also common to the barbiturates.
   b. Leukopenia and thrombocytopenia.
   c. Systemic lupus erythematosus.
   d. Acute psychotic reactions.

C. HYDANTOINS

1. All hydantoins are highly fat-soluble and are insoluble in water.
2. Though two major hydantoin derivatives exist, namely **phenytoin (diphenylhydantoin)** and **mephenytoin**, the former is the most widely used.
3. **Phenytoin**
   a. Phenytoin (Dilantin) exerts its anticonvulsant action without producing CNS depression.
   b. It is believed to act by promoting the extrusion of sodium from cortical neuronal fibers. The altered ion concentration is presumed to block the spread of the seizure discharge.
   c. Because phenytoin is a very weak acid (pK_a 8.3), its gastrointestinal absorption is variable, incomplete, and slow. Nearly all (90 percent) is bound to plasma proteins. The drug is metabolized by the drug microsomal metabolizing system and is excreted first in the bile, then the urine. A genetic defect in phenytoin metabolism has been reported.
   d. The main therapeutic usefulness of phenytoin is in the treatment of grand mal epilepsy, for which it is effective in 80 percent of the cases. It also has some value in treating simple and complex partial seizures.
   e. It may exacerbate petit mal epilepsy.
   f. Generally, tolerance to the anticonvulsant action of phenytoin is not problematic.
   g. Untoward effects include
      (1) Gastrointestinal irritation; therefore, it should be taken with meals.
      (2) Ataxia and diplopia.
      (3) Blood dyscrasias.
      (4) Hypersensitivity reactions, including Stevens-Johnson syndrome and systemic lupus erythematosus. The drug should be stopped if a rash occurs.
      (5) Gingival hyperplasia, hirsutism, increased collagen proliferation, and bone growth.
      (6) Hepatitis.
      (7) Cardiovascular collapse and CNS depression, which may occur with intravenous administration exceeding 50 mg/min.
      (8) Drug interactions: Increased plasma concentrations of phenytoin can occur due to inhibition of its inactivation by concurrent administration of chloramphenicol, isoniazid, dicumarol, disulfiram, and certain sulfonamides.
      (9) Fetal malformations: Phenytoin is teratogenic.
4. **Mephenytoin** has a much higher incidence of blood dyscrasias than phenytoin and greater CNS depressant activity, which limit its usefulness. It has been used in the treatment of grand mal, psychomotor, and focal seizures.

D. SUCCINIMIDES

1. **Ethosuximide** is considered the drug of first choice in the treatment of petit mal epilepsy.
   a. It may exacerbate grand mal epilepsy.
   b. Ethosuximide is absorbed from the gastrointestinal tract. Eighty percent is metabolized in the hepatic microsomal metabolizing system; twenty percent is unchanged. Both unchanged drug and hepatic metabolites appear in the urine.
   c. Untoward effects include
      (1) Gastrointestinal reactions—anorexia and nausea.
      (2) CNS effects–drowsiness, headache, and hiccup; extrapyramidal symptoms and photophobia have been reported.
      (3) Hypersensitivity reactions, as for phenytoin.

2. Both **methsuximide** and **phensuximide** have been useful antiepileptic agents, with adverse experience profiles similar to that of ethosuximide. They appear to have a lower efficacy than the prototype agent ethosuximide.

E. BENZODIAZEPINES

1. Many of these agents are sedative–hypnotics and mild tranquilizers (see VI C). Some are also very effective in seizure control.

2. Benzodiazepines enhance a variety of GABA-mediated synaptic systems involving both presynaptic and postsynaptic inhibition.

3. **Diazepam**, given intravenously, is now considered a drug of choice for status epilepticus. It should be used with great caution in patients who have received barbiturates. It is also effective against all other types of seizures, particularly petit mal and other minor motor seizures. Its usefulness as a long-term antiepileptic agent is limited by the development of refractoriness within a few months.

4. **Clonazepam** is useful in the treatment of absence seizures and myoclonic seizures in children.
   a. It is absorbed well from the gastrointestinal tract and its central effects develop rapidly.
   b. Its chief therapeutic limitation is the development of tolerance, which can be overcome by increasing the dose. At higher doses, however, sedation is induced.

5. **Clorazepate** is a useful adjunctive drug in the treatment of complex partial seizures.

6. When any benzodiazepine is used intravenously, cardiovascular and respiratory collapse can occur.

F. OTHER ANTICONVULSANTS

1. **Carbamazepine** is an iminostilbene and is related chemically to the tricyclic antidepressants.
   a. It is particularly useful in the treatment of temporal lobe epilepsy, especially if this is accompanied by a mixed-seizure pattern. In addition, it is useful in the treatment of trigeminal neuralgia.
   b. Its anticonvulsant actions are similar to those of phenytoin.
   c. Serious untoward effects include
      (1) Diplopia, ataxia, and nausea.
      (2) Bone marrow depression, including aplastic anemia.
      (3) Congestive heart failure.
      (4) Atropine-like symptoms.

2. **Valproic acid** (dipropylacetic acid) had been used as a solvent in the screening of certain compounds for antiepileptic activity. It was itself found to possess antiseizure activity.
   a. Sodium valproate has proved most effective in seizure states having a subcortical focus (e.g., absence seizures). It has also been somewhat effective in grand mal seizures but much less so in partial seizures.
   b. Valproic acid is rapidly absorbed from the gastrointestinal tract. Its mechanism of anticonvulsant action is unclear but is thought to occur by inhibition of GABA transaminase, the enzyme responsible for the breakdown of GABA. Valproate antagonizes pentylenetetrazol-induced convulsions, suggesting an additional postsynaptic site of action.
   c. Untoward effects are uncommon but include
      (1) Pancreatitis and hepatic failure, especially when the drug is used in combination with other antiseizure medication.
      (2) Anorexia and nausea.
      (3) Sedation and ataxia.

(4) Drug interactions, including a 40 percent rise in plasma phenobarbital concentration with concurrent administration.

IV. ANTIPARKINSONIAN AGENTS

A. LEVODOPA (L-DOPA)

1. In the treatment of parkinsonism a dopamine deficiency in the striatum needs to be corrected.
   a. Dopamine does **not** cross the blood–brain barrier; thus, levodopa, the precursor of dopamine, is given instead.
   b. Levodopa is formed from L-tyrosine and is an intermediate in the synthesis of catecholamines.
   c. Levodopa itself has minimal pharmacologic activity, in contrast to its decarboxylated product, dopamine.
2. Objective improvement usually occurs by 3 weeks after therapy is begun.
3. The effects on bradykinesia and rigidity are more rapid and complete than the effects on tremor. Other motor defects in Parkinson's disease improve. The psychological well-being of the patient is also improved.
4. Tolerance to both the beneficial and untoward effects occurs with time; thus, the therapeutic benefit is more impressive during the first few years of therapy.
5. Levodopa is well absorbed from the small bowel. However, 95 percent is rapidly decarboxylated in the periphery. Peripheral dopamine is metabolized in the liver to dihydroxyphenylacetic acid (DOPAC) and homovanillic acid (HVA), which are then excreted in the urine.
6. Since the decarboxylation of levodopa increases peripheral concentrations of dopamine, prominent α- and β-adrenergic effects are seen, but these effects are significantly less severe than those seen with epinephrine, norepinephrine, or isoproterenol.
7. Principal untoward effects include
   a. Anorexia, nausea, and vomiting, upon initial administration, which often limit the initial dosage.
   b. Cardiovascular untoward effects: tachycardia, arrhythmias, and orthostatic hypotension.
   c. Mental disturbances, including delusions and hallucinations.
   d. A decrease in prolactin secretion.
   e. Dyskinesia upon long-term administration.
8. **Drug interactions**
   a. Pyridoxine reduces the beneficial effects of levodopa by enhancing its extracerebral metabolism. The decarboxylation of levodopa to dopamine is mediated by a pyridoxine-dependent enzyme.
   b. Phenothiazines, reserpine, and butyrophenones antagonize the effects of levodopa because they lead to a junctional blockade of dopamine action.
   c. Therapy with monoamine oxidase inhibitors must be stopped 14 days prior to the initiation of levodopa therapy.
   d. Anticholinergic agents act synergistically with levodopa, further improving many of the symptoms of parkinsonism.

B. CARBIDOPA

1. Carbidopa is an inhibitor of dopa decarboxylase. Since it is unable to penetrate the blood–brain barrier, it acts to reduce the peripheral conversion of levodopa to dopamine. As a result
   a. Levodopa blood levels are increased and drug half-life is lengthened.
   b. The dose of levodopa can be significantly reduced and therefore the associated untoward effects are reduced.
   c. A shorter latency period precedes the occurrence of beneficial effects.
2. Untoward effects are similar to those seen with high doses of levodopa.
3. If the patient has been taking levodopa, it should be withheld for 8 hours before starting carbidopa, and the dosage of levodopa should be reduced by 75 percent.
4. **Sinemet** is the trade name of a preparation that combines carbidopa and levodopa in fixed proportions (1:10 and 1:4).

C. AMANTADINE

1. Amantadine is an antiviral agent used in the prophylaxis of influenza A_2. (See Chapter 12, XIII A).
2. It is believed to stimulate the release and re-uptake of dopamine from dopaminergic nerve terminals in the nigrostriatum.
3. Amantadine is more efficacious in parkinsonism than the anticholinergic atropine derivatives (see E, below), but is less effective than levodopa.
4. Tolerance is observed in 6 to 8 weeks.
5. Amantadine is well absorbed orally and is excreted unchanged in the urine.
6. Untoward effects are infrequent; however, long-term use can produce livedo reticularis in the lower extremities.

D. BROMOCRIPTINE

1. An ergot derivative, bromocriptine mimics the action of dopamine.
2. Bromocriptine is expensive but probably provides additional therapeutic benefit when added to levodopa therapy.
3. Untoward effects such as hallucinations, hypotension, and livedo reticularis are more common with bromocriptine than with levodopa; however, it induces less dyskinesia than levodopa.

E. ANTICHOLINERGIC AGENTS

1. Since the deficiency of dopamine in the striatum augments the excitatory cholinergic system in the striatum, the blockade of this system by anticholinergic agents such as trihexyphenidyl helps to alleviate the motor dysfunction. also Benztropine
2. Improvement in the parkinsonian tremor is more pronounced than improvement in bradykinesia and rigidity.
3. Side effects such as mental confusion and hallucinations, due to central muscarinic toxicity, can occur as well as peripheral atropine-like toxicity (e.g., cycloplegia, urinary retention, and constipation).
4. **Antihistamines** (e.g., diphenhydramine) are less effective therapeutically but are better tolerated than anticholinergic agents.

V. ANTIPSYCHOTIC AGENTS NEUROLEPTICS

A. GENERAL CONSIDERATIONS

1. These agents are prescribed for the management of psychotic symptoms.
2. They are useful in both acute and chronic psychoses and in nonpsychotic individuals who are delusional or excited. They improve mood and behavior without producing excessive sedation.
3. As a group these agents produce little physical dependence or habituation but, notably, are capable of causing reversible and irreversible extrapyramidal symptoms.

B. PHENOTHIAZINES (Table 3-2)

1. **Chemistry**. The phenothiazines have a three-ring structure in which two benzene rings are linked by a sulfur and a nitrogen atom (Fig. 3-4). Differences within this group result from substitution on the nitrogen.
2. **Effects on the CNS**
   a. The psychotic patient has fewer hallucinations and delusions. Improvements in behavior are most often noted with long-term therapy.
      (1) Tolerance to these effects is rarely seen.
      (2) The antipsychotic effects are believed to be due to antagonism of dopaminergic neurotransmission in the limbic, nigrostriatal, and hypothalamic systems.
   b. Extrapyramidal symptoms (parkinsonian symptoms, akathisia, tardive dyskinesia) occur most often with chronic administration.

Table 3-2. The Phenothiazines

Drug	Major Use	Frequency of Untoward Effects	
		Orthostatic Hypotension	Extrapyramidal Symptoms
Chlorpromazine (Thorazine)	Antipsychotic Antiemetic	Moderate	Moderate
Thioridazine (Mellaril)	Antipsychotic	Moderate	Low
Triflupromazine (Vesprin)	Antipsychotic	Moderate	High
Fluphenazine (Prolixin)	Antipsychotic	Low	High
Prochlorperazine (Compazine)	Antiemetic	Low	Low–moderate
Promethazine (Phenergan)	Antihistaminic	Moderate	Low

(1) These effects arise, presumably, because of antidopaminergic effects in the basal ganglia.

(2) Phenothiazines having the greatest antihistaminic and anticholinergic properties will exhibit the fewest extrapyramidal symptoms.

c. Most phenothiazines are antiemetic, antagonizing agents such as apomorphine which stimulate the chemoreceptor trigger zone. In high doses, phenothiazines may directly depress the medullary vomiting center.

d. Phenothiazines are capable of altering temperature-regulating mechanisms. Normally they produce hypothermia; however, in a hot climate they can cause hyperthermia because of failure to lose body heat.

e. Since phenothiazines depress the hypothalamus, endocrine alterations may occur.

(1) This includes the release of lactogenic hormone (prolactin), inducing lactation.

(2) Abnormal pigmentation can occur because of an increased release of melanocyte-stimulating hormone from the pituitary.

(3) Decreased urinary concentrations of gonadotropins can cause galactorrhea and gynecomastia.

(4) In addition, phenothiazines decrease corticotropin release and secretion of pituitary growth hormone.

(5) Weight gain and increased appetite are seen with phenothiazine use.

f. The **neuroleptic effect** of the antipsychotic drugs consists of emotional quieting, reduced physical movement, and a potential for neurologic side effects.

(1) The neurologic effects include characteristic extrapyramidal and parkinsonian movement disorders.

(2) In contrast to the type of emotional quieting produced by CNS depressants and hypnotics, the intellectual functioning of the patient is little affected by the neuroleptics.

3. Peripheral effects

a. An α-adrenergic blocking activity is seen, especially with the prototypic phenothiazine, chlorpromazine.

b. Adrenergic potentiation, especially with chronic administration, is probably a result of the ability of phenothiazines to inhibit the re-uptake of norepinephrine.

c. Anticholinergic effects can result in blurred vision, constipation, dry mouth, decreased sweating, and, rarely, urinary retention. Miosis is seen with chlorpromazine and is probably due to α-adrenergic blockade. Other phenothiazines can produce mydriasis.

d. Chlorpromazine is a potent local anesthetic.

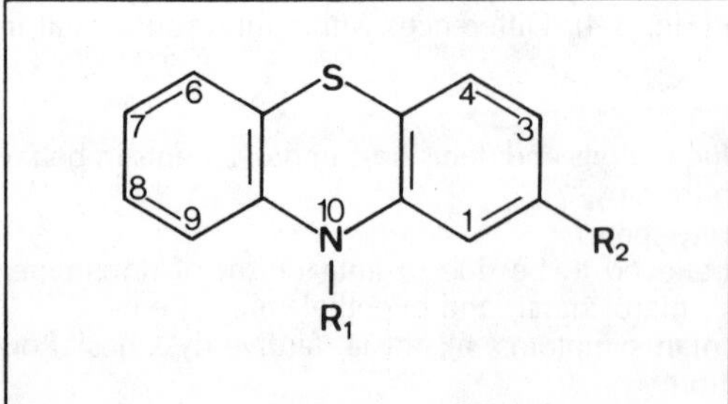

Figure 3-4. The phenothiazine nucleus.

e. Antihistaminic activity is seen with most phenothiazine derivatives.
f. Inhibition of ejaculation without interference with erection can be observed, especially with thioridazine.
g. Inhibition of antidiuretic hormone (ADH) secretion by chlorpromazine can result in a weak diuretic effect.
h. Orthostatic hypotension can occur as a result of both the central action of phenothiazines and inhibition of norepinephrine uptake mechanisms. In addition chlorpromazine has an antiarrhythmic effect upon the heart.
i. Phenothiazines are known to enhance the pharmacologic actions of barbiturates, narcotics, and ethyl alcohol.

4. **Pharmacokinetics**
   a. The phenothiazines are erratically absorbed from the gastrointestinal tract.
   b. They are highly protein-bound and enter the fetal circulation.
   c. Their biologic effects last 24 hours, allowing once-daily dosing.
   d. Phenothiazines are metabolized in the hepatic microsomal system by hydroxylation, followed by conjugation with glucuronic acid. In addition, the formation of sulfoxides is an important metabolic pathway.
   e. At least five metabolites ultimately appear in the urine.

5. **Therapeutic uses**
   a. Phenothiazines are used chiefly in the treatment of psychotic disorders, including mania, paranoid states, schizophrenia, and psychoses associated with chronic alcoholism (alcoholic hallucinosis).
   b. In addition, several phenothiazines have proven effective in the treatment of nausea and vomiting of certain etiologies, such as drug-induced nausea.
   c. Some phenothiazines, due to their H_1 antihistaminic activity, are useful as antipruritics.
   d. Chlorpromazine has proved useful in the control of intractable hiccup.

6. **Untoward effects**
   a. **CNS effects** include
      (1) Parkinsonian syndrome—Patients display rigidity and tremor at rest.
      (2) Acute dystonic reactions—These may be seen with initial drug therapy; patients display facial grimacing and torticollis.
      (3) Tardive dyskinesia—This motor disorder may be seen with chronic therapy; patients display sucking and smacking of the lips and other involuntary facial movements. The dyskinesia may persist far after discontinuation of therapy.
      (4) Lethargy and drowsiness.
   b. **Cardiovascular effects** include orthostatic hypotension, which can result in syncope, and reflex tachycardia.
   c. **Allergic reactions** most often occur during the first few months of therapy.
      (1) Cholestatic jaundice can occur; it resolves with discontinuation of drug therapy.
      (2) Blood dyscrasias (e.g., agranulocytosis) and eosinophilia can occur but are rare.
      (3) Various forms of dermatitis may occur, including a photosensitivity reaction that resembles a severe sunburn.
   d. Children exhibit extrapyramidal symptoms and, less commonly, may develop jaundice, blood dyscrasias, or hyperpyrexia.
   e. Somnolence and hypotension are prominent untoward effects of acute intoxication.

C. **THE THIOXANTHENE DERIVATIVES** are similar chemically and pharmacologically to the phenothiazine derivatives. They differ chemically in that a carbon is substituted for a nitrogen in the central ring of the phenothiazine nucleus (position 10). The thioxanthenes in clinical use are **chlorprothixene** and **thiothixene**.

D. **BUTYROPHENONES**

1. The prototype is **haloperidol**, which resembles the phenothiazine derivatives pharmacologically.

2. It has potent antiemetic properties, antagonizing stimulation of the chemoreceptor trigger zone.

3. Significant extrapyramidal symptoms are associated with its use.

4. Another butyrophenone, **droperidol**, can be combined with a potent narcotic analgesic such as fentanyl to produce neuroleptanalgesia. This combination is known by the trade name Innovar (see Chapter 4, III B 1).

VI. ANTIANXIETY AGENTS

A. GENERAL CONSIDERATIONS. Unlike the antipsychotic agents, these agents are used to treat anxiety or neurosis. They are not used in the treatment of psychosis. Many of these drugs, therefore, are known as **antianxiety agents**, or "minor" tranquilizers.

1. In addition, antianxiety agents have sedative and even hypnotic properties, and also possess some central skeletal muscle relaxant activity.
2. They have a habituation and physical dependence liability.
3. Generally, the antianxiety agents have a lower incidence of untoward effects than the antipsychotic agents, including a lower incidence of extrapyramidal effects.

B. MEPROBAMATE

1. Meprobamate is a propyl alcohol derivative (propanediol carbamate).
2. It depresses the CNS in a fashion similar to the barbiturates, especially phenobarbital, but is shorter-acting.
3. It is capable of promoting sleep but, like phenobarbital, it decreases the REM phase of sleep.
4. The skeletal muscle relaxant activity demonstrated by meprobamate is probably a combination of its sedative effect and specific central skeletal muscle relaxant activity.
5. Meprobamate is well absorbed from the gastrointestinal tract and its peak serum concentration is reached in about 1½ hours. Metabolism occurs in the liver and the inactive metabolites are excreted via the kidney.
6. At one time meprobamate was a widely used antianxiety agent; however, it has largely been replaced by the benzodiazepines.
7. **Untoward effects** include
   a. Drowsiness, often seen with full therapeutic doses.
   b. Blood dyscrasias, including purpura, but these are rare.
   c. Habituation and physical dependence with long-term administration. Withdrawal from drug therapy should therefore be gradual.

C. BENZODIAZEPINES

1. The first benzodiazepine developed was **chlordiazepoxide** (Fig. 3-5). Others include **diazepam, lorazepam, oxazepam, clorazepate, prazepam,** and the sedative hypnotic **flurazepam** (see II B 7).
2. The **CNS effects** of benzodiazepines include
   a. Depression of the CNS, in particular the limbic system. In addition, they are thought to potentiate the effects of GABA in the CNS. Both actions probably contribute to the antianxiety effect of benzodiazepines. They are also effective hypnotics, and flurazepam is promoted as such.

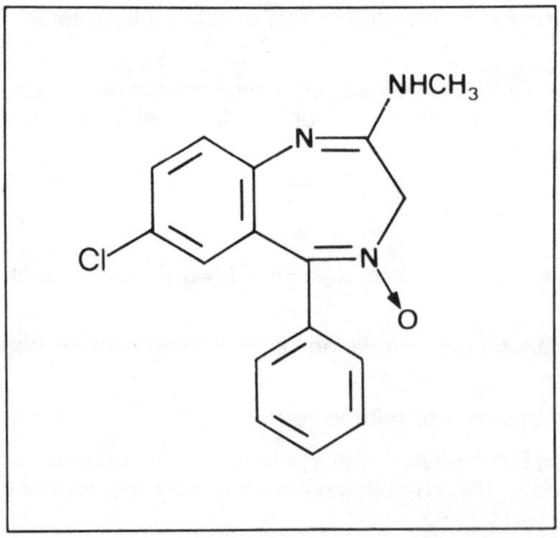

Figure 3-5. Chlordiazepoxide.

b. An increase in the seizure threshold. Benzodiazepines are useful as anticonvulsants, especially diazepam in status epilepticus. They prevent convulsions caused by strychnine or pentylenetetrazole.

3. At therapeutic doses there are minimal effects on the cardiovascular system.

4. Although the benzodiazepines, especially diazepam, are widely used as central skeletal muscle relaxants, their effectiveness has not been firmly established.

5. **Pharmacokinetics**
   a. Diazepam is rapidly absorbed from the gastrointestinal tract, reaching peak serum concentrations in 1 hour. There is a secondary peak at 6 to 12 hours after an oral dose, presumably due to enterohepatic circulation. The distributive half-life is 2.5 hours, while the elimination half-life is 1.5 days.
   b. Chlordiazepoxide and oxazepam are slowly absorbed from the gastrointestinal tract, and peak serum concentrations are not reached for several hours.
   c. Benzodiazepines are highly protein-bound in the plasma.
   d. Most benzodiazepines are metabolized in the hepatic microsomal metabolizing system to active metabolites, with the exception of lorazepam and oxazepam. The latter two, because of their short duration of action, are safer agents when the patient is elderly or has altered hepatic function.
   e. Benzodiazepines are excreted via the kidney as glucuronide-conjugated or oxidized metabolites.

6. **Therapeutic uses** include
   a. Treatment of anxiety.
   b. Anesthetic premedication.
   c. Use as amnestics, such as in cardioversion.
   d. Use as sedative–hypnotics.
   e. Management of seizure disorders.
   f. Treatment of alcohol withdrawal syndromes.
   g. Use as central skeletal muscle relaxants.

7. **Untoward effects** include
   a. Ataxia, drowsiness, and sedation. Additive depressant effects are seen when benzodiazepines are combined with other agents possessing CNS depressant activity.
   b. Paradoxically increased anxiety, including psychoses, especially with high doses.
   c. Reversible confusion in the elderly.
   d. Menstrual irregularities, including anovulation.

8. Overdoses, although frequent, are seldom fatal. Treatment is supportive. Owing to the high plasma-protein–binding characteristics of benzodiazepines, the benefit from dialysis is limited.

9. Habituation and physical dependence can develop and withdrawal symptoms can follow the abrupt discontinuation of high-dose, long-term therapy. Because of the long half-life of certain benzodiazepines, withdrawal symptoms may not occur until a week after discontinuation of therapy.

VII. MOOD-ALTERING DRUGS

A. LITHIUM CARBONATE

1. Lithium is used in the treatment of mania and does not produce psychotropic effects in normal persons. It has no effect on schizophrenia.

2. The mechanism by which lithium acts in the control of mania is unknown but it is probably related to incomplete ion substitution for cations such as sodium and potassium at the cellular membrane.

3. Lithium ion is well absorbed from the gastrointestinal tract and eventually reaches equilibrium between plasma and tissues. It is eliminated by renal excretion; 80 percent of the lithium is reabsorbed in the proximal tubule. The ion is secreted into breast milk.

4. Since lithium has a low therapeutic index, serum concentrations must be carefully maintained between 0.8 and 1.5 mEq/liter.

5. The major therapeutic indications are the treatment of acute mania and the prevention of recurrent bipolar manic-depressive illness.

6. Untoward effects

a. High serum lithium levels are associated with anorexia, vomiting, diarrhea, excessive thirst, and polyuria. The latter two symptoms probably involve the ability of lithium to inhibit the action of antidiuretic hormone on renal adenylate cyclase. This ultimately can result in a syndrome resembling diabetes insipidus.

b. Epileptic seizures have been reported as well as somnolence, confusion, and psychomotor disturbances.

c. The use of lithium in early pregnancy can result in cardiovascular anomalies in the newborn.

d. Adverse cardiovascular effects include hypotension and cardiac arrhythmias.

e. Chronic lithium use can result in thyroid enlargement.

f. Lithium intoxication can be reversed by osmotic diuresis or, in more severe cases, by dialysis.

B. ANTIDEPRESSANT AGENTS

1. General considerations

a. Depression is an alteration of mood characterized by sadness, worry, and anxiety. The patient may suffer from losses of weight, libido, and enthusiasm.

b. Most antidepressants are believed to improve mood by increasing catecholamine stores.

c. There are various pharmacologic modalities that may be useful, and selection often depends on the patient's history and symptomatology.

2. Monoamine oxidase (MAO) inhibitors

a. **Chemically**, these consist of two major groups, the hydrazides and the nonhydrazides.

(1) The **hydrazide derivatives** include **isocarboxazid, phenelzine,** and **iproniazid**. The latter is no longer used because of its hepatotoxicity.

(2) The prototypic **nonhydrazide** is **tranylcypromine**, which structurally (Fig. 3-6) resembles dextroamphetamine.

b. **Mechanism of action**

(1) The MAO inhibitors form stable complexes with the enzyme monoamine oxidase, irreversibly inactivating it and thereby preventing the oxidative deamination of biogenic amines such as norepinephrine, epinephrine, dopamine, serotonin, and tyramine.

(a) These biogenic amines are thus increased significantly in the brain, intestines, heart, and blood.

(b) The increase of biogenic amine levels in the brain is thought to underlie the observed antidepressant effects.

(2) The nonhydrazide, tranylcypromine, by way of its amphetamine-like action, will release norepinephrine centrally. This probably accounts for the rapidity by which tranylcypromine works, in contrast to the other MAO inhibitors, which have latency periods of 2 to 3 weeks.

c. **Effects on the CNS**

(1) Besides their effect on depression, MAO inhibitors are effective in sleep disorders, including narcolepsy. They suppress REM sleep.

(2) Except for tranylcypromine, which has a stimulant effect on the electroencephalogram (EEG), other MAO inhibitors have minimal EEG effects.

d. **Cardiovascular effects**

(1) Hypotension, especially postural, can result from the ability of MAO inhibitors to affect ganglionic transmission and reduce the release of norepinephrine in certain organ systems. This effect is believed to be due to the uptake and release of "false transmitters" such as tyramine.

(2) MAO inhibitors can interact with foods containing a high tyramine content, such as cheese, beer, and chicken liver.

(a) The high concentrations of tyramine absorbed from these foods cannot undergo oxidative deamination.

C_6H_5–CH–CH–NH_2 (CH and CH bridged by CH_2)

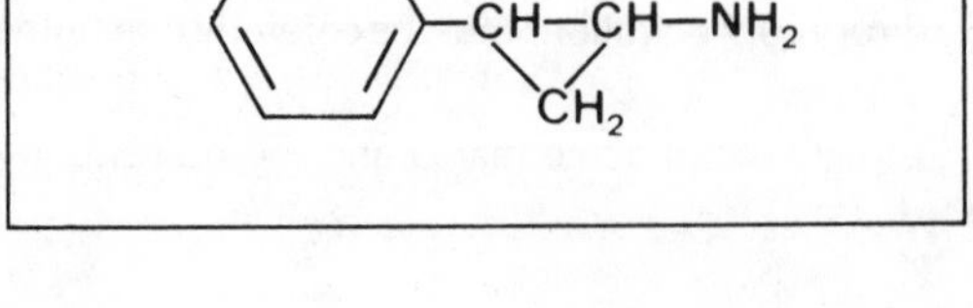

Figure 3-6. Tranylcypromine.

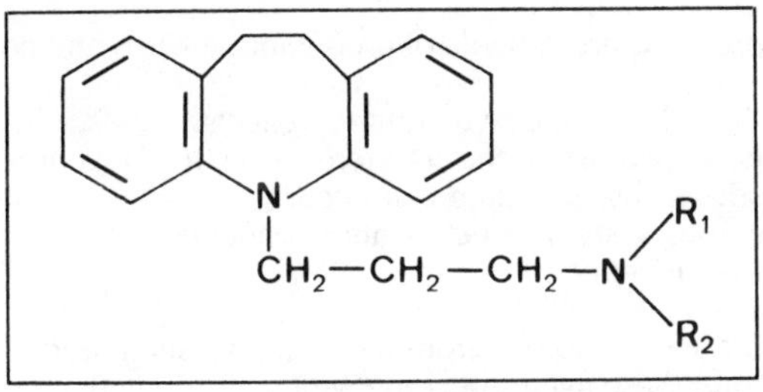

$$\text{[tricyclic ring: two benzene rings joined by } -CH_2-CH_2- \text{ bridge and N]} - CH_2-CH_2-CH_2-N(R_1)(R_2)$$

Figure 3-7. The basic structure of tricyclic antidepressants.

(b) The tyramine can therefore induce the release of large amounts of stored catecholamines from nerve terminals. This can precipitate a **hypertensive crisis,** which is the most serious untoward effect of MAO inhibitors.

e. Hepatic effects

(1) MAO inhibitors interfere with the detoxification of many drugs.

(2) They enhance the action of general anesthetics, sedatives, atropine-like agents, narcotics (especially meperidine, which can result in hyperpyrexia), and tricyclic antidepressants.

f. Pharmacokinetics

(1) All MAO inhibitors are rapidly absorbed from the gastrointestinal tract, but, inexplicably, the observed therapeutic response does not occur for 2 to 3 weeks.

(2) The hydrazide derivatives are cleaved, resulting in biologically active products. Inactivation occurs by acetylation, and in patients who are genetically slow acetylators, conventional doses of agents such as phenelzine may produce exaggerated effects.

(3) Enzyme regeneration terminates the drug effect; this frequently takes weeks after use of the drug is stopped.

(4) When switching antidepressant therapy, a minimum of 2 weeks' delay is required after termination of MAO-inhibitor therapy (see VII B 3 i (9), below).

g. Therapeutic uses. MAO inhibitors have been used to treat depression, phobic–anxiety states, and narcolepsy. Their use is now limited because more efficacious and less toxic agents are available.

h. Untoward effects

(1) Hydrazide-derived MAO inhibitors can cause hepatocellular damage.

(2) Excessive CNS stimulation, resulting in insomnia and convulsions, has occurred.

(3) Overdosage can result in agitation, headache, convulsions, hypotension, or hypertension. Treatment of overdosage is usually supportive. Since the effects of MAO inhibitors are lengthy, patients should be observed in the hospital for at least 1 week.

3. Tricyclic antidepressants

a. Chemically, the tricyclic antidepressants and their desmethyl derivatives are similar to the phenothiazines. The basic structure is shown in Figure 3-7.

b. Specific agents

(1) **Imipramine** is closely related to the phenothiazines.

(2) **Amitriptyline** is thought to be better tolerated than imipramine in older psychotic or depressed patients.

(3) **Desipramine**, the monodesmethyl derivative of imipramine, is less sedating than its parent compound.

(4) **Nortriptyline**, like desipramine, produces less sedation than its parent compound amitriptyline.

(5) **Doxepin** is also effective in treating depression when anxiety is present.

c. Mechanism of action

(1) Tricyclic antidepressants potentiate the action of biogenic amines, presumably by blocking the inactivating re-uptake of the amines after release from the presynaptic neuron. It is thought that the demethylated antidepressants are more selective in blocking the uptake of norepinephrine.

(2) In addition, the tricyclic antidepressants possess antimuscarinic action and block the re-uptake of serotonin.

d. Effects on the CNS

(1) The nondepressed individual experiences sleepiness when a tricyclic antidepressant is administered. In addition, anxiety and untoward anticholinergic effects may be experienced.

(2) In the depressed patient, an elevation of mood occurs 2 to 3 weeks after administration begins. The latency period can be as long as 4 weeks.

(3) High doses of tricyclic antidepressants are capable of producing seizures and coma.

e. **Cardiovascular effects**

(1) Orthostatic hypotension and arrhythmias are two common effects.

(2) Tachycardia in response to the hypotension and interference with atrioventricular conduction similar to that produced by quinidine can occur.

f. The most common **autonomic nervous system effect** is anticholinergic. Amitriptyline possesses the most potent antimuscarinic effects.

g. **Pharmacokinetics**

(1) The tricyclic antidepressants are well absorbed from the gastrointestinal tract.

(2) Because of their lipophilic nature, these agents become widely distributed and have relatively long half-lives. They are metabolized in the microsomal metabolizing system. Hydroxylation, *N*-demethylation, and conjugation with glucuronic acid are the major metabolic pathways.

(3) The demethylated metabolites of both amitriptyline and imipramine have antidepressant activity.

(4) Excretion of metabolites is via the kidney.

h. **Therapeutic uses**

(1) These agents are considered the treatment of choice for severe endogenous depression (characterized by regression and inactivity). In overall efficacy, the various tricyclic antidepressants are equivalent at appropriate dosages.

(2) Enuresis has been successfully treated with imipramine.

(3) Obsessive-compulsive neurosis accompanied by depression, and phobic–anxiety syndromes, chronic pain, and neuralgia may respond to tricyclic agents; it should be noted that these indications are investigational.

i. **Untoward effects**

(1) The untoward effects often resemble those seen with phenothiazines, owing to the common structural features of the two groups of drugs.

(2) Anticholinergic effects can be prominent and occur both peripherally and centrally. Amitriptyline produces the highest incidence of antimuscarinic effects. Because of these actions, caution is required in treating patients with prostatic hypertrophy and glaucoma.

(3) Sweating is common, although its mechanism is unknown.

(4) The elderly may suffer from dizziness and muscle tremor.

(5) As with phenothiazines, cardiac arrhythmias can occur; in addition, hypotension is frequent.

(6) Manic excitement and delirium can be produced in patients with bipolar manic-depressive illness.

(7) Other, less frequent, untoward effects include skin rashes, cholestatic jaundice, and orgasmic impotence.

(8) Acute poisoning is often treated with activated charcoal, although gastric lavage and physostigmine have been used successfully as adjuncts. Vital functions need to be supported and constantly monitored.

(9) The combination of a MAO inhibitor with a tricyclic antidepressant should be avoided, since hyperpyrexia, convulsions, and coma can result.

VIII. CNS STIMULANTS

A. AMPHETAMINE (β-Phenylisopropylamine)

1. **CNS effects**

a. In addition to its peripheral sympathomimetic action (see Chapter 2, II G), amphetamine is a powerful CNS stimulant, presumably acting by releasing biogenic amines from storage sites in the nerve terminals.

b. It stimulates the medullary respiratory center and has analeptic action, counteracting the central depression produced by other drugs (e.g., barbiturates).

c. Increased alertness, decreased sense of fatigue, increased motor and speech activity, and elevation of mood are often produced.

d. Large doses or prolonged usage are usually followed by fatigue and mental depression.

2. **Untoward effects**

a. Some individuals experience dysphoria, headache, confusion, dizziness, fatigue, or delirium.

b. Blood pressure is usually raised and cardiac arrhythmias may occur.

c. The toxic dose of amphetamine shows wide variation. Overdosage results in psychotic reactions, marked cardiovascular effects such as hypertension or hypotension and circulatory collapse, and, eventually, convulsions and coma.

d. Treatment of acute intoxication is facilitated by acidification of the urine to increase excretion.

3. **Therapeutic uses**
   a. Amphetamine has been used as an anorectic in weight control of obese individuals because it decreases the appetite and consequently lowers food intake. Since tolerance develops rapidly, psychologically driven food intake is not affected, and because of the significant abuse potential, this therapeutic use is of questionable merit.
   b. The stimulant effect of amphetamine is useful in the treatment of narcolepsy.
   c. A paradoxical calming effect is produced with long-term therapy in many abnormally hyperactive children (hyperkinetic syndrome).

4. **Dextroamphetamine** and **methamphetamine** are preferred to amphetamine because of their increased CNS action and reduced peripheral effects.

B. COCAINE

1. Cocaine is benzoylmethylecgonine; its sole clinical use is as a local anesthetic applied in direct contact to nerve tissue (see Chapter 4, II C 1).

2. Although not intended for internal use or injection clinically, cocaine is abused because of its marked systemic effect in stimulating the CNS. This effect appears to be due to the potentiation of the action of catecholamines in the CNS.

3. Euphoria, dysphoria, or excitement may be produced. At higher doses, central depression occurs, followed by respiratory failure.

IX. NARCOTIC ANALGESICS

A. GENERAL CONSIDERATIONS

1. **Analgesia** is the relief of pain without the loss of consciousness.

2. The chief action of opiates and similar compounds is to impair the normal sensory awareness and response to tissue injury.

3. Opiates are derived from the poppy plant. The exudate of the seed capsule contains morphine, codeine, thebaine, and papaverine.

4. The term *opioid* refers to both naturally occurring opiates and synthetic drugs with similar actions.

B. MECHANISM OF ACTION

1. Through the use of ligand-binding techniques, opiate receptors of several types have been quantitated and localized within the CNS. These receptors are found in the following sites:
   a. The limbic system, including the amygdaloid nucleus and the hypothalamus.
   b. The medial and lateral thalamus, and the area postrema, which is the site of the chemoreceptor trigger zone governing nausea and emesis.
   c. The nucleus tractus solitarii, which is the location of the cough center.
   d. The substantia gelatinosa and, to a lesser degree, other areas of the spinal cord.

2. Endogenous ligands known as **enkephalins** are pentapeptides that are localized in some nerve endings. Their distribution closely parallels the distribution of opiate receptors. It is thought that the enkephalins may be involved in the modulation of the pain response.

3. In addition, longer polypeptides called **endorphins** possess potent analgesic activity and are found in the pituitary and hypothalamus.

4. It is presently assumed that the opioids act by mimicking these endogenous ligands.

C. MORPHINE AND RELATED OPIOIDS

1. **Morphine** (Fig. 3-8) is a member of the phenanthrene series of alkaloids.
   a. **Effects on the CNS**
      (1) Analgesia and increased tolerance of pain are the most prominent effects of morphine. Consciousness is not lost, and the patient can usually still locate the source of pain. Some patients become euphoric. If morphine is given to a person who is pain-free, dysphoria, anxiety, or mental clouding may be produced.
      (2) Morphine stimulates the chemoreceptor trigger zone, producing nausea and vomiting. In most cases, after the first therapeutic dose, subsequent doses of morphine do not produce vomiting.

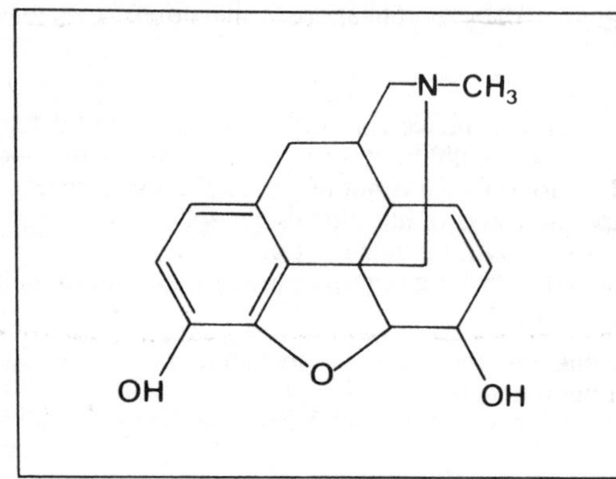

Figure 3-8. Morphine.

(3) Morphine produces miosis by stimulating the Edinger-Westphal nucleus, and pin-point pupils are indicative of toxic dosage prior to asphyxia. Miosis can be blocked with atropine.
(4) Morphine is a powerful respiratory depressant which acts by reducing the responsiveness of the respiratory centers in the brain stem to blood levels of carbon dioxide.
  (a) Both alveolar and serum P_{CO_2}, are increased because of the depression of medullary responsiveness.
  (b) Because of the depressed respiration and increased arterial CO_2, cerebral vasodilation can occur, causing an increase in intracranial pressure.
(5) Morphine is believed to stimulate the release of antidiuretic hormone (ADH), producing oliguria.
(6) It is a potent cough suppressant.
(7) Morphine has a biphasic, dose-dependent effect on body temperature. Low doses of morphine cause a decrease in body temperature; higher doses cause an increase.

b. Cardiovascular effects. Orthostatic hypotension can occur, due to vasomotor medullary depression and histamine release.

c. Gastrointestinal effects
(1) Constipation results from the ability of morphine to block intestinal propulsive peristalsis and stomach motility. In addition, spasmodic nonpropulsive contractions of gastrointestinal smooth muscle are produced.
(2) Both biliary and pancreatic secretions are decreased.
(3) Constriction at the sphincter of Oddi causes an increase in biliary pressure.

d. Other systemic effects
(1) Morphine increases detrusor muscle tone in the urinary bladder, producing a feeling of urinary urgency. Vesical sphincter tone is also increased, making voiding difficult.
(2) Prolongation of labor can occur by an undefined uterine mechanism.
(3) Bronchoconstriction can occur because morphine causes the release of histamine and causes vagal stimulation.
(4) Cutaneous vasodilation secondary to histamine release can result in pruritus and sweating.

e. Tolerance and dependence
(1) Tolerance may develop to the analgesia, the euphoria, and the respiratory depression.
(2) Tolerance to the miosis and gastrointestinal effects (i.e., delayed gastric emptying and constipation) also develops, but to a much lesser extent.
(3) Physical addiction occurs, although the morphine withdrawal syndrome is not as severe as barbiturate withdrawal.

f. Pharmacokinetics
(1) Morphine is well absorbed from the gastrointestinal tract. A greater analgesic effect is noted when the drug is administered intramuscularly or intravenously.
(2) Morphine is metabolized in the liver, where it is transformed into inactive metabolites by conjugation with glucuronide.
(3) Ninety percent of a given dose is excreted in the urine; the remaining 10 percent in the feces. This latter component is derived from bile as conjugated morphine.

g. Therapeutic uses
(1) Analgesia, such as the relief of pain from myocardial infarction, terminal illness, surgery, and obstetrical procedures, is the major use of morphine.
(2) It is also used for the acute treatment of dyspnea due to pulmonary edema, in which morphine produces decreased peripheral resistance and increased capacity of peripheral and splanchnic vascular compartments.

(3) Because of their constipating effects, the morphine-like drugs can be useful in treating severe diarrhea.

h. **Untoward effects**

(1) Respiratory depression is the most important untoward effect and is dose-dependent.
(2) Nausea and sometimes dysphoria can occur.
(3) Increased biliary tract pressure can occur and caution should be exercised in gallbladder disease.
(4) Long-term chronic administration can result in physical dependence, and pinpoint pupils are a consistent finding in addiction.
(5) Allergic reactions can occur, and skin rashes are a common manifestation.
(6) Morphine should be avoided in the asthmatic patient due to its bronchoconstrictive action.
(7) Some phenothiazines are capable of producing antianalgesia when combined with an opiate such as morphine, whereas other phenothiazines can enhance the action of morphine.

2. **Codeine**

a. The 3-methyl ether of morphine, codeine, can be obtained from opium or synthesized by methylation of morphine.
b. Although the pharmacologic effects of codeine are similar to those of morphine, it has about one-twelfth the analgesic potency of morphine, and it is generally used for somewhat milder pain.
c. Codeine has a high oral–parenteral potency ratio.
d. An oral dose of 30 mg of codeine will produce equivalent analgesia to 600 mg of aspirin.
e. Codeine is also very useful as a cough suppressant but care should be exercised in administering it to sedated patients because of the risk of respiratory depression.
f. Codeine produces less sedation or respiratory depression than morphine, and fewer gastrointestinal effects.
g. Addiction liability is lower than with morphine and the effects of withdrawal are less severe than with morphine.

3. **Hydrocodone and oxycodone**

a. These codeine derivatives possess an analgesic potency closer to that of morphine.
b. Their potential for causing respiratory depression is also greater than that of codeine; this is especially true of oxycodone.
c. They possess a significant addiction liability.
d. Hydrocodone bitartrate is used in combination with other agents in some proprietary analgesic–antipyretic mixtures (e.g., Hycodan).
e. The oxycodone found in certain analgesic–antipyretic mixtures will produce analgesia equivalent to that of morphine.

4. **Heroin**

a. Heroin is diacetylated morphine.
b. Heroin has a more rapid onset and shorter duration of action than morphine.
c. It has an analgesic potency greater than that of morphine: 3 mg of heroin is equivalent to 10 mg of morphine.
d. Heroin is not used clinically in the United States.

5. **Hydromorphone**

a. Hydromorphone is ten times more potent than morphine in producing analgesia, with correspondingly more respiratory depressant activity.
b. Hydromorphone is less nauseating and constipating than morphine.
c. It is highly physically addicting.
d. Hydromorphone can be administered orally, parenterally, or rectally.

6. **Levorphanol** produces effects similar to those of morphine but with a lower incidence of nausea and vomiting.

D. MEPERIDINE AND CONGENERS

1. **Meperidine**, a phenylpiperidine derivative, is an entirely synthetic analgesic.

a. It is about one-eighth as potent as morphine, 100 mg of meperidine being equivalent to 15 mg of morphine.
b. Meperidine is well absorbed by all routes of administration and is better absorbed orally than morphine is. Excretion is mainly in the urine.
c. Meperidine causes respiratory depression and possesses addiction liability, although withdrawal effects are less severe than with morphine.

d. Meperidine causes histamine release and smooth muscle spasm, including bronchospasm.
e. It possesses weak atropine-like activity and tends to cause mydriasis. In toxic doses the pharmacologic effects are in part atropine-like.
f. With intravenous administration, the incidence of untoward effects is increased. Repeated intramuscular administration can produce tissue irritation.
g. Meperidine has no gastrointestinal or antitussive action.

2. Diphenoxylate, a derivative of meperidine, is available in combination with atropine (e.g., Lomotil).
a. Its principal use is to control diarrhea because of its opioid-like constipating effect.
b. In the recommended dosage it causes few morphine-like subjective effects and possesses a low addiction liability.
c. Due to the atropine in the combination, untoward effects such as dry mouth and blurred vision curtail overdosage.

3. Fentanyl, like diphenoxylate, is a congener of meperidine.
a. It has 80 times the analgesic potency and respiratory depressant properties of morphine.
b. When combined with droperidol it produces dissociative or neuroleptic anesthesia.
c. Its principal use is in anesthesia, where it is administered parenterally and has a rapid onset and short duration of action.
d. High doses of fentanyl are capable of producing muscular rigidity.

E. METHADONE AND CONGENERS

1. Methadone is a modified diphenylheptane; its structure is shown in Figure 3-9.
a. This synthetic analgesic has pharmacologic properties similar to those of morphine, but it is more effective orally than morphine.
b. The duration of analgesia with methadone is equal to that of morphine, although the half-life of methadone is longer. This can result in cumulative toxicity.
c. Methadone is well absorbed from the gastrointestinal tract, undergoes extensive biotransformation in the liver, and is excreted in both the urine and bile.
d. Its principal uses are in analgesia, in the suppression of withdrawal symptoms due to opiate addiction, and in treatment of heroin users.
(1) In methadone maintenance, opiate addicts receive periodic oral doses of methadone.
(2) In appropriate doses, methadone will satisfy the craving for heroin without producing euphoria or somnolence.
(3) Because of cross-tolerance, the effects of other self-administered opiates will be blocked.
e. Untoward effects are similar to those caused by morphine.
f. Both tolerance and physical dependence can occur with methadone administration.
g. Methadone withdrawal is less severe than the withdrawal from other opiates.

2. Propoxyphene is a structural analog of methadone with a spectrum of pharmacologic activity similar to that of codeine.
a. Propoxyphene is not an anti-inflammatory agent and thus is less effective in treating pain associated with inflammation. In analgesic potency, it closely resembles codeine. The combination of aspirin and codeine is less costly, however, than aspirin and propoxyphene.

$CH_3{-}CH_2{-}C({=}O){-}C(C_6H_5)_2{-}CH_2{-}CH(CH_3){-}N(CH_3)_2$

Figure 3-9. Methadone.

b. The water-soluble hydrochloride is absorbed more rapidly than the water-insoluble napsylate.
c. The *N*-demethylated metabolites are slowly excreted in the urine.
d. Propoxyphene is capable of depressing respiration about one-third as much as codeine.
e. The incidence of abuse is comparable to that seen with codeine.
f. Physical dependence and tolerance can occur but are usually seen only after chronic high-dose administration.

F. OPIOID ANTAGONISTS AND AGONIST–ANTAGONISTS

1. **Pentazocine** is a benzomorphan derivative with moderate agonistic and weak antagonistic activity.
   a. Due to its antagonistic activity pentazocine is capable of precipitating withdrawal in addicts.
   b. Although pentazocine is similar to morphine in pharmacologic properties, it has one-fifth the analgesic potency. A dose of 50 mg, given parenterally, produces analgesia equivalent to 10 mg of morphine; given orally, 50 mg is equivalent to 60 mg of codeine.
   c. Pentazocine is well absorbed from the gastrointestinal tract as well as from subcutaneous and intramuscular sites. Pentazocine is biotransformed in the liver and excreted via the kidney.
   d. **Untoward effects**
      (1) Pentazocine can produce nalorphine-like psychotomimetic effects such as anxiety and hallucinations.
      (2) There may be less nausea associated with its use than with other opioids.
      (3) Analgesic doses are capable of increasing the pulmonary artery pressure and cardiac work.
      (4) Respiratory depression with higher doses is less pronounced than with comparable doses of morphine.
   e. Tolerance to the analgesia can develop.
   f. Pentazocine possesses both physical dependence potential and abuse potential.

2. **Butorphanol** has actions similar to those of pentazocine.
   a. As with pentazocine, but in contrast to morphine, as the analgesic dose is increased, respiratory depression is not increased proportionately.
   b. Pulmonary artery pressure and myocardial work are increased at analgesic doses.
   c. Unlike pentazocine, butorphanol does not precipitate a withdrawal syndrome in opioid addicts.

3. **Nalbuphine**, although structurally similar to naloxone, is equivalent (on a weight basis) to morphine in producing analgesia.
   a. Its antagonistic properties are weak.
      (1) Nalbuphine has one-fourth the antagonistic activity of nalorphine.
      (2) It is capable of producing a withdrawal state in the opioid addict.
   b. Nalbuphine produces respiratory depression, but doses beyond 30 mg produce no further depression.
   c. Unlike pentazocine and butorphanol, nalbuphine does not cause untoward cardiac effects.
   d. Nalbuphine possesses abuse potential, and physical dependence has been reported.

4. **Naloxone** is an *N*-allyl derivative of oxymorphone and is considered a **pure opioid antagonist** with no agonist activity.
   a. Naloxone does not appear to antagonize endogenous opioids such as endorphins and enkephalins.
   b. The sedative effects, respiratory depression, and untoward cardiovascular effects of opioid agonists are reversed within 1 to 2 minutes after parenteral administration of naloxone. There may be an "overshoot," producing increased respiration for a short period of time.
   c. The duration of the antagonistic effect is dose-dependent and usually lasts 1 to 4 hours.
   d. If naloxone is administered to patients addicted to morphine-like opioids, a withdrawal syndrome is easily precipitated.
   e. Tolerance to the antagonistic effects does not develop.
   f. Naloxone is usually administered parenterally. It is metabolized in the liver via glucuronide conjugation.
   g. During labor, mothers who have received opioids prior to the birth may be given a dose of naloxone just prior to delivery in order to minimize neonatal respiratory depression. Alternatively, naloxone can be administered to the neonate via the umbilical vein.

5. **Nalorphine**
   a. Nalorphine is capable of antagonizing the effects of morphine, but in the absence of opioids it produces morphine-like actions. Nalorphine is thus a **partial agonist**.
   b. Smaller doses may antagonize opioid effects better than larger ones.
   c. As with naloxone, a withdrawal syndrome can be precipitated in addicted individuals.
   d. Unpleasant mental effects (e.g., dysphoria, hallucinations) are so prominent that nalorphine is not used as an analgesic.
   e. The opioid antagonists are primarily used for the treatment of opioid-induced respiratory depression.

G. NONOPIOID ANTITUSSIVES

1. **Dextromethorphan** is the *d* isomer of the codeine analog of levorphanol (see IX 2 a, 6).
2. In contrast to the *l* isomer, dextromethorphan does not possess analgesic or addictive properties, and its principal use is as a cough suppressant.
3. Although it is as effective as codeine in cough suppression it is not beset with codeine's untoward effects.
4. At high doses, CNS depression may occur.

STUDY QUESTIONS

Directions: Each question below contains five suggested answers. Choose the **one best** response to each question.

1. A patient comes into your office. Examination reveals that the patient has a parkinsonian tremor and tardive dyskinesia. Chronic use of which of the following drugs would yield these symptoms?

(A) Meprobamate
(B) Codeine
(C) Chloral hydrate
(D) Chlorpromazine
(E) Phenobarbital

2. Which of the following statements best characterizes lithium?

(A) It produces a noticeable calming effect even in normal persons
(B) It is indicated in psychotic agitated depressive states
(C) It is difficult to correlate therapeutic effects with plasma levels of the agent
(D) It has the potential to inhibit the action of antidiuretic hormone on renal adenylate cyclase
(E) It is useful in the treatment of hypocalcemic disorders

3. Grand mal–type seizures, tremors, and psychosis are often observed during rapid withdrawal in persons addicted to

(A) barbiturates
(B) opiates
(C) chloral hydrate
(D) benzodiazepines
(E) meprobamate

4. Which of the following statements concerning the nonbarbiturate sedative–hypnotic drugs is true?

(A) They produce a sleep state which resembles normal physiologic sleep
(B) They offer lower abuse liability than barbiturates
(C) They are less toxic than barbiturates
(D) They do not appear to induce enyzmes which would alter tolerance to barbiturates
(E) They can be administered to patients with significant liver or kidney disease

5. Which of the following statements about sedative–hypnotics is true?

(A) Trichloroethanol is a pharmacologically active metabolite of chloral hydrate
(B) Methyprylon does not significantly suppress REM sleep
(C) Ethyl alcohol is a physiologic antagonist to the CNS depressant effects of ethchlorvynol
(D) Habituation and physical dependence do not develop with prolonged use of glutethimide
(E) Thiopental is a poor anesthetic induction agent

6. Monoamine oxidase inhibitors should not be used concurrently with

(A) α-adrenergic blocking agents
(B) narcotic analgesics
(B) sulfonamide antibiotics
(D) tricyclic antidepressants
(E) flurazepam

7. A feature common to all phenothiazines is

(A) a marked increase in blood pressure which occurs often during therapy with these agents
(B) akathisia, tremor at rest, and pill-rolling movements with prolonged use
(C) antidiuretic hormone stimulation
(D) a diminished response to CNS depressants such as barbiturates and minor tranquilizers
(E) a lack of allergic reactions

8. Propoxyphene is structurally related to

(A) heroin
(B) morphine
(C) meperidine
(D) methadone
(E) fentanyl

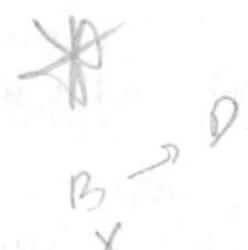

9. A patient being treated for pathologic depression presents with the following drug-induced symptoms: insomnia, hypertension, and all the autonomic side effects associated with amphetamine. Which agent is the patient most likely to be taking?

(A) Tranylcypromine
(B) Imipramine
(C) Desipramine
(D) Amitriptyline
(E) Nortriptyline

10. The brief duration of action of an ultra-short-acting barbiturate is due to

(A) a rapid redistribution of the drug from the brain to other tissues
(B) a slow rate of biotransformation in the liver
(C) a low lipid solubility
(D) a high degree of binding to plasma proteins
(E) slow renal excretion of the drug

11. Among the nonbarbiturate sedative–hypnotics, a certain agent can produce a particularly hazardous condition involving severe CNS depression, hyperpyrexia, and profound cardiovascular shock upon acute overdosage. The agent capable of producing this condition is

(A) methyprylon
(B) glutethimide
(C) chloral hydrate
(D) ethchlorvynol
(E) methaqualone

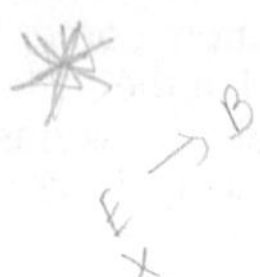

Directions: Each question below contains four suggested answers of which **one or more** is correct. Choose the answer

A if **1, 2, and 3** are correct
B if **1 and 3** are correct
C if **2 and 4** are correct
D if **4** is correct
E if **1, 2, 3, and 4** are correct

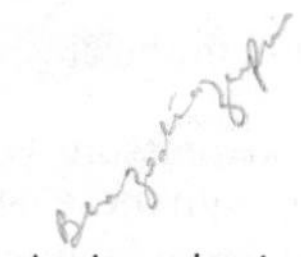

12. Antipsychotic agents have which of the following properties?

(1) They will block copper sulfate–induced vomiting at low doses
(2) They produce a parkinsonian syndrome in certain cases
(3) They stimulate the release of antidiuretic hormone
(4) They may produce α-adrenergic blockade

13. A hypertensive crisis might be seen with which of the following drug classes?

(1) Tricyclic antidepressants
(2) Barbiturates
(3) Narcotic analgesics
(4) Monoamine oxidase inhibitors

14. True statements concerning the drug therapy of seizure disorders include which of the following?

(1) Phenobarbital is an effective anticonvulsant in doses below the sedative–hypnotic range
(2) Phenobarbital is frequently of value in combination with phenytoin in controlling refractory grand mal seizures
(3) Phenytoin may exacerbate petit mal seizures
(4) Patients may be abruptly withdrawn from phenobarbital if refractoriness develops

15. Which of the following drugs might be effective in reducing the pain in a patient who is dying of cancer?

(1) Morphine
(2) Meperidine
(3) Hydromorphone
(4) Diphenoxylate

16. Which side effects might be observed in a patient who has been taking chlorpromazine for 1 month?

(1) Extrapyramidal symptoms
(2) Hypotension
(3) Lethargy
(4) Weight gain

ANSWERS AND EXPLANATIONS

1. The answer is D. *(V B 2 b)* The presenting symptoms of this patient are compatible with chronic administration of a phenothiazine such as chlorpromazine. Patients often display rigidity and tremor at rest and sucking and smacking of the lips.

2. The answer is D. *(VII A)* Lithium is used in the treatment of mania and does not produce psychotropic effects in normal persons. Therapeutic effects correlate well with plasma levels. It can inhibit the action of antidiuretic hormone on renal adenylate cyclase which results in excessive thirst and polyuria.

3. The answer is A. *(II A 7 b)* Rapid withdrawal of barbiturates in persons addicted to these drugs may result in grand mal seizures, severe tremors, vivid hallucinations, and psychosis. Withdrawal should therefore never be abrupt.

4. The answer is D. *(II B)* The nonbarbiturate sedative–hypnotics reduce REM sleep. Agents such as methaqualone have significant abuse potential. Some (e.g., glutethimide) can be quite toxic. They do not induce liver enzymes but should not be administered to patients with significant liver and kidney disease.

5. The answer is A. *(II A 2, B)* Trichloroethanol is the pharmacologically active metabolite of chloral hydrate. Methyprylon significantly suppresses REM sleep. Ethyl alcohol is a CNS depressant and is not a physiologic antagonist of ethchlorvynol. Glutethimide does possess habituation and physical dependence liabilities. Thiopental is an excellent anesthetic induction agent.

6. The answer is D. *(VII B 3 i (9))* Of agents listed in the question, monoamine oxidase inhibitors should not be used with tricyclic antidepressants: Their interaction has produced hyperpyrexia, hypertension, convulsions, and coma.

7. The answer is B. *(V B)* Phenothiazines can produce orthostatic hypotension due to their α-adrenergic blocking activity. Inhibition of antidiuretic hormone (ADH) usually results in a weak diuretic effect. The addition of other CNS depressants to phenothiazine therapy can result in severe CNS depression. Allergic reactions can occur during the first few months of therapy. The parkinsonian syndrome is a characteristic untoward effect.

8. The answer is D. *(IX E 2)* Propoxyphene is a structural analog of methadone. It has, however, a spectrum of pharmacologic activity similar to that of codeine. Since it does not possess anti-inflammatory properties, it is less effective in treating pain associated with inflammation.

9. The answer is A. *(VII B)* Imipramine, desipramine, nortriptyline, and amitriptyline (all tricyclic antidepressants) produce untoward effects resembling those of the phenothiazines, including hypotension. Tranylcypromine chemically resembles amphetamine and produces autonomic side effects similar to those of amphetamine.

10. The answer is A. *(II A 5)* Ultra-short-acting barbiturates have a high lipid solubility, allowing rapid transport across the blood–brain barrier. Their brief duration of action results from their removal from the brain via distribution to other tissues.

11. The answer is B. *(II B)* Glutethimide can produce all of the untoward effects listed in the question. In addition, its plasma half-life during acute intoxication can be as long as 4 days. Even with hemodialysis a secondary rise in glutethimide plasma levels can result from additional intestinal absorption.

12. The answer is C (2, 4). *(V)* Antipsychotic agents (e.g., chlorpromazine) will block agents that stimulate the chemoreceptor trigger zone, but not the effects of copper sulfate, which is a direct gastrointestinal irritant. They inhibit the release of antidiuretic hormone (ADH) and can produce a syndrome resembling Parkinson's disease. A peripheral effect is α-adrenergic blockade.

13. The answer is D (4). *(II A, VII B, IX)* Tricyclic antidepressants, barbiturates, and narcotic analgesics can be associated with hypotension but not hypertension. Monoamine oxidase inhibitors can interact with certain foods (e.g., cheese, beer) which have a high tyramine content. Because tyramine cannot undergo oxidative deamination, catecholamines are released from nerve terminals, producing the hypertensive crisis.

14. The answer is A (1, 2, 3). *(III)* All of the statements are true except the fourth. If barbiturate therapy is withdrawn, it should be done gradually in order to prevent status epilepticus. Hallucinations, severe tremors, and psychosis can also occur.

15. The answer is A (1, 2, 3). *(IX C 1, 5, D)* The narcotic analgesics morphine, meperidine, and hydromorphone are effective in reducing the pain associated with cancer. Diphenoxylate, although classified as a narcotic analgesic, is used principally in the treatment of diarrhea and is not used as an analgesic.

16. The answer is E (all). *(V B 2, 3, 6)* Chlorpromazine can cause hypotension due to its α-adrenergic blocking properties. Lethargy and increased weight are untoward effects. The most distinguishing untoward effects seen with administration of a phenothiazine such as chlorpromazine are extrapyramidal symptoms.

4
Anesthetic Agents

I. INTRODUCTION

A. LOCAL ANESTHETICS

1. Local anesthetic agents, by blocking nerve conduction, produce a transient and reversible loss of sensation in a regionalized area of the body without producing a loss of consciousness.
2. Unlike general anesthetics, they normally do not cause central nervous system (CNS) depression.

B. GENERAL ANESTHETICS are agents which produce analgesia, amnesia, or hypnosis and, by themselves or in combination with other agents, are capable of producing unconsciousness and the absence of pain sensation in a manner compatible with the performance of surgery.

1. **Inhalation anesthetics** are agents for which transfer across the alveolus serves as the portal of entry into the body. These agents can depress the central nervous system.
2. **Intravenous anesthetics** are most often used for induction of anesthesia (e.g., thiopental) before administration of more potent anesthetic agents. However, they are also applicable for certain procedures of longer duration.
   a. **Neuroleptanesthesia** is induced by combining a powerful narcotic analgesic with a neuroleptic agent together with the inhalation of nitrous oxide and oxygen.
   b. **Dissociative anesthesia**, such as that caused by ketamine, produces rapid analgesia and amnesia while maintaining laryngeal reflexes.
   c. **Barbiturate anesthesia** is rarely used.
3. **Preanesthetic medications** may include sedatives, opioids, tranquilizers, and anticholinergic agents.

II. LOCAL ANESTHETICS

A. MECHANISM OF ACTION

1. Local anesthetics reduce the rate of rise of the action potential as well as the rate of repolarization, and thus slow the propagation of nerve impulses.
2. The threshold for electrical excitability gradually increases until complete block of conduction occurs.
3. They block nerve conduction by interfering with the permeability of the cell membrane to sodium in response to partial depolarization, and thus they stabilize the membrane at the resting potential.
4. Two theories have been advanced to explain the mechanism of interference with membrane permeability.
   a. The **specific receptor theory** postulates that the local anesthetic binds to Na^+ channels, and thus interferes with the normal passage of Na^+ through the membrane.
   b. The **membrane expansion theory** hypothesizes that local anesthetics, because of their lipophilicity, incorporate into the cell membrane, preventing the opening of pores and thus interfering with the passage of electrolytes.
5. The smallest unmyelinated fibers, which conduct impulses for pain, temperature, and autonomic activity, conduct slowly and are the first to be blocked by local anesthetics.

B. CHEMISTRY AND STRUCTURE–ACTIVITY RELATIONSHIP

1. Structurally, all local anesthetics consist of a hydrophilic amino group, linked through a connecting group to a lipophilic aromatic residue.
2. If the **connecting link** between the intermediate group and aromatic residue is an **ester group**, the site of metabolism is hydrolysis by plasma pseudocholinesterase; if the link is an **amide bond**, hydrolysis occurs in the liver.
3. In general, the greater the length of the connecting and amino groups, the greater the potency and the toxicity of the local anesthetic (see Table 4-1).
4. Local anesthetics are weak bases and as such are usually water-insoluble. The drug may be dispensed as a crystal, but more usually is prepared as an acidic salt solution which is highly water-soluble and stable.
5. At tissue pH, depending upon the pK_a of the agent, the drug will exist as either an uncharged tertiary or secondary amine or a positively charged ammonium cation. The former state is lipophilic and crosses connective tissue and enters nerve cells; the cation is thought to block the generation of action potentials via a membrane–receptor complex.

C. AGENTS

1. **Cocaine**
   - **a.** This drug is an ester of benzoic acid.
   - **b.** In addition to local anesthetic activity, **pharmacologic effects** of cocaine include:
     - **(1)** Central nervous system stimulation, producing euphoria and sometimes dysphoria. The initial effect is followed by post-stimulatory depression.
     - **(2)** Major actions on the cardiovascular system. Cocaine blocks the uptake of catecholamines at adrenergic nerve terminals, causing sympathetically mediated tachycardia and vasoconstriction leading to hypertension. (The vasoconstriction also decreases intraoperative mucous membrane bleeding.)
     - **(3)** Hyperpyrexia.
   - **c.** Cocaine is degraded by plasma esterases.
   - **d.** Tolerance, abuse, and poisoning can occur with cocaine overuse.
   - **e. Preparations and uses. Cocaine hydrochloride** is used in 4 to 10 percent concentrations as well as crystals for topical anesthesia of the nose, pharynx, and tracheobronchial tree.
2. **Procaine**
   - **a.** This local anesthetic is an ester of diethylaminoethanol and para-aminobenzoic acid.
   - **b. Pharmacologic effects**, in addition to local anesthetic activity, include a procaine–sulfonamide antagonism. The metabolic product of procaine hydrolysis is para-aminobenzoic acid, which inhibits the action of sulfonamides.
   - **c.** Procaine is well absorbed following parenteral administration and is rapidly metabolized by pseudocholinesterase.
   - **d.** The drug lacks topical activity.
   - **e.** Procaine administration causes minimal systemic toxicity and no local irritation.
   - **f. Preparations and uses. Procaine hydrochloride** is available with and without epinephrine. **Epinephrine** decreases the rate of anesthetic absorption in the bloodstream and so approximately doubles the duration of anesthesia produced by a given dose.
     - **(1)** A 1 to 2 percent solution is used for nerve block and infiltration anesthesia.
     - **(2)** A 5 to 20 percent solution is used for spinal anesthesia.
3. **Tetracaine**
   - **a.** This local anesthetic is an ester and a derivative of para-aminobenzoic acid.

Table 4-1. Pharmacodynamic Properties of Local Anesthetics

Agent	Linkage	Potency	Toxicity
Procaine	Ester	1	1
Lidocaine	Amide	4	2
Mepivacaine	Amide	2	2
Bupivacaine	Amide	16	10
Tetracaine	Ester	16	10
Etidocaine	Amide	16	10
Dibucaine	Amide	15	15

b. It is many times more potent and more toxic than procaine. Its onset of action is approximately 5 minutes and its duration of action is between 2 to 3 hours.

c. **Preparations and uses**
   (1) **Tetracaine hydrochloride is** a commonly used local anesthetic for spinal anesthesia and in this context usually is combined with 10 percent dextrose to increase the specific gravity so that the solution is heavier than cerebrospinal fluid.
   (2) A 2 percent solution is used topically on mucous membranes.

4. **Lidocaine**
   a. This drug is an amide local anesthetic and an acetanilid derivative.
   b. Its **pharmacologic effects** include:
      (1) Rapid onset of anesthesia.
      (2) Minimal local irritation.
      (3) A greater potency and longer duration of action than procaine.
      (4) Moderate topical activity.
   c. Lidocaine is rapidly absorbed after parenteral administration and is metabolized in the liver by microsomal mixed-function oxidases.
   d. Its major **clinical uses** are as a local anesthetic and, intravenously, as an antiarrhythmic agent (see Chapter 5, III E).
   e. **Preparations**
      (1) **Lidocaine hydrochloride** can be administered with or without epinephrine.
      (2) A 0.5 percent solution is used for infiltrative anesthesia.
      (3) A 1 to 2 percent solution is used for topical mucosal and nerve block anesthesia.
      (4) For spinal anesthesia, the concentration of lidocaine used is 5 percent or less.
      (5) For anesthetic use, lidocaine is available as an ointment, jelly, cream, and topical solution.
      (6) Lidocaine is also available as a solution for intravenous use.

5. **Dibucaine**
   a. This drug is a substituted amide which is a quinoline derivative.
   b. Dibucaine is a potent anesthetic with a long duration of action.
   c. It has a very high systemic toxicity.
   d. Dibucaine currently is used only as a topical anesthetic.
   e. **Preparations and uses. Dibucaine hydrochloride** is used for anesthesia of mucous membranes in a 0.2 percent concentration.

6. **Prilocaine**
   a. Like lidocaine, prilocaine is an amide local anesthetic. Its onset and duration of action are slightly longer than those of lidocaine.
   b. The major disadvantage of prilocaine is the production of methemoglobinemia and a shift of the oxygen-dissociation curve for hemoglobin to the left.
   c. **Preparations and uses. Prilocaine hydrochloride** has been used for infiltrative, regional, and spinal anesthesia and is available in a 1 to 3 percent solution.

7. **Etidocaine**
   a. Pharmacologically, etidocaine is similar to lidocaine except for its greater potency and longer duration of action.
   b. It is **used** clinically in epidural, infiltrative, and regional anesthesia. The drug usually blocks motor fibers before sensory fibers.
   c. **Preparations. Etidocaine hydrochloride** is available both with and without epinephrine, in concentrations ranging from 0.5 to 1.5 percent.

8. **Mepivacaine**
   a. Like lidocaine, mepivacaine is an amide-type local anesthetic.
   b. Pharmacologically, mepivacaine is similar to lidocaine. However, it does not have antiarrhythmic activity. In onset of action mepivacaine is more rapid than lidocaine and its duration of action is about 20 percent longer. Therefore, epinephrine is rarely used with this drug.
   c. Major **uses** are for infiltrative and regional nerve block anesthesia. It also can be used for spinal anesthesia.
   d. **Preparations. Mepivacaine hydrochloride** is used in concentrations ranging from 1 to 4 percent.

9. **Bupivacaine**
   a. An amide local anesthetic, bupivacaine is structurally similar to mepivacaine.
   b. It is more potent and has a longer duration of action than mepivacaine, lasting for more than 24 hours in some situations, possibly as a result of increased tissue binding. The onset of action is slower than that of mepivacaine.

c. Toxicity is similar to that of tetracaine; however, cardiac arrest has recently been reported in association with a 0.75 percent solution of bupivacaine used for obstetrical epidural anesthesia.

d. **Preparations and uses. Bupivacaine hydrochloride** is used mainly for regional nerve block anesthesia in concentrations ranging from 0.25 to 0.75 percent.

D. ADVERSE SYSTEMIC EFFECTS OF LOCAL ANESTHETICS result from absorption of toxic amounts of these agents into the bloodstream. Adding epinephrine, a vasoconstrictor, to the optimal concentration of a local anesthetic reduces the rate of systemic absorption of the anesthetic and so can decrease systemic toxicity.

1. Seizures, the result of absorption of the local anesthetic and stimulation of the CNS, are the most serious adverse effect. Convulsions, if they occur, are treated with basic supportive measures including ventilation and oxygenation, and with intravenous diazepam.
2. Respiratory failure secondary to CNS depression is a late stage of intoxication.
3. A quinidine-like effect on the myocardium can be produced by local anesthetics.
4. Hypotension is a late effect which can occur as the result of myocardial depression and peripheral arterial vasodilation; affected patients are treated with appropriate parenteral vasopressor agents.
5. Allergic reactions to local anesthetic agents rarely occur.

III. GENERAL ANESTHETICS

A. INHALATION ANESTHETICS

1. General information

a. The relationship between the administered dose of an inhalation anesthetic and the quantitative effect produced is described as the **minimum alveolar concentration (MAC)** of the anesthetic at 1 atmosphere that will produce loss of movement in 50 percent of subjects exposed to a noxious stimulus. MAC is used as the **measure of potency** for all inhalation anesthetics.

b. The concentration of an inhalation anesthetic in blood or tissue is the product of its solubility and partial pressure. The solubility of an agent is expressed most commonly in terms of a blood:gas or a tissue:blood partition coefficient.

(1) An agent with a **blood:gas partition coefficient** of 2 will reach twice the concentration in the blood phase as in the gas phase when the partial pressure is the same in both phases (i.e., at equilibrium). Very soluble agents (e.g., ether) have a blood:gas partition coefficient as high as 12; relatively insoluble agents (e.g., nitrous oxide) have a coefficient of less than 1. **The lower the blood:gas partition coefficient of an anesthetic, the more rapid the induction of anesthesia** with that agent, because high blood solubility constantly lowers the alveolar gas pressure.

(2) Most inhalation agents are equally soluble in lean tissue and in blood (so that the tissue:blood partition coefficient often approximates 1). On the other hand, most anesthetics have a far greater concentration in fatty tissues than in blood at equilibrium.

2. Halothane

a. Pharmacologic characteristics

(1) Halothane, with a MAC of 0.75 percent, is a potent anesthetic agent.

(2) Halothane lacks significant analgesic potency and thus is most frequently used with another anesthetic.

b. Effects on organ systems

(1) Respiratory effects

(a) Respirations become rapid and shallow during halothane anesthesia.

(b) Halothane reduces the minute volume.

(c) It causes a reduction in the ventilatory response to carbon dioxide. This effect appears to be due to depression of central chemoreceptors.

(d) Halothane produces bronchiolar dilation.

(2) Cardiovascular effects

(a) Halothane causes a decrease in arterial blood pressure that is dose-dependent.

(b) Cutaneous blood flow may increase as blood vessels dilate.

(c) Myocardial contractility is depressed with halothane administration.

(d) Halothane interferes with the action of norepinephrine and thus antagonizes the sympathetic response to arterial hypotension.

(e) Halothane anesthesia depresses cardiac sympathetic activity, which can result in a slow heart rate.
(f) Although arrhythmias are uncommon, halothane can increase the automaticity of the heart. This condition is exacerbated by adrenergic agonists, cardiac disease, hypoxia, and electrolyte abnormalities.

(3) Effect on the CNS
(a) As halothane anesthesia deepens, fast, low-voltage electroencephalographic waves are replaced by slow, high-voltage waves.
(b) Cerebral blood vessels dilate, increasing cerebral blood flow and cerebrospinal fluid pressure. A maldistribution of cerebral blood flow and altered metabolism can occur.
(c) Shivering during recovery is common.

(4) Effects on the kidneys
(a) At a level of 1 MAC, halothane causes renal blood flow and glomerular filtration to drop to about 50 percent of normal.
(b) These effects are mitigated by adequate hydration.

(5) Effects on the liver
(a) Halothane depresses liver function. This effect is rapidly reversed when administration of the anesthetic is stopped.
(b) A low incidence of **hepatic necrosis** that cannot be attributed to known etiologies is associated with halothane anesthesia.
(i) Two to five days postoperatively, an affected patient develops fever, anorexia, and vomiting. This syndrome is known as **halothane hepatitis.**
(ii) Eosinophilia and biochemical abnormalities characteristic of hepatitis occur.
(iii) The incidence of halothane hepatitis is 1 in 35,000 administrations of the anesthetic.
(iv) The syndrome occurs most often after repeated administration of halothane.
(v) A toxic or immunogenic product may result from halothane administration and may be responsible for an immune response that leads to halothane hepatitis.

(6) Effects on muscle
(a) Halothane causes skeletal muscle relaxation by both central and peripheral mechanisms.
(b) It appears to increase the sensitivity of end-plates to the action of competitive neuromuscular blocking agents.
(c) It relaxes uterine smooth muscle.
(d) Halothane, like all potent inhalation agents, can trigger malignant hyperthermia, a potentially fatal condition believed to be autosomal dominant, in which, in response to anesthesia, a sudden, rapid rise in body temperature and signs of increased muscle metabolism occur.

c. Elimination
(1) Approximately 70 percent of halothane is eliminated unchanged in exhaled gas in the first 24 hours after administration.
(2) Approximately 5 percent is biotransformed by the cytochrome P-450 system in the endoplasmic reticulum of the liver.

d. Therapeutic use
(1) Halothane is a highly potent, nonflammable general anesthetic with a relatively high blood:gas partition coefficient; thus induction of and recovery from anesthesia with this agent may be prolonged.
(2) Halothane is not irritating to the larynx, and thus induction of anesthesia with this agent is smooth and bronchospasm is uncommon.
(3) Halothane administration is often supplemented with thiopental for induction of anesthesia. Nitrous oxide, oxygen, and muscle relaxants are normally used with halothane.

3. Enflurane

a. Pharmacologic characteristics
(1) Enflurane has a MAC of 1.68 percent.
(2) Enflurane causes mild stimulation of salivation and tracheobronchial secretions. It suppresses laryngeal reflexes.

b. Effects on organ systems

(1) Respiratory effects
(a) Enflurane produces dose-dependent respiratory depression.
(b) With enflurane at 1 MAC, respiratory responses to hypoxia and hypercapnia are less than with halothane.
(c) Enflurane causes bronchodilation and inhibits bronchoconstriction.

(2) Cardiovascular effects
- **(a)** Dose-dependent depression of the arterial blood pressure and depressed baroreceptor responses are similar to those caused by halothane.
- **(b)** Dose-dependent myocardial depression also occurs and is similar to that caused by halothane.
- **(c)** Bradycardia usually does not occur with enflurane, and cardiac output is not decreased as much as with halothane.
- **(d)** Enflurane causes a lower incidence of arrhythmias and less sensitization of the myocardium to catecholamines than does halothane.

(3) Effects on the CNS
- **(a)** Enflurane anesthesia can lead to an electroencephalographic pattern characteristic of seizure activity or to frank seizures.
  - **(i)** The seizures are self-limited and can be prevented by avoiding both high concentrations of enflurane and hyperventilation, which leads to hypocapnia.
  - **(ii)** Enflurane is contraindicated in patients who have known seizure disorders.
- **(b)** Enflurane causes cerebral vasodilation and increased intracranial pressure as long as the arterial blood pressure remains normal.

(4) Effects on the kidneys
- **(a)** At a level of 1 MAC, enflurane anesthesia causes a reduction in renal blood flow and glomerular filtration that is similar to that caused by halothane.
- **(b)** Although fluoride is a metabolic product of enflurane biotransformation, it poses little if any danger of renal toxicity.

(5) Effects on the liver
- **(a)** Liver impairment has been reported but usually is reversible.
- **(b)** Hepatic necrosis also has been reported, especially after repeated administration of enflurane.

(6) Effects on muscle
- **(a)** Enflurane provides adequate muscular relaxation for most surgical procedures. The agent acts directly on the neuromuscular junction.
- **(b)** Enflurane relaxes uterine smooth muscle.

c. Elimination
- **(1)** Approximately 80 percent of enflurane is eliminated unchanged as expired gas.
- **(2)** Because enflurane's oil:gas partition coefficient is less than that of other halogenated anesthetics, enflurane leaves fatty tissues more rapidly.
- **(3)** About 5 percent of enflurane is metabolized in the liver. Free fluoride ion is released.

d. Therapeutic use
- **(1)** Enflurane is a potent general anesthetic that causes a lower incidence of arrhythmias than halothane.
- **(2)** Enflurane is a better skeletal muscle relaxant than halothane but, unlike halothane, can cause seizure activity.

methoxy Fluane : nephrotoxicity ; induces microsomes ; induction ↑ toxicity

4. Isoflurane

a. Pharmacologic characteristics
- **(1)** Isoflurane, a volatile anesthetic, is an isomer of enflurane and has similar physical properties.
- **(2)** It produces significant respiratory depression.
- **(3)** Because of hypercapnia resulting from respiratory depression, cardiac output may increase.
- **(4)** Peripheral vascular resistance is decreased by isoflurane, resulting in a fall in arterial blood pressure.
- **(5)** Isoflurane does not sensitize the heart to catecholamines and rarely causes cardiac arrhythmias.
- **(6)** It is a good muscle relaxant.

b. Therapeutic use. Unlike enflurane, isoflurane does not cause seizure activity; unlike halothane, isoflurane does not sensitize the myocardium to epinephrine or induce aryhthmias.

5. Nitrous oxide

a. Pharmacologic characteristics
- **(1)** Nitrous oxide (N_2O) is an inorganic inert gas that supports combustion.
- **(2)** The MAC for nitrous oxide is 105.2 percent, meaning that hyperbaric conditions would be required to reach 1 MAC with this drug. For maintaining anesthesia, a concentration of 75 to 80 percent nitrous oxide is required.
- **(3)** Nitrous oxide is not effective for anesthesia as a single agent, and attempts made to use

it in this manner are associated with a high risk of hypoxia. To achieve "complete" anesthesia with this agent, administration of opioids to supplement analgesia, the use of thiopental for narcosis, and a neuromuscular blocking agent for muscular relaxation are all required.

(4) When nitrous oxide is combined with more potent inhalation agents, such as enflurane or halothane, it provides significant analgesia.

b. Effects on organ systems

(1) Respiratory effects

(a) The effects of nitrous oxide on respiration are minimal when a concentration of 50 percent is used.

(b) However, when nitrous oxide is combined with thiopental or another anesthetic agent for induction of anesthesia, the respiratory stimulant response to carbon dioxide is depressed more than when thiopental or the other anesthetic agent is used alone.

(2) Cardiovascular effects. When nitrous oxide is combined with a potent inhalation anesthetic, activation of the sympathetic nervous system results; blood pressure and total peripheral vascular resistance rise and cardiac output is reduced.

c. Elimination

(1) Nitrous oxide is eliminated primarily as an expired gas.

(2) The amount of nitrous oxide subject to biotransformation is not known.

d. Therapeutic use

(1) Nitrous oxide is an important and powerful **analgesic** that is well tolerated. Its onset of action is rapid, as is recovery from its effects. Because of this it is frequently used for outpatient dental procedures.

(2) Nitrous oxide is used as a supplement to more potent anesthetic agents, and, in this capacity, is probably the most widely used general anesthetic agent.

e. Untoward effects

(1) Because of its high partial pressure in blood and its low blood:gas partition coefficient, nitrous oxide diffuses into air-containing body cavities and can increase the pressure or expand the volume of gas in air pockets. This action can result in:

(a) Distention of the bowel.

(b) Expansion or rupture of a pulmonary cyst.

(c) Rupture of the tympanic membrane in an occluded middle ear.

(2) When nitrous oxide is dissolved in blood, it can enlarge the volume of air emboli.

(3) Leukopenia has been reported with chronic nitrous oxide abuse.

(4) Diffusion hypoxia can occur at the termination of nitrous oxide anesthesia if a patient abruptly begins to breathe room air. This hypoxia is caused by a rapid outward diffusion of nitrous oxide from tissues into the bloodstream and then into the alveoli, where it decreases alveolar tension and consequently lowers arterial oxygen levels. This problem can be avoided by administration of 100 percent oxygen for a short period at the termination of nitrous oxide anesthesia.

6. Diethyl ether

a. Pharmacologic characteristics. Diethyl ether is a highly flammable and explosive anesthetic agent which essentially has been replaced by halogenated anesthetics.

b. Effects on organ systems

(1) Respiratory effects

(a) Increased sympathetic activity produced by diethyl ether results in bronchodilation.

(b) The respiratory response to carbon dioxide, although reduced, is maintained spontaneously by reflex excitation at peripheral sites.

(2) Cardiovascular effects

(a) Although diethyl ether is a myocardial depressant, cardiac output and arterial blood pressure are maintained because of sympathetic activation.

(b) Vagal blockade also occurs with diethyl ether administration, resulting in tachycardia.

(3) Effects on the kidneys. Diethyl ether is a strong stimulant of antidiuretic hormone.

(4) Effects on the liver. Sympathetic activation results in increased hepatic glycogenolysis.

(5) Effects on muscle

(a) Diethyl ether is a good skeletal muscle relaxant because it causes central nervous system depression at synaptic pathways in the spinal cord.

(b) In addition, diethyl ether has a curare-like action, allowing a lower dose of neuromuscular blockers; several aminoglycoside antibiotics augment this effect.

c. Untoward effects. When used as a sole agent to induce anesthesia, diethyl ether causes increased salivary secretions, vomiting, and laryngospasm.

B. INTRAVENOUS ANESTHETICS

1. Neuroleptanesthesia

a. General considerations

(1) When a neuroleptic agent is combined with a powerful narcotic, **neuroleptanalgesia** is produced. The addition of nitrous oxide and oxygen to this combination produces **neuroleptanesthesia**.

(2) The agents most frequently used to achieve neuroleptanalgesia are **droperidol** (a butyrophenone derivative—see Chapter 3, V D) and **fentanyl citrate** (an opioid—see Chapter 3, IX D 3). A combination of the two drugs is available as a premixed compound called **Innovar**.

b. Effects on organ systems

(1) **Respiratory effects**

(a) Droperidol slightly decreases the respiratory rate but increases tidal volume.

(b) Fentanyl reduces both respiratory rate and tidal volume.

(c) The marked respiratory depressant effect of the two drugs outlasts the analgesic effect.

(2) **Cardiovascular effects**

(a) Droperidol can produce mild α-adrenergic blockade, causing some hypotension.

(b) Fentanyl has a parasympathomimetic effect that can cause bradycardia and hypotension.

(c) Innovar can cause bradycardia. However, it rarely causes other cardiac arrhythmias, and in general it has little effect on the cardiovascular system.

c. Therapeutic use

(1) Fentanyl should be administered as a slow intravenous infusion (given over 5 to 10 minutes) since rapid injection may cause respiratory muscle spasm.

(2) Respiratory depression is a frequent occurrence, and adequate ventilation and oxygenation may require use of mechanical measures.

(3) After induction of neuroleptanalgesia, nitrous oxide administration is begun. Supplementary fentanyl may be required for prolonged analgesia because fentanyl has a short duration of action.

d. Untoward effects

(1) Confusion and mental depression are the most common complaints after neuroleptanesthesia.

(2) Extrapyramidal symptoms occur rarely.

2. Dissociative anesthesia

a. General considerations

(1) Dissociative anesthesia is a state similar to neuroleptanalgesia in which anesthetized patients feel totally dissociated from their surroundings. **Phencyclidine** was the original dissociative anesthetic; the structurally similar **ketamine** is the only drug used at present to produce this state.

(2) Ketamine produces profound analgesia and amnesia.

(3) It has no effect on laryngeal reflexes.

(4) Skeletal muscle tone, heart rate, arterial blood pressure, and cerebrospinal fluid pressure can be increased by ketamine.

(5) The respiratory cycle is maintained near normal.

b. Therapeutic use

(1) Premedication with atropine reduces salivary secretions; premedication with a narcotic analgesic decreases the dose of ketamine needed for anesthesia.

(2) Ketamine is used mainly for children and young adults, for diagnostic procedures of short duration.

c. Untoward effects

(1) Because of its hallucinogen-like structure, ketamine frequently produces unpleasant dreams, especially in adults. Recovery from ketamine anesthesia often is accompanied by emergence delirium and psychomotor activity.

(2) Contraindications to the use of ketamine include psychiatric disorders, a history of cerebrovascular disease (to avoid the risk of hypertension-induced stroke), and respiratory infections.

3. Barbiturates

a. Thiopental is the barbiturate most frequently used for general anesthesia. It provides rapid and pleasant induction and thus often is used before administration of stronger agents. It can be used alone to provide anesthetic for short procedures, but thiopental and other barbiturates are poor analgesics.

b. Once a barbiturate has been injected, little can be done to facilitate its removal. Termination of its effects depends on redistribution of the drug from brain to other tissues and, to a lesser extent, on biotransformation.

c. The pharmacology and clinical uses of barbiturates is presented in Chapter 3, II A.

C. **PREANESTHETIC MEDICATIONS** can foster an uncomplicated anesthetic and operative course by improving the rapidity and smoothness of induction, reducing anxiety, providing analgesia and amnesia, and compensating for the salivation, bradycardia, and some of the other side effects of anesthesia. Agents used as preanesthetic medications include sedatives, opioids, tranquilizers, and anticholinergic agents.

1. When **barbiturates** are used as preoperative sedatives, **secobarbital** and **pentobarbital** are the drugs most frequently employed. These agents produce less postoperative nausea and vomiting than opioids.

2. **Opioids** such as **morphine** or **fentanyl** often are given to patients who are to be anesthetized with general anesthetics of fairly low potency, such as the combination of nitrous oxide and thiopental. In addition, they can be administered with a barbiturate or diazepam for regional anesthesia. In both instances, they provide analgesia.

3. **Phenothiazine** derivatives, such as **promethazine** and the antihistamine **hydroxyzine**, often are administered concomitantly with opioids because they potentiate the analgesic effect without increasing side effects.

4. **Tranquilizers** such as **diazepam** are useful in a wide variety of anesthetic situations. They can provide preoperative sedation, help to prevent and treat the central nervous system stimulation caused by local anesthetics, and provide amnesia.

5. **Anticholinergic agents**. **Atropine** and **scopolamine**, as well as the quaternary ammonium compound **glycopyrrolate**, are used routinely to decrease the flow of saliva.

6. The pharmacology, therapeutic uses, and undesirable effects of barbiturates, opioids, and tranquilizers are discussed in Chapter 3; the anticholinergic agents are discussed in Chapter 2, VI.

STUDY QUESTIONS

Directions: Each question below contains five suggested answers. Choose the **one best** response to each question.

1. Thiopental sodium has which of the following features?

(A) It provides adequate anesthesia for any surgical procedure
(B) It provides excellent analgesia and muscle relaxation
(C) It provides a smooth rapid induction of sleep
(D) It is usually not supplemented with another agent such as nitrous oxide
(E) It can only be administered orally

2. All of the following statements concerning general inhalation anesthetics are true EXCEPT

(A) they may profoundly depress myocardial force of contraction
(B) they can cause temporary depression of renal and hepatic function
(C) they may cause respiratory depression to the extent that respiratory acidosis will ensue unless ventilation is artificially supported
(D) they are chemically inert and as such not metabolized
(E) they are capable of depressing electron transport in mitochondria

3. A patient with known asthma comes to the operating room for lower-extremity surgery. He has severe hepatitis but needs the surgery. The anesthetic of choice should be

(A) enflurane
(B) halothane
(C) a spinal anesthetic
(D) isoflurane
(E) nitrous oxide

4. All of the following statements about procaine are true EXCEPT

(A) it is nonaddictive
(B) it is nontoxic in the normal dose range
(C) it has a short duration of action
(D) it is metabolized by acetylcholinesterase
(E) it is metabolized in the blood

5. The local anesthetic with the longest duration of action is

(A) procaine
(B) bupivacaine
(C) lidocaine
(D) mepivacaine
(E) tetracaine

Directions: Each question below contains four suggested answers of which **one or more** is correct. Choose the answer

A if **1, 2, and 3** are correct
B if **1 and 3** are correct
C if **2 and 4** are correct
D if **4** is correct
E if **1, 2, 3, and 4** are correct

6. Properties of inhalation anesthetics are found to correlate well (directly *or* inversely) with an index of solubility (a ratio) called a "partition coefficient." Which of the following pharmacological factors relate to the blood/gas partition coefficient?

(1) Anesthetic efficacy
(2) MAC (potency)
(3) Respiratory rate
(4) Induction rate

7. An incorrect toxic dose of lidocaine was administered locally into the dorsalis pedis artery. Which of the following effects may have occurred?

(1) Convulsions
(2) Respiratory depression
(3) Hypotension
(4) Increased inotropic effect

8. A patient who has an untreatable hepatic carcinoma must undergo foot surgery. Which of the following local anesthetic agents would be deleterious based on this history?

(1) Lidocaine
(2) Dibucaine
(3) Mepivacaine
(4) Procaine

9. Which of the following drugs and drug properties are correctly matched?

(1) Cocaine—inhibits the re-uptake of norepinephrine
(2) Procaine—is metabolized by glucuronide conjugation
(3) Lidocaine—is an amide
(4) Mepivacaine—is usually administered with epinephrine

10. Correct statements concerning nitrous oxide (N_2O) include which of the following?

(1) The common N_2O concentration required for the maintenance of anesthesia is 5 percent
(2) It has the ability to produce surgical anesthesia when used alone
(3) It is a weak analgesic
(4) It can produce bowel distention

ANSWERS AND EXPLANATIONS

1. The answer is C. *(III B 3)* Thiopental alone does not provide adequate analgesia or muscle relaxation, and for most surgical procedures it must be supplemented with another inhalation anesthetic agent. It does provide a smooth rapid induction of sleep and is administered parenterally. It is the barbiturate most commonly used for general anesthesia.

2. The answer is D. *(III A)* All general inhalation anesthetics are myocardial depressants. They can temporarily depress renal and hepatic function. Unless ventilation is supported, respiratory acidosis can occur. They can depress electron transport in mitochondria. Many anesthetics like halothane are metabolized in the liver cytochrome P-450 system.

3. The answer is C. *(II C; III A 2–5)* Enflurane, halothane, and isoflurane, an isomer of enflurane, all have hepatotoxic potential and therefore should not be used in this patient. Nitrous oxide is not adequate alone for surgery. Considering that is is lower-extremity surgery, spinal anesthesia would be the anesthetic of choice.

4. The answer is D. *(II B 2, C 2)* Procaine is metabolized by pseudocholinesterase, not acetylcholinesterase. The metabolic products of procaine hydrolysis are para-aminobenzoic acid and diethylaminoethanol.

5. The answer is B. *(II C)* The duration of action (shortest to longest) is procaine > lidocaine > tetracaine > mepivacaine > bupivacaine. Bupivacaine is an amide local anesthetic whose long duration of action is possibly a result of increased tissue binding.

6. The answer is C (2, 4). *(III A1)* The minimum alveolar concentration (MAC) necessary to anesthetize 50 percent of the patients relates to the blood:gas partition coefficient. This MAC is also a good index of potency. The induction rate is inversely proportional to the blood:gas partition coefficient because low blood:gas partitioning means only limited amounts of anesthetic must enter the blood. Moreover, the blood:tissue partition coefficient is usually not greater than 2 with the exception of fat so that blood levels grossly approximate total body load.

7. The answer is A (1, 2, 3). *(II D)* Lidocaine toxicity can cause convulsions, followed by a CNS depression that results in respiratory depression and hypotension. Local anesthetic toxicity can also produce myocardial depression (a negative inotropic effect).

8. The answer is B (1, 3). *(II B 2, C 2, 4, 5, 8)* Both lidocaine and mepivacaine are metabolized in the hepatic microsomal system. Dibucaine is a surface anesthetic and would not enter the general circulation to be metabolized, while procaine is metabolized by pseudocholinesterase.

9. The answer is B (1, 3). *(II B 2, C 1, 2, 4, 8)* Cocaine indeed inhibits the re-uptake of norepinephrine at the nerve terminal. Procaine is metabolized by pseudocholinesterase. Lidocaine is an amide local anesthetic. Mepivacaine has a rapid onset, and its duration of action is sufficiently long so that a vasoconstrictor such as epinephrine is not usually coadministered.

10. The answer is D (4). *(III A 5)* Nitrous oxide is not potent. The most common N_2O:O_2 mixture is 70 percent:30 percent, and concentrations of 5 percent would be ineffective. When used alone, N_2O is not adequate for surgical anesthesia. Nitrous oxide has significant analgesic properties that are useful in surgical applications. Because of its high partial pressure in blood, nitrous oxide diffuses into air-containing cavities, such as the bowel, and can cause distention.

5
Cardiovascular Agents

I. INTRODUCTION. This chapter discusses four major groups of drugs that have a selective action on the cardiovascular system. **Cardiac glycosides** exert a positive inotropic force on the heart. They are used principally for the treatment of congestive heart failure. **Antiarrhythmic agents** (quinidine, procainamide, disopyramide, lidocaine, phenytoin, propranolol, bretylium) are used both for treatment and for prevention of cardiac arrhythmias. **Antianginal drugs** (nitrates, β-adrenergic antagonists, and the new calcium-antagonist agents) relieve the symptoms of angina pectoris. **Antihypertensive drugs** (diuretic agents, vasodilators, antiadrenergic agents, and renin–angiotensin blockers) are used in the treatment of primary hypertension.

II. CARDIAC GLYCOSIDES

A. CHEMISTRY

1. Cardiac glycosides are the combination of an aglycone, or genin, and one to four sugars.
   a. The **aglycone (genin)** is chemically similar to bile acids and to steroids such as adrenocortical and sex hormones. It is the pharmacologically active portion of the glycosides.
   b. The **sugars** modify the water- and lipid-solubility of the glycoside molecule and thus affect its potency and duration of action.
2. Glycosides are obtained from dried leaves of the foxglove, *Digitalis purpurea* (digitoxin) or *Digitalis lanata* (digitoxin, digoxin), and from the seeds of *Strophanthus gratus* (ouabain).
3. The term **digitalis** is frequently used to refer to the entire group of cardiac glycosides, as is the case in some paragraphs that follow.

B. PHARMACOKINETICS

1. The most important property of digitalis and the other cardiac glycosides is their ability to increase the force of myocardial contraction (positive inotropic effect).
2. Cardiac glycosides also have effects on the electrophysiologic properties of the heart (conductivity, refractory period, automaticity).
3. In addition, glycosides have extracardiac effects on vascular smooth muscle, neural tissue, and other tissues.
4. Consideration of the effects of cardiac glycosides on the heart must include:
   a. The dose of the agent (therapeutic to toxic).
   b. The interaction of direct effects with reflex alterations in the autonomic and hormonal regulation of cardiovascular function.
   c. The underlying pathophysiology of the cardiovascular system prior to administration of the glycoside.

C. EFFECTS OF DIGITALIS GLYCOSIDES ON THE HEART.
A summary of the effects of cardiac glycosides on the heart is shown in Table 5-1.

1. **Myocardial contractility**
   a. Cardiac glycosides increase the contractility of cardiac muscle both by increasing the rate at which cardiac muscle tension is developed and by increasing the maximum force that is developed.
   b. In patients with congestive heart failure (CHF) a shift in the ventricular function curve with digitalis (and other glycosides) leads to an increase in cardiac output, a decrease in cardiac filling pressures, and decreases in heart size and venous and capillary pressures.

Table 5-1. Effects of Cardiac Glycosides on the Heart

	Atria	A–V Node	Ventricles
Direct effects	Contractility↑ ERP↑ Conduction velocity↓	ERP↑ Conduction velocity↓	Contractility ↑ ERP↓ Automaticity↑
Indirect effects	ERP↓ Conduction velocity↑	ERP↑ Conduction velocity↓	No effect
Effects on electrocardiogram	P changes	P–R interval↑	Q–T ; ↓ T and S–T depressed
Adverse effects	Extrasystole Tachycardia	A–V depression or block	Fibrillation Extrasystole Tachycardia

Note.—ERP = Effective refractory period. Arrows indicate changes: ↑ = increased; ↓ = decreased.

c. The **mechanism** by which cardiac glycosides exert their positive inotropic effect is unclear.

(1) Apparently digitalis does not affect myocardial contractile proteins or alter cellular mechanisms that provide chemical energy for contraction.

(2) At present, the most probable mechanism underlying the positive inotropic effect appears to be the ability of digitalis to inhibit the membrane-bound $Na^+ - K^+$-activated adenosine triphosphate (Na^+-K^+-ATPase). Inhibition of this enzyme results in intracellular accumulation of Na^+ (and loss of intracellular K^+).

(3) Theories relating this membrane phenomenon to myocardial contractility indicate a prominent role for the translocation of cellular Ca^{2+}:

(a) Accumulation of intracellular Na^+ results in slight movement of extracellular Ca^{2+} into the cell secondary to activation of a membrane Na^+–Ca^{2+} carrier.

(b) Displacement of membrane-bound Ca^{2+} by elevated intracellular Na^+ enhances the amount of free intracellular Ca^{2+} available.

(c) Digitalis may interfere with the ability of the sarcoplasmic reticulum to bind Ca^{2+}, thus making more Ca^{2+} available for interaction with contractile proteins.

2. **Electrical activity**

a. The electrophysiologic effects of cardiac glycosides vary in different parts of the heart.

b. Digitalis glycosides increase the vagal tone of the heart (indirect effects). They prolong the refractory period of the A–V node and decrease conduction velocity (direct and indirect effects) through the A–V node.

3. **Heart rate.** Digitalis tends to slow the heart rate (a negative chronotropic effect) in patients with congestive heart failure. The change in rate results from a decrease in sympathetic activity brought about by increased cardiac output. Tachycardia is seen with excessive doses of digitalis (see II H 5). In normal individuals, digitalis has little effect on the heart rate.

D. EXTRACARDIAC EFFECTS

1. When digitalis and its glycosides increase the cardiac output in patients who have congestive heart failure, a reduction in peripheral vascular resistance and venomotor tone occurs, as well as an increase in blood flow. (In normal individuals, however, digitalis produces venous and arterial constriction.)

2. Because digitalis increases the stroke volume in patients with congestive heart failure, systolic blood pressure may rise.

3. Diastolic pressure may fall because of improved circulation, increased tissue oxygenation, and diminished reflex vasoconstriction.

4. A diuretic effect occurs with digitalis administration because of improved myocardial contractility and decreased sympathetic activity, which result in increased renal blood flow and thus promote the excretion of salt and water.

E. THERAPEUTIC USES

1. Cardiac glycosides are of greatest value for treating **low-output cardiac failure**.

2. They are also of great value in the control of **atrial fibrillation and flutter** because of their ability to reduce the ventricular rate by prolonging the refractory period of conduction tissue. Digitalis may convert atrial flutter to atrial fibrillation.
3. **Paroxysmal atrial tachycardia** frequently responds to digitalis therapy, presumably as a result of reflex vagal stimulation.

F. PHARMACOKINETICS. A comparison of the salient features of the pharmacokinetics of the more commonly used cardiac glycosides is shown in Table 5-2.

1. **Digoxin** is the most commonly used digitalis glycoside.
   a. There is a wide variation in the bioavailability of different proprietary preparations of digoxin, and intestinal absorption of the drug may be as low as 40 percent.
   b. The serum half-life is normally about 34 hours but is significantly prolonged by impaired renal function.
   c. Digoxin is not metabolized, and it is eliminated principally by the kidneys in almost unchanged form.
2. **Digitoxin**
   a. Digitoxin is well absorbed from the gastrointestinal tract and does not have the problem of variable bioavailability seen with digoxin.
   b. The serum half-life of digitoxin is 5 to 7 days.
   c. Digitoxin is metabolized by the liver, and drugs that increase the activity of hepatic microsomal enzymes, such as phenobarbital and phenytoin, accelerate its metabolism.
   d. In contrast to digoxin, digitoxin is about 95 percent bound to plasma albumin.

G. DIGITALIZATION AND MAINTENANCE DOSAGE

1. Since digitalis glycosides are used almost exclusively either to restore adequate circulation in patients with CHF or to slow ventricular rate in patients with actual fibrillation or flutter, long-term therapy is frequently necessary to maintain therapeutic myocardial concentrations. The low margin of safety (see II, H below) increases the critical nature of dosage and administration.
2. **Digoxin**
   a. If there is no urgent need for a desired effect, an oral **digitalizing dose** is first administered, and then the maintenance dose is adjusted on the basis of clinical and laboratory assessment. Usually, a steady-state level is achieved in five half-lives (about 8 days).
   b. When digitalization must be achieved rapidly, digoxin can be administered intravenously over a period of several minutes. The maximal effect of an intravenous dose is reached in 1 to 5 hours after administration.
3. **Digitoxin**
   a. The total oral loading dose of digitoxin is divided into doses given every 6 hours and administered over the course of 36 to 48 hours.
   b. The maximum effect of a dose of digitoxin is reached approximately 9 hours after oral administration.
   c. Once optimal benefit has been achieved, the maintenance dose usually is adjusted to 10 percent of the digitalizing dose.
   d. Although digitoxin is available for intravenous administration, its long latency period precludes its use in emergency situations.

H. UNTOWARD EFFECTS

1. Digitalis glycosides have a low margin of safety, and intoxication due to an excess of the drug is a common and potentially fatal problem. In most patients with heart failure, the lethal dose of a digitalis glycoside is likely to be only five to ten times the minimal effective dose.

Table 5-2. Pharmacokinetics of Commonly Used Cardiac Glycoside Preparations

Drug	GI Absorption	Protein Binding	$T_{1/2}$	Principal Metabolic Route	Serum Concentration (ng/ml)
Digoxin	Approx. 70%	<30%	36 hr	Kidney	Therapeutic: 0.5–2.5 Toxic: >2
Digitoxin	90%–100%	97%	5–7 days	Liver	Therapeutic: 20–35 toxic: >45

2. The therapeutic:toxic ratio does not vary from one glycoside to another, and the only difference among the drugs lies in the *duration* of toxicity.

3. Intoxication is most frequently precipitated by depletion of potassium stores due to diuretic administration, but it also can occur as a result of the accumulation of maintenance glycoside doses taken over a long period of time.
   a. Hypokalemia leading to digitalis intoxication also may occur as a consequence of
      (1) Prolonged administration of corticosteroids.
      (2) Protracted vomiting.
      (3) Protracted diarrhea.
   b. Decreased renal function and hypothyroidism predispose to digitalis toxicity because they result in excessive accumulation of the glycoside.

4. When the concentrations of digoxin and digitoxin rise above 2 ng/ml and 35 ng/ml of blood, respectively, signs of systemic toxicity often appear, and therapy must be discontinued.

5. **Signs of toxicity** include:
   a. Anorexia (often the earliest sign).
   b. Nausea and vomiting.
   c. Headache, fatigue, malaise, neuralgias, and delirium.
   d. Vision changes, including abnormal color perception.
   e. Gynecomastia (rare).
   f. **Cardiac effects:**
      (1) Premature ventricular beats and ventricular tachycardia and fibrillation.
      (2) A–V dissociation and block.
      (3) Sinus arrhythmia and sinoatrial block.
      (4) Paroxysmal and nonparoxysmal atrial tachycardia, often with A–V block.

I. TREATMENT OF UNTOWARD EFFECTS

1. Digitalis and potassium-depleting diuretics are discontinued.

2. Potassium chloride is administered orally or by slow, careful intravenous infusion if hypokalemia is present; potassium is *not* given, however, if severe A–V block is found or if serum K^+ levels are high.

3. Because hypomagnesemia may accompany hypokalemia, magnesium replacement may be necessary.

4. Phenytoin can be given for ventricular and atrial arrhythmias.

5. Lidocaine also can be used to treat ventricular tachyarrhythmias.

6. Propranolol can be used for ventricular and supraventricular tachycardia, but *not* in the presence of A–V block.

7. Atropine can be used to control sinus bradycardia and various degrees of A–V block.

8. Cholestyramine binds to cardiac glycosides and has been used experimentally to hasten their elimination.

9. Purified digoxin-specific antibody fragments have been used recently to reverse advanced life-threatening digitalis intoxication.

10. Electrical conversion often is hazardous in the treatment of digitalis-induced arrhythmias because it can precipitate ventricular fibrillation.

III. ANTIARRHYTHMIC DRUGS

A. GENERAL CONSIDERATIONS

1. **Cardiac arrhythmias**
   a. Cardiac arrhythmias are abnormalities in the rate, regularity, or site of origin of the cardiac impulse, or a disturbance in conduction of the impulse such that the normal sequence of activation of atria and ventricles is altered.
   b. Arrhythmias may be due to
      (1) Faulty impulse initiation.
      (2) Faulty impulse conduction.
      (3) Combinations of the above.
   c. The change in the impulse upsets the normal relationship which exists between the duration of the refractory period and the conduction velocity in myocardial tissue. Changes in the normal relationship between refractoriness and conduction velocity may be critical,

considering the heterogeneity of electrophysiologic and mechanical properties of the heart.

2. **Automaticity**
   a. Automaticity is the ability of a cardiac cell to spontaneously reach threshold potential and generate impulses.
   b. In the cardiac cells, the resting potential depolarizes during phase 4 until a threshold potential is reached and an action potential is initiated.
   c. In man, the sinoatrial node is the normal pacemaker since it has the steepest slope of phase 4 and the most rapid firing rate. However, specialized atrial conduction fibers, distal cells of the A–V node, and His–Purkinje fibers are latent pacemakers.
   d. Abnormalities in cardiac rhythms arise from alterations in the site of normal automaticity and abnormal generation of impulses.
   e. Most antiarrhythmic agents depress the automaticity (i.e., decrease the rate of phase 4 depolarization) of latent pacemakers more effectively than of the sinoatrial node.
   f. Inhibition of automaticity may also be due to a decreased threshold potential or decreased excitability of pacemaker cells.

3. **Conduction velocity**
   a. Conduction velocity is the speed at which a stimulus of an action potential is propagated.
   b. It is a function of
      (1) The maximum rate of depolarization of phase 0.
      (2) The threshold potential.
      (3) The resting membrane potential.
   c. Depolarization of the membrane is associated with a decrease in conduction velocity.
   d. The **effective refractory period** (ERP) is the period of repolarization during which no normal action potential can be elicited. Shortening of the ERP during tachycardia may produce arrhythmia, and an effective antiarrhythmic mechanism may be a prolongation of the action potential duration.
   e. Disturbances in cardiac conductance may underlie supraventricular or ventricular arrhythmias.
   f. In areas of injured myocardium, conduction may be slow and/or refractoriness shortened, resulting in the **reentry** of aberrant impulses and hence a cardiac arrhythmia.

B. QUINIDINE

1. **Chemistry**. Quinidine, an alkaloid isolated from cinchona bark, is the *d* isomer of quinine.

2. **Pharmacokinetics**
   a. Quinidine is well absorbed after oral administration. It exerts a maximum effect within 1 to 2 hours after administration by this route.
   b. Quinidine is rarely given intramuscularly since it may cause local pain and its absorption is inconsistent.
   c. Approximately 80 percent of the drug is bound to plasma albumin.

3. **Actions on the heart**. At high concentrations, quinidine has direct effects on most cells of the heart. At lower concentrations, indirect (anticholinergic) effects may significantly contribute to the overall action of quinidine on the heart (see Table 5-3).
   a. **Responsiveness, conduction, and refractoriness**. The major effect of quinidine is to reduce the maximal rate of rise ($\dot{V}_{max}$) of depolarization during phase 0 at all transmembrane voltages in atrial, ventricular, and Purkinje fibers. Thus, conduction velocity decreases and ERP increases in all of these tissues.
   b. Automaticity is decreased in ventricular tissue by depression of the slope of phase 4. Quinidine has little effect on automaticity of the sinus node.

4. **Electrocardiographic effects** (see Table 5-4)
   a. Because quinidine depresses conduction in the bundle of His and Purkinje fibers, it produces progressive prolongation of the QRS complex.
   b. Prolongation of the Q–T interval and alterations in T waves are related to delayed repolarization.
   c. Prolongation of the P–R interval is caused by the direct effect of the drug on A–V conduction and the refractoriness of the A–V system.

5. **Extracardiac effects.** Quinidine can depress vascular smooth muscle tone, in part by α-receptor blockade. This may contribute to a reduction in peripheral vascular resistance.

6. **Therapeutic uses** (see Table 5-5)
   a. **Supraventricular arrhythmias**
      (1) Quinidine is primarily used chronically and prophylactically to prevent recurrences of

Table 5-3. Effects of Antiarrhythmic Drugs on Electrophysiologic Properties of the Heart

Drug	Automaticity: Sinus Node	Automaticity: Purkinje Fibers	Effective Refractory Period: A–V Node	Effective Refractory Period: Purkinje Fibers	Membrane Responsiveness (Purkinje Fibers)
Quinidine, Procainamide, Disopyramide	→	↓	↑→↓	↓	↓
Lidocaine, Phenytoin	→	↓	↑→↓	↓	↓
Propranolol	↓	↓	↑	↑	↓

Note.—Arrows indicate changes: ↑ = increased; ↓ = decreased; → = no change.

paroxysmal supraventricular tachycardia due to A–V nodal reciprocating tachycardia or to Wolff-Parkinson-White syndrome.

(2) Quinidine can also be used to convert atrial flutter or fibrillation to normal sinus rhythm, but direct-current cardioversion is now the procedure of choice for this problem, and quinidine is now more frequently used to prevent recurrence of this arrhythmia.

b. Ventricular arrhythmia. Quinidine is very useful for long-term treatment of ventricular premature depolarization or to prevent recurrences of ventricular tachycardia after cardioversion of this arrhythmia.

7. Route of administration

a. Quinidine is usually given orally three or four times a day.

b. For intravenous use, the dose must be diluted in glucose solution and injected slowly, and the patient's electrocardiogram must be carefully monitored.

8. Untoward effects

a. Cardiotoxicity includes A–V block, ventricular tachyarrhythmias, and depression of myocardial contractility.

(1) A 50 percent increase in the QRS complex indicates the need for a prompt reduction in dosage.

(2) Ventricular arrhythmias are life-threatening, and if the therapist can distinguish this adverse effect of quinidine from the underlying disease, treatment (besides cessation of quinidine) may be either of the following:

(a) Sodium lactate or sodium bicarbonate, catecholamines (see Chapter 2, II A 7 a (4) and II B 3), or glucagon.

(b) Removal of quinidine by dialysis.

b. Diarrhea, vomiting, nausea, and anorexia are the most common side effects and, when severe, may force discontinuation of quinidine.

Table 5-4. Major Effects of Antiarrhythmic Drugs on Electrocardiogram

Drug	QRS	Q–T	P–R
Quinidine, Procainamide	↑	↑	→↑
Disopyramide	↑	↑	=
Lidocaine, Phenytoin	→	↓	→↑↓*
Propranolol	→	↓	→↑*

Note.—Arrows indicate changes: ↑ = increased; ↓ = decreased; → = no change.

*P–R intervals: All antiarrhythmias have a variable response, usually with little observable effect. However, lidocaine hardly ever affects the P–R interval, while phenytoin and propranolol usually increase the P–R interval.

Table 5-5. Therapeutic Usefulness of Antiarrhythmic Drugs in Treatment of Common Cardiac Arrhythmias

Arrhythmia	Treatment of Choice	Alternatives
I. Supraventricular		
Atrial fibrillation or flutter	Digitalis to control ventricular rate, DC shock for conversion	Quinidine to suppress recurrences after DC shock
Paroxysmal atrial or nodal tachycardia	Vagotonic maneuver; digitalis	Quinidine, procainamide, disopyramide, and propranolol may all be useful, especially prophylactically
II. Ventricular		
Ventricular premature depolarization	Lidocaine	Procainamide, quinidine, or disopyramide for prolonged suppression
Ventricular tachycardia	DC shock	Lidocaine or procainamide
III. Digitalis-induced	Lidocaine or phenytoin	Procainamide is somewhat useful; propranolol is useful but has high incidence of adverse effects

c. Quinidine can cause cinchonism. Mild symptoms of this condition include tinnitus, hearing loss, vomiting, and diarrhea; severe symptoms include headache, diplopia, photophobia, altered perception of color, confusion, and psychosis.

d. Sensitivity phenomena, including thrombocytopenia, can occur.

e. Quinidine, especially when administered intravenously, can cause hypotension because of a decrease in arteriolar resistance. When arterial pressure declines by 20 mm Hg or more, the drug should be stopped.

C. PROCAINAMIDE

1. Chemistry. Procainamide differs from procaine only in that it contains an amide structure rather than an ester linkage; this difference protects it from enzymatic hydrolysis and frees it from most of the central nervous system effects of procaine.

2. Pharmacokinetics

a. Procainamide may be administered orally, intravenously, or intramuscularly.

b. It is rapidly absorbed after oral administration and, when capsules are used, normally has a peak effect in about 1 hour. However, absorption of the drug from the gastrointestinal tract may be impaired immediately after an acute myocardial infarction.

c. The half-life of procainamide is approximately 3 hours.

d. Approximately 15 percent of the drug is bound to plasma proteins.

e. Procainamide is eliminated by both hepatic metabolism and renal excretion, and renal failure can produce toxicity.

(1) There is a rather marked variation among individuals in the rate of acetylation and excretion.

(2) From 50 to 60 percent of an administered dose is excreted unchanged in the urine.

3. Actions on the heart (see Table 5-3)

a. The direct cardiac effects of procainamide are quite similar to those of quinidine.

b. Procainamide decreases automaticity and lengthens the duration of the action potential and the refractory period in the atria and ventricles.

c. It slows conduction in the atrium, A–V node, and ventricle.

4. **Electrocardiographic effects** are also very similar to those of quinidine (see Table 5-4).
   a. Prolongation of the QRS complex is the most consistent finding.
   b. At high doses, prolongation of the P–R interval or heart block may appear.

5. **Extracardiac effects**
   a. Procainamide, especially when given intravenously, can cause a drop in blood pressure, probably from peripheral vasodilation.
   b. Unlike quinidine, procainamide does not have α-adrenergic blocking properties.

6. **Therapeutic uses** (see Table 5-5)
   a. The clinical uses of procainamide are similar to those of quinidine. However, patients may respond to one drug after failing to respond to the other.
   b. **Ventricular arrhythmias.** Procainamide is particularly effective in promptly abolishing ventricular premature depolarizations and paroxysmal ventricular tachycardia.
   c. **Supraventricular arrhythmia.** Procainamide is now believed to be as effective as quinidine for the treatment of atrial arrhythmias; however, higher doses of procainamide than of quinidine may be necessary.

7. **Route of administration**
   a. Procainamide may be given orally, both initially and for maintenance.
   b. The intravenous dose, which is reserved for life-threatening situations, must be administered slowly. When the arrhythmia has been interrupted, infusion is stopped.

8. **Untoward effects**
   a. Acute procainamide toxicity can cause ventricular arrhythmia, ventricular fibrillation, and cardiac depression (see III B 8 a, above).
   b. Nausea, vomiting, diarrhea, and anorexia fairly frequently result from oral administration of procainamide, but they occur much less commonly than with quinidine therapy.
   c. Mental confusion and psychosis have been reported but occur less commonly than with the chemically similar compounds procaine and lidocaine.
   d. Hypersensitivity reactions are much more common than with quinidine.
      (1) Fever, joint and muscle pain, and skin rashes can occur.
      (2) Fatal agranulocytosis has occurred.
      (3) A systemic lupus erythematosus–like syndrome, which is reversible on discontinuation of procainamide, develops in as many as 30 percent of patients taking procainamide for long periods of time. As many as 70 percent of patients taking procainamide develop positive antinuclear antibody tests.
   e. Hypotension can result, especially following intravenous administration.

D. DISOPYRAMIDE

1. **Pharmacokinetics**
   a. Disopyramide is well absorbed (83 percent) following oral administration.
   b. The free plasma concentration is a nonlinear function of the total amount of drug in the plasma. It varies from 5 to 75 percent as the total increases from 0.1 to 8 μg/ml.
   c. Approximately 50 percent of a dose of disopyramide is excreted in the urine in unchanged form. Disappearance from the plasma is a function of both renal and hepatic clearance.
   d. The half-life of disopyramide in plasma is 5 to 7 hours but may be prolonged in patients with renal disease.

2. **Actions on the heart** (see Table 5-3). Disopyramide has both direct and indirect actions on the heart which resemble those of quinidine.
   a. **Responsiveness, conduction, and refractoriness**
      (1) Disopyramide reduces membrane responsiveness, amplitude of the action potential, and excitability of atrial and ventricular muscle.
      (2) Accordingly, conduction velocity is decreased and ERP is increased in these tissues.
      (3) Unlike either quinidine or procainamide, disopyramide produces a greater reduction in the maximum rate ($\dot{V}_{max}$) of phase 0 depolarization at depressed membrane potentials than at normal resting membrane potentials.
   b. **Automaticity**. Concentrations of disopyramide which do not affect conduction velocity or ERP can reduce automaticity in atrial and ventricular tissue.

3. **Electrocardiographic changes** are similar to but milder than those of quinidine and procainamide (see Table 5-4).

4. **Extracardiac effects**. Disopyramide has a mild atropine-like action. It is neither an α- nor a β-receptor antagonist.

5. **Therapeutic uses** (see Table 5-5)
   a. Disopyramide is approved in the United States for treatment of ventricular arrhythmias as an alternative to quinidine and procainamide.
   b. It may be as effective as quinidine and procainamide against supraventricular arrhythmias, but it has not been approved for this use.
   c. Disopyramide is approved only for oral administration in the United States.

6. **Untoward effects**
   a. Major untoward effects are related to the action of disopyramide on the heart and may include conduction disturbances, congestive heart failure, or hypotension. Disopyramide has a negative inotropic action that can be especially troublesome in patients with preexisting ventricular failure.
   b. Other adverse effects relate to its anticholinergic action. These effects include dry mouth, constipation, blurred vision, and urinary retention. Consequently, patients with glaucoma or with conditions causing urinary retention should not take the drug.

E. LIDOCAINE

1. **Chemistry**. Lidocaine is an amide local anesthetic (see Chapter 4, II C 4).

2. **Pharmacokinetics**
   a. Lidocaine is rapidly metabolized by the hepatic microsomal enzyme system, with 70 percent of the amount that enters the liver being metabolized in a single pass. Reductions in hepatic blood flow or function will reduce lidocaine plasma clearance.
   b. Oral administration of lidocaine results in a very low plasma concentration because of the high percentage of the drug that is removed by hepatic metabolism before reaching the general circulation.
   c. Lidocaine has an elimination half-time of approximately 1½ hours.
   d. Approximately 70 percent of the drug is bound to plasma albumin.

3. **Actions on the heart** (see Table 5-3)
   a. **Automaticity**. Lidocaine does *not* affect sinus nodal pacemaker discharge. It will depress the rate of phase 4 depolarization of Purkinje and atrial muscle fibers and thus depress automaticity at these sites.
   b. **Responsiveness, conduction, and refractoriness**
      (1) Lidocaine has very little effect on these electrophysiologic properties of the atria.
      (2) In the His–Purkinje system, lidocaine reduces action potential amplitude and membrane responsiveness.
      (3) The $\dot{V}_{max}$ of phase 0 depolarization in normal Purkinje fibers is not as greatly depressed with lidocaine as it is with procainamide or quinidine. However, the $\dot{V}_{max0}$ is severely depressed in fibers with reduced resting membrane potentials and elevated extracellular K^+.
      (4) Lidocaine decreases the duration of the action potential and shortens the ERP of Purkinje fibers.

4. **Electrocardiographic effects**. Unlike quinidine and procainamide, lidocaine produces very few changes in electrocardiograms (see Table 5-4).

5. **Extracardiac effects**. Lidocaine has little effect on autonomic tone.

6. **Therapeutic uses** (see Table 5-5). The use of lidocaine as an antiarrhythmic agent is limited, even though lidocaine is very effective in treating ventricular arrhythmias. Because of its rapid onset and short duration of action, the drug is particularly useful in treating these arrhythmias when they arise in emergency situations, such as:
   a. Open-heart surgery.
   b. Digitalis intoxication.
   c. Myocardial infarction.

7. **Route of administration**. Lidocaine hydrochloride (Xylocaine) can be administered intravenously or intramuscularly.
   a. The usual intravenous dose is given until the arrhythmia is abolished.
   b. Lidocaine also can be given by continuous intravenous infusion. Because its half-life is short, a steady-state plasma concentration can be reached quickly by this method.
   c. Lidocaine may be given intramuscularly to achieve rapid plasma levels during emergencies.

8. **Untoward effects**
   a. Central nervous system side effects of lidocaine can include drowsiness, paresthesias, decreased auditory function, convulsions, and respiratory arrest.

b. Circulatory collapse can occur in patients with an acute myocardial infarction after a rapid, large intravenous injection.

F. **PHENYTOIN** (diphenylhydantoin) is closely related in structure to phenobarbital and is effective in treating epileptic seizures (see Chapter 3, III C). As an antiarrhythmic agent, phenytoin resembles lidocaine in many respects.

1. **Pharmacokinetics**
   a. Phenytoin is slowly and somewhat variably absorbed following oral administration.
   b. It is inactivated by microsomal enzymes in the liver, with considerable variability in this process among individuals.
   c. The plasma half-time for elimination is prolonged with increasing doses and is about 17 hours for a single 300-mg dose.
   d. Approximately 90 percent of a dose of phenytoin is bound to plasma proteins.

2. **Actions on the heart** (see Table 5-3). The prominent effects of phenytoin on the heart are very similar to the effects of lidocaine.

3. The **electrocardiographic effects** of phenytoin, like those of lidocaine, are minimal (see Table 5-4).

4. **Extracardiac effects**. Phenytoin exerts a depressant action on the sympathetic centers in the central nervous system that may contribute to its antiarrhythmic effects.

5. **Therapeutic uses** (see Table 5-5). Phenytoin is most useful in treating ventricular arrhythmias. It is particularly useful for ventricular arrhythmias associated with digitalis toxicity or acute myocardial infarction.

6. **Route of administration**
   a. Phenytoin is most frequently administered by intermittent intravenous injection, until either a therapeutic effect is achieved or a toxic effect results.
   b. Orally, therapy is initiated with a loading dose, followed by maintenance oral therapy.

7. **Untoward effects**
   a. Central nervous system side effects are the most common problems encountered and include nystagmus, vertigo, and loss of mental acuity.
   b. Large intravenous doses can alter hemodynamic function and produce both a fall in cardiac output and hypotension.

G. **PROPRANOLOL** is a β-adrenergic receptor blocking agent and is discussed in this context in Chapter 2, III B 1. Its antiarrhythmic action is featured here, while its uses in treating angina and hypertension are discussed later in this chapter.

1. **Pharmacokinetics** (see Chapter 2, III B 1 b)

2. **Actions on the heart.** The antiarrhythmic effects of propranolol are due primarily to β-receptor blockade but also result from a direct membrane effect (see Table 5-3).
   a. **Automaticity**. Propranolol, by blocking β-receptors in the sinoatrial node and blocking sympathetic and hormonal influences on this structure, depresses sinoatrial node firing and causes bradycardia. Automaticity is also depressed in Purkinje fibers.
   b. **Responsiveness and conduction velocity** are not greatly affected by propranolol.
   c. **Duration of action potential and refractoriness**. The major effect of propranolol which underlies its use as an antiarrhythmic agent is that it causes a substantial increase in the ERP of the A–V node due to β-blockade. The refractoriness of the sinoatrial node and of atrial and ventricular muscle is not greatly affected, whereas the ERP of Purkinje fibers is shortened substantially.
   d. Hemodynamic effects are discussed in Chapter 2, III B 1.

3. **Electrocardiographic effects**. Propranolol prolongs the P–R interval by its action on the A–V node (see Table 5-4)

4. **Therapeutic antiarrhythmic uses** (see Table 5-5)
   a. Propranolol is used to control supraventricular tachyarrhythmias, including atrial fibrillation, atrial flutter, and paroxysmal supraventricular tachycardia. By decreasing conduction through the A–V node, propranolol decreases the response of the ventricles to atrial flutter and fibrillation but does *not* usually convert these arrhythmias to sinus rhythm.
   b. Propranolol is useful in ventricular arrhythmias that are due to enhanced adrenergic stimulation (from emotional stress, exercise).
   c. Propranolol is sometimes used to abolish ventricular arrhythmias caused by digitalis excess, but it can cause conduction problems in this context, resulting in A–V dissociation. Furthermore, propranolol, by itself, can depress myocardial contractility.

5. **Route of administration**
   a. For intravenous administration, propranolol hydrochloride is given slowly, with additional doses usually given every 3 to 5 minutes.
   b. Oral medication usually is begun with relatively small divided doses. The total amount may need to be increased significantly to produce a therapeutic effect.

6. **Untoward effects**
   a. Because propranolol decreases sympathetic activity, it can produce severe hypotension, significantly worsen congestive heart failure, and cause cardiac arrest.
   b. Because it impairs A–V conduction and depresses ventricular pacemaker activity, propranolol can produce asystole.
   c. Propranolol can induce significant bronchospasm in asthmatic patients and can mask signs and symptoms of acute hypoglycemia.
   d. Sudden withdrawal of the drug can produce angina, arrhythmias, and infarction.

H. BRETYLIUM

1. **Mechanism of action**
   a. Bretylium, a quaternary ammonium salt, is an adrengeric neuronal blocking agent (see Chapter 2, III C 3). It accumulates in postganglionic adrenergic nerve terminals, where it initially stimulates norepinephrine release but then inhibits the release of norepinephrine in response to neuronal stimulation. Bretylium does not impair the postsynaptic response to exogenous catecholamines.
   b. The drug also has direct electrophysiologic effects on the heart.

2. **Pharmacokinetics**
   a. Oral absorption of bretylium is poor; however, it is well absorbed after intramuscular administration.
   b. The drug is excreted unchanged in the urine.
   c. Its elimination half-time is approximately 6 to 10 hours.

3. **Actions on the heart**
   a. **Automaticity.** Bretylium does not directly affect automaticity. It is the only antiarrhythmic agent discussed here which does not affect automaticity in His–Purkinje systems.
   b. **Excitability and threshold.** Resting membrane potentials are not greatly affected in any cardiac cell. However, bretylium increases the ventricular fibrillation threshold.
   c. **Responsiveness, conduction, and refractoriness.** In therapeutic doses bretylium does not affect either responsiveness or conduction in cardiac tissue. Bretylium prolongs the duration of action potentials and the ERP of atrial and ventricular muscle and the A–V node.

4. **Electrocardiographic effects.** Bretylium decreases the sinus rate and increases the P–R and Q–T intervals.

5. **Therapeutic uses.** Bretylium is reserved for life-threatening ventricular arrhythmias that are refractory to other therapy. Its use is confined to intensive care units.

6. **Route of administration**
   a. Bretylium tosylate is for short-term use only, and is administered with patients in the supine position.
   b. For **intravenous use,** the drug usually is diluted and infused over 10 to 20 minutes.
   c. For immediately life-threatening arrhythmias, undiluted bretylium can be injected intravenously every 15 to 30 minutes.
   d. For **intramuscular use,** undiluted bretylium is used.

7. **Untoward effects**
   a. Intravenous bretylium causes orthostatic hypotension and some degree of supine hypotension.
   b. Nausea and vomiting can occur with rapid intravenous administration.

IV. ANTIANGINAL AGENTS AND OTHER VASODILATORS.

The nitrates, the β-adrenergic antagonists, and the new calcium antagonists are drugs that are useful in treating the pain resulting from ischemic heart disease. They provide symptomatic treatment of angina pectoris but do not affect the course of the disorder. Several vasodilators that have not proved useful in the treatment of angina are also briefly discussed in this section.

A. NITRATES

1. **Chemistry**
   a. The term **nitrates** will be used in this chapter to encompass both **nitrites** (esters of nitrous acid) and **nitrates** (polyol esters of nitric acid).

b. Glyceryl trinitrate **(nitroglycerin)** is the prototype of this group.
c. Nitroglycerin and amyl nitrite are volatile liquids at room temperature. Other nitrates (isosorbide dinitrate, pentaerythritol tetranitrate, erythrityl tetranitrate) are solids.

2. Mechanism of action and effects on the heart

a. The nitrates relax all smooth muscle, including vascular smooth muscle.
b. They reduce venous tone, thereby increasing venous capacitance and decreasing venous return to the heart.
c. They decrease peripheral arteriolar resistance.
d. The major effect of the nitrates on the heart is to reduce myocardial oxygen requirements relative to myocardial oxygen delivery.

(1) The arterial dilation produced by nitrates causes a reduction in the mean systemic arterial pressure, which reduces the afterload of the heart and thus diminishes the oxygen requirements of the heart.
(2) The venous dilation produced by nitrates results in increased peripheral pooling of blood (decreased preload), which decreases ventricular end-diastolic pressure and volume. This reduction in ventricular pressure and size results in a decreased myocardial wall tension and, therefore, in decreased oxygen requirements.
(3) In addition, the decrease in left ventricular end-diastolic pressure (LVEDP) reduces tissue pressure around subendocardial vessels, favoring the redistribution of coronary blood flow to this area.

e. Nitrates are believed to dilate the large epicardial and collateral coronary arteries selectively, an action that favors the distribution of blood to ischemic areas. (They do *not* increase the total coronary blood flow in patients with atherosclerosis.)

3. Extracardiac effects

a. Vasodilation of cerebral vessels produced by nitrates results in increased intracerebral pressure and sometimes in headache.
b. The nitrates dilate vessels in the skin, resulting in flushing.
c. They relax bronchial and biliary tract smooth muscle, with the latter action resulting in a reduction of biliary pressure.

4. Therapeutic uses

a. The primary therapeutic use of nitrates is to treat attacks of angina pectoris and, in anticipation of attacks, to prevent their occurrence.
b. Paroxysmal nocturnal dyspnea can be relieved with nitroglycerin by improving left ventricular pressure and reducing pulmonary pressure.

5. Pharmacokinetics

a. The nitrates can be absorbed through the mucous membranes and the skin, and from the gastrointestinal tract and the lungs.

(1) Sublingual administration produces rapid onset (2 to 5 minutes) and short duration of action (less than 30 minutes) and thus provides the best treatment for acute attacks of angina.
(2) Oral preparations, which often come in a sustained-release form, can provide more prolonged prophylaxis against angina than sublingual forms.

b. The nitrates are broken down in the liver by a glutathione-dependent organic nitrate reductase and are excreted in the form of various nitrites and nitrates.

6. Route of administration

a. Nitroglycerin (glyceryl trinitrate) is usually given sublingually. However, for longer-lasting effects, nitroglycerin may be administered either orally or topically (transdermally) via ointment or patch.
b. Nitroglycerin may also be given intravenously in medical emergencies.
c. Nitroglycerin tablets quickly lose potency when stored in contact with cotton, paper, or plastic and should be kept in a dark glass container.

7. Tolerance. When nitrates are appropriately administered intermittently, tolerance does not occur.

8. Untoward effects

a. Headache is a common early side effect of nitrates that usually decreases after the first few days of treatment (i.e., patients usually develop a tolerance to headache).

(1) Temporarily discontinuing the drugs for a few days causes a recurrence of susceptibility to headache (as well as to the direct vascular effect of the drugs) when the nitrates are readministered.
(2) Decreasing the dose of nitrates is sometimes beneficial for headache.

b. Dizziness, weakness, and cerebral ischemia associated with postural hypotension occasionally occur.

c. Nitrite ions, when present in large amounts, can oxidize enough hemoglobin to methemoglobin to result in hypoxia.
d. Death can occur with acute nitrate poisoning from circulatory collapse or respiratory failure.

B. PROPRANOLOL

1. Mechanism of action
a. The β-adrenergic blocking action of propranolol (see Chapter 2, III B 1) decreases sympathetic stimulation of the heart and thus reduces the heart rate, especially during exercise, and decreases myocardial contractility. These effects in turn decrease the oxygen requirements of the myocardium, both during exercise and at rest.
b. Propranolol may also decrease arterial pressure.

2. Therapeutic uses
a. Propranolol is used prophylactically to decrease the severity and frequency of anginal attacks.
b. Propranolol can be administered concomitantly with nitroglycerin, in which case it reduces the amount of nitroglycerin needed to control angina.
(1) However, no data conclusively show a synergistic effect of these drugs.
(2) The two drugs do tend to counteract some of each other's "nontherapeutic" effects; for example, the ability of nitroglycerin to reduce ventricular end-diastolic pressure mitigates the tendency of propranolol to increase end-diastolic pressure.
c. Propranolol should *not* be used for Prinzmetal's (variant) angina, which is caused by coronary vasospasm.

3. Untoward effects
a. As noted in III G 6, propranolol can worsen congestive heart failure and can precipitate bronchospasm in patients with bronchial asthma.
b. Bradycardia and hypotension can occur.
c. Renal plasma flow and glomerular filtration rate may be reduced.

4. Route of administration. Propranolol is usually administered orally for the treatment of angina.

C. CALCIUM ANTAGONISTS—VERAPAMIL AND NIFEDIPINE

1. Verapamil and nifedipine belong to a new class of antianginal drugs, the **calcium channel blockers**.
a. These drugs selectively inhibit calcium ion influx into heart muscle (i.e., they block the slow inward channel for Ca^{2+}) or inhibit Ca^{2+} influx into vascular smooth muscle.
b. They do not change the serum calcium concentration.

2. **Mechanism of action and effects on the heart**. By their inhibition of Ca^{2+} influx into myocardial and vascular smooth muscle cells, calcium antagonists have diverse effects on the cardiovascular system.
a. The calcium antagonists dilate the main coronary arteries and coronary arterioles, and, by inhibiting coronary artery spasm, they increase myocardial oxygen delivery in patients with Prinzmetal's angina.
b. The drugs dilate peripheral arterioles and reduce the total peripheral vascular resistance, thereby reducing the oxygen requirements of the myocardium.
c. The more precise mechanisms of action of the calcium antagonists as antianginal agents remains to be determined.
d. Both drugs slow A–V and sinoatrial node conduction and prolong the ERP within the A–V node in isolated heart tissue, but verapamil seems to have a greater effect than nifedipine on these parameters in clinical situations.

2. **Extracardiac actions**. Verapamil (but not nifedipine) produces nonspecific sympathetic antagonism and has a local anesthetic effect.

3. **Therapeutic uses**
a. For both verapamil and nifedipine the major areas of therapeutic benefit appear to be in the treatment of both Prinzmetal's (variant) angina and classic exertional angina.
b. Repeated attacks of ventricular fibrillation, complicating attacks of variant angina, respond to verapamil. The antiarrhythmic action is probably secondary to a reduction of the myocardial ischemia induced by the coronary vasospasm.

4. **Pharmacokinetics**
a. Both drugs are rapidly and almost fully absorbed after oral administration.

b. Peak blood levels of nifedipine occur in about 30 minutes; peak levels of verapamil occur in 1 to 2 hours.

c. Both drugs are highly bound by serum proteins.

d. Verapamil undergoes extensive first-pass biotransformation in the liver. Approximately 70 percent of a dose of verapamil is excreted as metabolites in the urine; approximately 80 percent of nifedipine and its metabolites are excreted in the urine.

5. Route of administration. Calcium antagonists may be given orally; for use in medical emergencies, they are also available in intravenous form.

6. Untoward effects

a. The calcium antagonists, perhaps especially when used in combination with β-adrenergic blocking agents, can produce or aggravate the following:

(1) Hypotension.

(2) A–V block.

(3) Congestive heart failure.

(4) Asystole.

b. Most of their adverse effects are mild; dizziness and peripheral edema are among the more common.

c. Treatment with verapamil increases serum levels of digitalis during the first week of therapy and thus can cause digitalis toxicity.

D. VASODILATORS

1. Nylidrin

a. Nylidrin is an adrenergic vasodilator. It acts primarily on the vascular bed of skeletal muscle by β-receptor stimulation.

b. Because it is a cardiac stimulant, nylidrin is **contraindicated** in progressive angina pectoris, acute myocardial infarction, and paroxysmal tachycardia.

c. The efficacy of nylidrin in increasing the blood supply in vasospastic disorders has not been proven.

2. Papaverine

a. This drug, which is an isoquinoline opium alkaloid, relaxes all smooth muscle structures in vitro. Papaverine relaxes the smooth muscle of large blood vessels and decreases total peripheral resistance in vivo, apparently through an effect on arterioles, but is a much weaker vasodilator than the nitrates. The drug is a potent inhibitor of phosphodiesterase.

b. Papaverine has not convincingly been shown to be of therapeutic value for angina or for any other condition, and when it is given intravenously it can produce a quinidine-like effect that results in sudden death.

3. Dipyridamole

a. By inhibiting the uptake of adenosine into erythrocytes and other tissues, dipyridamole allows metabolically released adenosine, which is a coronary vasodilator, to accumulate in the plasma. The drug decreases coronary vascular resistance and increases coronary blood flow and coronary sinus oxygen saturation. (Dipyridamole also inhibits in vitro platelet aggregation and can be used to prevent the formation of thromboemboli in patients with prosthetic cardiac valves.)

b. Dipyridamole has not been proved to be superior to placebo treatment for angina; it does not prevent the appearance of electrocardiographic signs of myocardial ischemia during exercise tolerance tests.

V. ANTIHYPERTENSIVE AGENTS

A. GENERAL CONSIDERATIONS

1. Because the etiology of essential hypertension is still unknown, drug therapy for this condition is empiric and often rather nonspecific.

2. The classes of drugs most commonly used to treat primary hypertension include diuretic agents, vasodilators, antiadrenergic agents, and renin–angiotensin blockers. These drugs have different sites and mechanisms of action, and thus may potentially be used in combination to affect several aspects of the pathophysiology of hypertension.

3. Clinical usage

a. For **mild hypertension**, initial drug therapy usually consists of either a thiazide diuretic or a β-adrenergic blocking agent (e.g., propranolol—see Chapter 2, III B1). If these drugs when used alone are ineffective or cause troublesome side effects, a combination of the two can be employed, or the diuretic can be administered in combination with methyldopa, clonidine, guanethidine, or reserpine.

b. **Moderate to severe hypertension** is treated similarly to mild hypertension except that single-agent therapy is rarely used and arterial vasodilators often are added to the combination therapy. Simultaneous administration of an appropriate sympathetic blocking drug is usually required to prevent reflex sympathetic responses to the vasodilator (such as tachycardia).

c. In **hypertensive emergencies**, parenteral therapy is indicated, usually with nitroprusside or diazoxide. Oral therapy should be started as soon as possible because parenteral therapy is not suitable for long-term management of hypertension.

B. DIURETIC AGENTS (see Chapter 6) are useful antihypertensive drugs when employed alone, as well as when used in combination therapy, where they potentiate the action of other hypotensive drugs. Although the exact mechanism of their antihypertensive action is unknown, it is believed to result from their ability to produce a negative sodium balance.

1. The **thiazides** are the most frequently used diuretics. Their early hypotensive effect is related to a reduction in blood volume; their long-term effect is related to a reduction in peripheral vascular resistance.

2. **Furosemide** and **ethacrynic acid** produce greater diuresis than the thiazides, but they have a weaker antihypertensive effect and can cause severe electrolyte imbalance. Because they retain their effectiveness in the presence of impaired renal function, they are useful in cases where renal function is so impaired that the thiazides can no longer promote sodium excretion.

3. **Spironolactone** and **triamterene** have modest hypotensive and diuretic effects, and are useful in combination with a thiazide diuretic, whose effects they potentiate and where they minimize potassium loss. Spironolactone is useful in treating patients whose hypertension is due to mineralocorticoid excess (see Chapter 6, IX).

C. ARTERIOLAR VASODILATORS

1. This group of antihypertensive drugs directly relaxes arteriolar smooth muscle and thus decreases peripheral vascular resistance and arterial blood pressure.
   a. However, the beneficial effect of these drugs on peripheral vascular resistance can be partially negated by the increased reflex sympathetic activity they produce, which can result in increased heart rate, stroke volume, and cardiac output.
   b. These drugs also can increase plasma renin activity as a result of increased reflex sympathetic discharge, causing a pressor effect.
   c. Finally, this group of drugs often causes sodium and water retention and thus expansion of the extracellular fluid and plasma volume.

2. **Hydralazine**. This phthalazine derivative has a greater effect on arterioles than on veins (which minimizes the incidence of postural hypotension). It may reduce diastolic more than systolic blood pressure.
   a. **Pharmacokinetics**
      (1) Hydralazine is well absorbed orally.
      (2) It is subject to extensive first-pass hepatic metabolism after oral administration.
      (3) It is extensively metabolized by several pathways, including acetylation, the rate of which is subject to genetic variation among individuals.
      (4) Some 85 percent is bound to plasma.
      (5) Its duration of effect ranges from 2 to 6 hours.
   b. **Therapeutic uses**
      (1) Hydralazine is used to treat moderate to severe hypertension.
      (2) For long-term treatment, it is administered orally, in combination with a β-adrenergic blocking agent and a diuretic agent—the former to prevent tachycardia and increased renin secretion due to reflex sympathetic stimulation, the latter to prevent sodium and water retention.
   c. **Route of administration.** Hydralazine hydrochloride can be given orally or intramuscularly.
   d. **Untoward effects**
      (1) Headache, anorexia, nausea, dizziness, and sweating occur frequently but tend to diminish as hydralazine is administered over a period of time.
      (2) Hydralazine can worsen coronary artery disease because of the myocardial stimulation it produces.
      (3) Hydralazine can cause a reversible lupus-like syndrome, especially when more than 400 mg per day are administered to slow acetylators of the drug (usually Caucasians). 

3. **Minoxidil**
   a. **Pharmacologic properties**
      (1) Minoxidil, a piperidinopyrimidine derivative, directly relaxes arteriolar smooth muscle.
      (2) It decreases peripheral vascular resistance more than hydralazine does.
      (3) It decreases renal vascular resistance while preserving renal blood flow and the glomerular filtration rate.
   b. **Pharmacokinetics**
      (1) Minoxidil is at least 90 percent absorbed following oral administration.
      (2) Approximately 90 percent of the drug is excreted as metabolites in the urine.
      (3) Although the plasma half-life averages around 4 hours, the duration of action may be significantly longer, since it is affected by hepatic blood flow and function.
   c. **Therapeutic uses**
      (1) Minoxidil is indicated for the treatment of severe hypertension that does not respond adequately to more conventional antihypertensive therapy.
      (2) It may be particularly useful for severe hypertension coupled with renal functional impairment.
      (3) Like hydralazine, minoxidil should be used in combination with a β-adrenergic blocking agent and a diuretic to avert increased sympathetic activity and salt and water retention.
   d. **Route of administration.** Minoxidil is administered orally in single or divided doses.
   e. **Untoward effects**
      (1) Like hydralazine, minoxidil can produce side-effects related to increased reflex sympathetic stimulation and to sodium and water retention.
      (2) Pericardial effusion and tamponade can occur, especially in patients with inadequate renal function.
      (3) Hirsutism occurs for unknown reasons; it is not associated with virilism or other endocrine abnormalities.

4. **Diazoxide** is chemically similar to the thiazide diuretics, but it causes sodium and water retention rather than diuresis.
   a. **Pharmacologic actions**
      (1) Diazoxide exerts its vasodilator effect principally on arterioles and has little effect on capacitance vessels.
      (2) It causes a fall in both systolic and diastolic pressure, accompanied by an increase in both heart rate and cardiac output.
      (3) The drug relaxes other smooth muscle in addition to vascular muscle.
      (4) It inhibits the release of insulin.
   b. **Pharmacokinetics**
      (1) Diazoxide is used as an antihypertensive drug in intravenous form only.
      (2) It has a rapid onset of action (3 to 5 minutes), and a given amount injected quickly produces a greater hypertensive effect than the same amount injected slowly.
      (3) The drug is extensively bound to serum proteins.
      (4) The plasma half-life averages 28 hours, but the antihypertensive effects usually last only 4 to 12 hours.
   c. **Therapeutic uses.** Intravenous diazoxide is one of two major drugs used for hypertensive emergencies (see D 1 c, below). (Diazoxide can be used orally to treat hypoglycemia that is caused by hyperinsulinemia).
   d. **Route of administration.** Diazoxide is given by rapid injection into a peripheral vein. Administration is started with a bolus dose which can be repeated at 5- to 15-minute intervals until the desired effect on blood pressure is attained.
   e. **Untoward effects**
      (1) Diazoxide can cause severe hypotension.
      (2) Its reflex sympathetic stimulation can cause angina and worsen myocardial ischemia.
      (3) Diazoxide inhibits the release of insulin from the pancreas and can produce hyperglycemia.
      (4) It can produce edema due to significant retention of sodium and water.

D. **ARTERIAL AND VENOUS VASODILATORS.** These drugs reduce both arterial resistance and venous tone and markedly decrease arterial blood pressure.

1. **Sodium nitroprusside**
   a. **Pharmacologic actions**
      (1) Nitroprusside acts directly on arterial and venous smooth muscle but has little effect on other smooth muscle.
      (2) It decreases blood pressure in both the supine and upright positions.
      (3) The increased venous capacitance that it produces results in decreased cardiac preload and thus decreases myocardial oxygen demand for a given output.

(4) Nitroprusside causes a slight increase in heart rate and decrease in cardiac output except when heart failure is present; in the latter case, the heart rate may decrease and the cardiac output increase.
(5) Renal blood flow is maintained with nitroprusside, and renin secretion is increased.

b. Pharmacokinetics
(1) Onset of action occurs within 1 minute of intravenous administration, and effects cease within 5 minutes of stopping an infusion.
(2) The drug is rapidly inactivated by hepatic enzymes, first to cyanide and then to thiocyanate.

c. Therapeutic uses
(1) Nitroprusside, like diazoxide, is used for short-term, rapid reduction of blood pressure in hypertensive emergencies. It is preferable to diazoxide for treating hypertensive emergencies in patients with coronary insufficiency or pulmonary edema because, in contrast to diazoxide, it reduces cardiac preload (by increasing venous capacitance) and thus myocardial oxygen demand.
(2) Nitroprusside can also be used to produce controlled hypotension to minimize bleeding during surgery.
(3) Nitroprusside can improve left ventricular function (lower ventricular filling pressure) in patients with acute myocardial infarction, and has beneficial hemodynamic effects in the treatment of acute congestive heart failure.

d. Route of administration
(1) Sodium nitroprusside is administered only as an intravenous infusion with sterile 5 percent dextrose in water. Once prepared, the solution must be protected from light and used within 4 hours.
(2) Blood pressure must be monitored continuously while the drug is being given.

e. Untoward effects
(1) Hypotension, nausea, diaphoresis, headache, restlessness, palpitations, and retrosternal pain can occur secondary to excessive, rapid vasodilation.
(2) The rate of conversion of nitroprusside from its metabolite cyanide to thiocyanate is dependent on the availability of sulfur (usually as thiosulfate). Rarely, when high doses of nitroprusside are administered for a prolonged period and sulfur stores are low, cyanide toxicity can occur.
(3) Because thiocyanate is cleared slowly by the kidneys, it can accumulate during prolonged nitroprusside therapy, especially in patients with poor renal function. A thiocyanate concentration of greater than 10 mg/100 ml can cause weakness, nausea, muscle spasms, and psychosis, as well as hypothyroidism due to interference with iodine transport.
(4) A case of methemoglobinemia following prolonged infusion of nitroprusside has been reported.

2. **Prazosin.** This quinazoline derivative is now thought to be a selective postsynaptic α_1-adrenergic receptor blocking agent that causes vasodilation of both the arteries and veins.

a. Pharmacologic actions
(1) Prazosin reduces peripheral vascular resistance and lowers arterial blood pressure in both supine and erect positions.
(2) Unlike nonselective α-adrenergic blockers, it does not usually produce reflex tachycardia.
(3) It does not increase plasma renin activity.
(4) Prazosin seems to produce minimal changes in cardiac output, renal blood flow, and glomerular filtration rate.
(5) Fluid retention occurs during long-term therapy.

b. Pharmacokinetics
(1) Prazosin is highly bound to plasma protein.
(2) Its plasma concentration peaks in about 3 hours. Plasma half-life is usually 2 to 3 hours but can be prolonged by congestive heart failure.
(3) Prazosin is extensively metabolized, may undergo significant first-pass metabolism, has a bioavailability around 60 percent, and is probably excreted in the feces and bile.

c. Therapeutic uses. Prazosin is used to treat mild to moderate hypertension. It may be more effective in conjunction with a diuretic or an α-adrenergic blocking agent than when used alone.

d. Route of administration. Prazosin hydrochloride (Mini-press) is given orally, two or three times daily.

e. Untoward effects
(1) Dizziness, headache, drowsiness, and palpitations can occur but often disappear with continued therapy and rarely cause discontinuation of the drug.
(2) Following the initial dose of prazosin, especially if the dose is larger than 1 mg, postural

hypotension and syncope can occur, probably due to decreased venous return to the heart.

(3) Tests for antinuclear factor may become positive with prazosin therapy.

E. CENTRALLY ACTING ANTIADRENERGIC AGENTS. Clonidine and methyldopa act centrally on the vasomotor centers of the brain and are predominantly α-receptor agonists.

1. Clonidine. This imidazoline derivative is thought to stimulate α-adrenergic receptors (probably presynaptic α_2-receptors) in the vasomotor centers of the brain, resulting in decreased sympathetic outflow to the peripheral vessels.

a. Pharmacologic effects

(1) Intravenous injection of clonidine causes an initial *increase* in both systolic and diastolic pressure; oral administration does not normally produce this hypertensive effect. The initial rise in blood pressure is caused by direct stimulation of peripheral α-adrenergic receptors, producing transient vasoconstriction. Clonidine also causes peripheral α-adrenergic blockade, and thus it is a partial agonist.

(2) The increase in blood pressure following intravenous injection is transient and is soon followed by a fall in blood pressure, resulting from a decrease in cardiac output and heart rate, usually not accompanied by a significant change in peripheral resistance. During long-term oral clonidine therapy, cardiac output tends to return to control values, and peripheral vascular resistance and heart rate are decreased.

(3) Vagal discharge is increased by clonidine in association with increased baroreceptor reflex sensitivity.

(4) Clonidine does not block the homeostatic control mechanisms of the peripheral autonomic system.

(5) It decreases plasma renin activity, primarily through a centrally mediated decrease in sympathetic stimulation of the juxtaglomerular cells of the kidney.

(6) Renal vascular resistance decreases, while renal blood flow remains essentially unchanged.

b. Pharmacokinetics

(1) The antihypertensive effects of clonidine develop within 30 to 60 minutes of oral administration, peak in 2 to 4 hours, and last for approximately 8 hours in normal subjects.

(2) The drug and its metabolites are excreted primarily in the urine.

c. Therapeutic uses

(1) Clonidine can be used to treat mild and moderate to severe hypertension.

(2) It can be used as a single agent or in combination with a diuretic and/or other antihypertensive agents.

(3) It cannot be administered to patients taking tricyclic antidepressants because these drugs block its hypotensive effect.

d. Route of administration

(1) Clonidine hydrochloride (Catapres) is given orally.

(2) It is often administered in two unequal doses, with the larger one given at bedtime to minimize problems resulting from the sedative effects of clonidine.

e. Untoward effects

(1) Dry mouth, drowsiness, and sedation are the most frequent problems and may require discontinuation of clonidine.

(2) Rebound hypertensive crises can result from abrupt cessation of clonidine when the drug is used as a single agent.

(3) Fluid retention often occurs, requiring concurrent diuretic therapy.

(4) Clonidine can cause or worsen depression.

2. Methyldopa

a. Mechanism of action

(1) Methyldopa is an effective inhibitor of L-aromatic amino acid decarboxylase and was initially thought to act as an antihypertensive agent by decreasing stores of norepinephrine in the sympathetic nervous system. However, as is now apparent, its primary mode of action is via a central effect.

(2) Methyldopa is metabolized by decarboxylation and β-hydroxylation in adrenergic neurons of the central nervous system. The metabolite, α-methylnorepinephrine, stimulates α-adrenergic receptors in the brain, inhibiting sympathetic outflow. This effect on the central nervous system is believed to be the principal mechanism by which methyldopa exerts its antihypertensive effect.

(3) Methyldopa reduces renal vascular resistance, possibly as a result of a α-methylnorepinephrine being a weaker vasoconstrictor than norepinephrine in renal beds, and is

thought to exert other direct actions on peripheral adrenergic neurons that contribute to its antihypertensive effect.

b. Pharmacologic actions

(1) Methyldopa decreases blood pressure and peripheral arteriolar resistance.

(2) It has little effect on cardiac output, renal blood flow, or glomerular filtration rate.

(3) It does not abolish sympathetic reflexes.

c. Pharmacokinetics

(1) Methyldopa is poorly absorbed (< 25 percent) following oral administration and may be subject to first-pass intestinal metabolism.

(2) Its peak effect is exerted 4 to 6 hours after administration, and its effect may last up to 24 hours.

(3) Methyldopa is excreted largely by the kidneys.

d. Therapeutic uses. Methyldopa is used orally to treat mild and moderate to severe hypertenson, usually in combination with a diuretic.

e. Route of administration

(1) Methyldopa (Aldomet) is given orally.

(2) Methyldopate hydrochloride (Aldomet ester hydrochloride) is administered in 5 percent dextrose solution by slow intravenous infusion.

f. Untoward effects

(1) Sedation is common, and although it may decrease with continued administration of methyldopa, mental acuity may remain decreased.

(2) Methyldopa can produce febrile episodes; these may be accompanied by alterations in liver function, which on rare occasions terminate in hepatic necrosis.

(3) A positive direct Coombs' test develops in as many as 25 percent of patients taking methyldopa for more than 6 months. Hemolytic anemia, usually reversible on discontinuation of the drug, occurs in a small percentage of these patients.

(4) Edema caused by salt and water retention can develop if a diuretic is not administered.

(5) Rebound hypertension can occur in association with sudden withdrawal of methyldopa but occurs less frequently than with clonidine.

(6) Orthostatic hypotension occurs more frequently than with clonidine but less frequently than with guanethidine.

(7) Lactation can occur in either sex, and impotence can occur in some men.

(8) Gastrointestinal disturbances can occur but usually are mild.

F. AGENTS THAT BLOCK POSTGANGLIONIC ADRENERGIC NEURONS (see also Chapter 2, III C). This group of drugs selectively inhibits sympathetic neuron function through interference with chemical mediation at ganglionic nerve endings; one or more mechanisms may be involved.

1. Reserpine

a. Mechanism of action

(1) Reserpine, a rauwolfia alkaloid, depletes catecholamine and serotonin stores in the peripheral and central nervous systems and causes impaired sympathetic nerve discharge (see Chapter 2, III C 1).

(a) It interferes with intracellular storage of catecholamines by inhibiting the binding of norepinephrine to neurosecretory vesicles at the vesicle membrane, both centrally and peripherally. Norepinephrine that diffuses from the storage site is degraded intracellularly by monoamine oxidase (MAO).

(b) Reserpine decreases the synthesis of norepinephine and increases its turnover rate.

(2) Reserpine also exerts a direct vasodilating effect on vascular smooth muscle when administered intra-arterially, and may have several other actions.

b. Pharmacologic actions

(1) Reserpine decreases blood pressure, usually decreases heart rate and cardiac output, and may decrease peripheral vascular resistance.

(2) In usual therapeutic doses, reserpine only partially inhibits cardiovascular reflexes.

(3) Reserpine exerts central actions that produce sedation.

c. Pharmacokinetics

(1) With oral administration, reserpine usually takes several days to several weeks to reach a maximum effect.

(2) A likely possibility for the breakdown of reserpine involves hydrolysis of the ester linkage and demethylation.

(3) Reserpine is concentrated in tissues with a high lipid content.

d. Therapeutic uses. Reserpine is used principally in low oral doses in combination with other antihypertensive agents (e.g., a thiazide diuretic and vasodilator) to control moderate hypertension.

e. **Route of administration**. Reserpine is usually given orally, but is also available for parenteral administration.

f. **Untoward effects**

(1) Reserpine regularly causes sedation and can cause severe depressive episodes, probably due to a reduction of biogenic amine levels in subcortical areas of the brain. It should not be administered to patients prone to depression.

(2) Because reserpine decreases sympathetic activity, unopposed parasympathetic activity can result in bradycardia, nasal congestion, and increased gastrointestinal activity. It is contraindicated for patients with active peptic ulcers.

(3) Controversy exists as to whether reserpine increases the incidence of breast cancer.

2. Guanethidine

a. **Mechanism of action**

(1) Guanethidine acts presynaptically to inhibit the release of neurotransmitter from peripheral adrenergic neurons, thus reducing the response to sympathetic nerve activation. Acutely, it produces sympathetic blockade before any appreciable decrease in norepinephrine stores has occurred; with chronic administration, it impairs the release of neurotransmitter from peripheral adrenergic neurons. (See Chapter 2, III C 2 for further discussion.)

(a) For guanethidine to exert an antihypertensive effect, it must be taken up and stored in adrenergic nerve terminals in a manner similar to norepinephrine uptake.

(b) Agents that prevent this uptake, such as cocaine and tricyclic antidepressants, inhibit the therapeutic effect of guanethidine.

(2) Unlike reserpine, guanethidine can inhibit the pressor action of indirectly acting amines such as tyramine.

(3) As with reserpine, the norepinephrine released by guanethidine is deaminated intraneuronally by MAO, but to a lesser degree than with reserpine.

(4) Although guanethidine displaces norepinephrine from storage granules and is subsequently released as a "false" neurotransmitter in response to stimulation of sympathetic nerves, this does not seem to be a primary mechanism of action.

(5) Guanethidine probably has some direct action on β-adrenergic receptors.

(6) The drug does not cross the blood–brain barrier like reserpine, and thus it does not affect serotonin and norepinephrine stores in the central nervous system.

(7) It is believed to decrease plasma renin activity.

b. **Pharmacologic actions**

(1) Initially, guanethidine displaces and releases enough unchanged norepinephrine to cause mild, transient hypertension and cardiac stimulation.

(2) Hypotension and bradycardia follow. Because guanethidine depresses vasoconstrictor reflexes, blood pressure is reduced significantly more in the erect position than in the supine. Venous return and cardiac output are decreased.

(3) Guanethidine has a direct inhibitory effect on skeletal muscle contraction.

(4) It increases the sensitivity of tissues to catecholamines.

c. **Pharmacokinetics**

(1) Absorption of guanethidine following oral administration varies from patient to patient and is low (3 to 30 percent).

(2) The drug has a long duration of action.

(3) Guanethidine is thought to be metabolized by hepatic enzymes and is excreted with its metabolites in the urine.

d. **Therapeutic uses**. Guanethidine is used in the treatment of moderate to severe hypertension, usually in combination with a thiazide diuretic or a diuretic and a vasodilator.

e. **Route of administration.** Guanethidine is given orally. The dose can be increased at intervals of not less than 5 days until either the desired effect is attained or untoward effects develop.

f. **Untoward effects**

(1) Significant orthostatic hypotension and syncope frequently occur, especially during exercise and when patients first arise in the morning.

(2) Salt and water retention occur but can be prevented or treated with a mild diuretic.

(3) Gastrointestinal hyperactivity occurs, probably as a result of the parasympathetic predominance that follows sympathetic blockade.

(4) Muscular aching and weakness can occur.

G. DRUGS THAT INTERFERE WITH THE RENIN–ANGIOTENSIN SYSTEM (see also Chapter 8, III C). The kidneys synthesize renin, which acts on a plasma globulin substrate to produce angiotensin I. This in turn is converted (by a peptidyl dipeptidase) to angiotensin II, a potent vasoconstrictor. Drugs in this group exert an antihypertensive effect by interfering with either the formation or the utilization of angiotensin II.

1. **Captopril**

a. **Mechanism of action**

(1) Captopril, which will be discussed in more detail in Chapter 8, III C 2, is a specific competitive inhibitor of peptidyl dipeptidase (angiotensin I–converting enzyme), the enzyme that converts angiotensin I to angiotensin II.

(a) Angiotensin II is a potent direct vasoconstrictor. (Thus, captopril inhibits vasoconstriction.)

(b) Angiotensin II stimulates the secretion of aldosterone, which promotes sodium and water retention. (Thus, captopril inhibits sodium and water retention and slightly increases serum potassium levels.)

(2) Because peptidyl dipeptidase is necessary to catalyze the degradation of bradykinin, captopril may increase the concentration of bradykinin, which is a potent vasodilator.

(3) Captopril exerts an antihypertensive effect in low-renin hypertension; the mechanism of action in this case is not explained.

b. **Pharmacologic actions.** The cardiovascular effects of captopril include a reduction in total peripheral resistance and mean arterial blood pressure, and either no change or an increase in cardiac output.

c. **Pharmacokinetics**

(1) Captopril is rapidly absorbed following oral administration and reaches peak blood levels within an hour.

(2) Approximately 95 percent of a dose is eliminated by the kidneys within 24 hours.

d. **Therapeutic uses**

(1) Captopril is indicated for the treatment of hypertensive patients who do not respond satisfactorily to or who develop unacceptable side effects from conventional combination antihypertensive therapy. It is effective for low-renin, as well as high-renin, hypertension.

(2) Captopril is effective when used alone, but it is often administered with a thiazide diuretic, in which case the antihypertensive effects appear to be additive. β-Blockers also can be used with captopril, but the effect produced appears to be less than additive.

(3) Captopril has recently been approved for the treatment of severe congestive heart failure.

e. **Route of administration**

(1) Captopril is given orally, one hour before meals.

(2) The initial dose can be increased at one- to two-week intervals.

f. **Untoward effects**

(1) Proteinuria can occur, especially in patients with compromised renal function. (Monthly monitoring of urinary protein levels is recommended for all patients taking captopril.)

(2) Neutropenia can occur, and in patients who have impaired renal function or serious autoimmune disease (e.g., systemic lupus erythematosus), captopril should be used with caution.

(3) Approximately 10 percent of patients treated with captopril develop reversible skin rashes and alteration in taste.

2. **Drugs that block receptors for angiotensin** (see also Chapter 8, III C 1). Saralasin, an angiotensin II analog, exemplifies the drugs that interfere with the renin–angiotensin system by this mechanism.

a. These drugs can be given only by intravenous infusion.

b. They are primarily used diagnostically to detect a renal cause of hypertension.

STUDY QUESTIONS

Directions: Each question below contains five suggested answers. Choose the **one best** response to each question.

1. All of the following untoward effects are correctly matched with the therapeutic agents EXCEPT

(A) quinidine—cinchonism
(B) procainamide—hypotension with intravenous administration
(C) lidocaine—systemic lupus erythematosus–like syndrome
(D) disopyramide—untoward anticholinergic effects
(E) bretylium—orthostatic hypotension

2. A 67-year-old male with a known history of recurrent ventricular tachycardia presents with joint and muscle pain, fatigue due to a hemolytic anemia, and a skin rash. He is taking several "heart pills." A likely cause of his signs and symptoms might be

(A) digoxin
(B) procainamide
(C) disopyramide
(D) minoxidil
(E) reserpine

3. Actions of nitroglycerin on the smooth muscle vasculature include all of the following EXCEPT

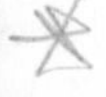

(A) vasodilation of cerebral vessels
(B) dilation of retinal vessels
(C) dilation of skin blood vessels
(D) constriction of meningeal blood vessels
(E) dilation of coronary arteries

4. All of the following statements about papaverine are true EXCEPT

(A) it is an isoquinoline opium alkaloid
(B) it exerts its smooth muscle relaxant activity by α-adrenergic blockade
(C) it is a potent inhibitor of phosphodiesterase
(D) it decreases total peripheral resistance by its effect on arterioles
(E) when injected intravenously, it produces quinidine-like effects

5. Captopril is an antihypertensive agent. Its mechanism of action includes specific competitive inhibition of the angiotensin I–converting enzyme. All of the following statements about captopril are true EXCEPT

(A) it reduces total peripheral resistance and mean arterial pressure
(B) currently it is indicated for patients who have failed to respond to multidrug regimens
(C) by inhibiting angiotensin II production, captopril increases aldosterone secretion
(D) the blood pressure–lowering effects appear to be additive with thiazide diuretics
(E) proteinuria is an important untoward effect requiring monthly monitoring of urinary protein levels

6. All of the following measures can be used in the treatment of digoxin-induced arrhythmias EXCEPT for

(A) stopping digoxin administration
(B) electrical conversion
(C) phenytoin administration
(D) lidocaine administration
(E) atropine administration

7. A patient with severe hypertension is being treated with an agent that stimulates presynaptic α_2 receptors in the vasomotor center of the brain. The patient might be taking

(A) guanethidine
(B) reserpine
(C) clonidine
(D) prazosin
(E) minoxidil

8. Ventricular arrhythmias that might result from open heart surgery, digitalis intoxication, or myocardial infarction would initially be *best* treated with

(A) lidocaine
(B) quinidine
(C) procainamide
(D) propranolol
(E) bretylium

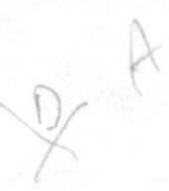

Directions: Each question below contains four suggested answers of which **one or more** is correct. Choose the answer

A if **1, 2, and 3** are correct
B if **1 and 3** are correct
C if **2 and 4** are correct
D if **4** is correct
E if **1, 2, 3, and 4** are correct

9. Therapeutic uses for propranolol include

(1) atrial fibrillation
(2) atrial flutter
(3) paroxysmal atrial tachycardia
(4) ventricular arrhythmias

10. Actions of digoxin on the heart include

(1) increased force of systolic contraction
(2) prolonged A–V nodal conduction time
(3) a decrease in ventricular size of the failing heart
(4) a positive chronotropic effect in the failing heart

11. A patient with hypertension, recurrent ventricular tachycardia, and congestive heart failure presents with anorexia, nausea, and color vision changes. Discontinuation of which of the following agents will most likely improve these untoward effects?

(1) Disopyramide
(2) Procainamide
(3) Clonidine
(4) Digoxin

12. True statements about the use of diuretic agents in the treatment of essential hypertension include which of the following?

(1) The early hypotensive effect of the thiazide diuretics is related to a reduction in peripheral vascular resistance
(2) Furosemide produces a greater diuresis than thiazide diuretics
(3) Triamterene, when combined with a thiazide diuretic, minimizes potassium loss but will decrease the overall diuretic effectiveness of the thiazide
(4) Ethacrynic acid has a weaker antihypertensive effect than the thiazide diuretics

13. Which of the following agents and untoward effects are correctly matched?

(1) Hydralazine—can induce a lupus-like syndrome
(2) Diazoxide—inhibits the release of insulin from the pancreas
(3) Clonidine—can cause fluid retention that often requires concurrent diuretic therapy
(4) Reserpine—augments sympathetic effects due to decreased parasympathetic activity

14. A 47-year-old male has been treated for essential hypertension for 6 months. The patient's hypertension is under control; however, he now complains of difficulty in doing mental work, vertigo, and impotence. Laboratory testing reveals a positive Coombs' test. Antihypertensive agents capable of causing these effects include

(1) prazosin
(2) captopril
(3) hydralazine
(4) methyldopa

ANSWERS AND EXPLANATIONS

1. The answer is C. *(III B 8 c, C 8 e, D 6 b, E 8, H 7 a)* All of the listed untoward effects are paired correctly with their respective therapeutic agents except for lidocaine. A systemic lupus erythematosus–like syndrome can be associated with procainamide administration. This syndrome is reversible on discontinuation of therapy but can develop in as many as 30 percent of patients taking procainamide for long periods of time.

2. The answer is B. *(III C 8 d (3)).* Procainamide is capable of producing a systemic lupus erythematosus–like syndrome, the signs and symptoms of which could be this patient's presenting problems. These untoward effects are reversible with time once the drug is discontinued.

3. The answer is D. *(IV A 2, 3)* Nitroglycerin relaxes all smooth muscle, including vascular smooth muscle. It dilates all blood vessels, including meningeal blood vessels. It reduces venous tone, thereby increasing venous capacitance and decreasing venous return to the heart.

4. The answer is B. *(IV D 2)* Papaverine does not possess α-adrenergic blocking activity. It is a nonspecific relaxant of all smooth muscle structures. It decreases total peripheral resistance through an effect on arterioles but is a much weaker vasodilator than are the nitrates.

5. The answer is C. *(V G I)* Captopril decreases the secretion of aldosterone by inhibiting the production of angiotensin II. In addition, vasoconstrictor properties associated with angiotensin II are inhibited. Captopril is a specific competitive inhibitor of peptidyl dipeptidase (angiotensin I–converting enzyme), the enzyme that converts angiotensin I to angiotensin II.

6. The answer is B. *(II I)* The use of phenytoin, lidocaine, or atropine for various digoxin-induced arrhythmias is considered to be appropriate therapy. Digoxin and potassium-depleting diuretics should be discontinued. Electrical conversion can be hazardous because it can precipitate ventricular fibrillation.

7. The answer is C. *(V E 1)* Clonidine, by stimulating presynaptic α_2 receptors in the vasomotor center of the brain, decreases sympathetic outflow to the peripheral vessels. Both guanethidine and reserpine are agents which block postganglionic adrenergic neurons. Prazosin is a selective postsynaptic α_1-adrenergic receptor blocker. Minoxidil directly relaxes arteriolar smooth muscle.

8. The answer is A. *(III E 6)* Lidocaine is the drug of first choice for ventricular arrhythmias that arise in an emergency situation. This drug is the best choice because of its rapid onset and short duration of action. Quinidine, procainamide, and bretylium can be useful in the treatment of ventricular arrhythmias but are not drugs of first choice. Propranolol is useful in ventricular arrhythmias that are due to enhanced adrengeric stimulation.

9. The answer is E (all). *(III G 4; Table 5-5)* Propranolol is used to control supraventricular tachyarrhythmias, including atrial fibrillation and flutter and paroxysmal supraventricular tachycardia. It is useful in ventricular arrhythmias that are due to enhanced adrengeric stimulation (from emotional stress, for example), and is also sometimes used to abolish digitalis-induced ventricular arrhythmias, but it can cause conduction problems in the latter context, resulting in A–V dissociation.

10. The answer is A (1, 2, 3). *(II C)* Digoxin will produce all of the effects listed in the question except that it tends to slow the heart rate, especially in the failing heart (a negative chronotropic effect). By improving cardiac output, digoxin produces a decrease in sympathetic activity.

11. The answer is D (4). *(II H 5)* The presenting symptoms are consistent with the symptoms of digoxin toxicity. When serum digoxin levels rise above 2 ng/ml, therapy with the glycoside should be discontinued until the level falls below this concentration.

12. The answer is C (2, 4). *(V B)* The early hypotensive effect seen with the use of thiazide diuretics is related to a reduction in blood volume, while their long-term effect is related to a reduction in peripheral vascular resistance. Both furosemide and ethacrynic acid produce a greater diuretic effect than the thiazides; however, they both have a weaker antihypertensive effect. Triamterene potentiates the overall diuretic effectiveness of the thiazides, and also minimizes their hypokalemic effects.

13. The answer is A (1, 2, 3). *(V C 2 d, 4 a, E 1 e, F 1 f)* All of the agents are correctly matched with an untoward effect except reserpine. Reserpine augments parasympathetic effects due to decreased sympathetic activity, which may result in bradycardia, increased gastrointestinal activity, and miosis.

14. The answer is D (4). *(V C 2 d, D 2 e, E 2 f, G 1 f)* An antihypertensive agent capable of producing the untoward effects described is methyldopa. In addition, methyldopa can cause sedation, extrapyramidal signs, postural hypotension, and hepatic dysfunction; rebound hypertension can occur with sudden withdrawal of methyldopa therapy.

6
Diuretic Agents

I. GENERAL CONSIDERATIONS

A. Diuretics are drugs that promote a net loss of sodium ions (Na^+) and water from the body, the net result being an increase in urine flow. Some drugs can increase urine flow by **nonrenal mechanisms** (e.g., increasing cardiac output in a patient with congestive heart failure), but these drugs are not generally regarded as diuretics.

B. Diuretics are frequently employed for the clinical management of disorders involving abnormal fluid distribution, such as edema, or for hypertension. They are also used to reduce the toxicity of ingested or administered substances. For example, mannitol, an osmotic diuretic, reduces the renal toxicity of the antitumor agent cisplatin, and acetazolamide is used to alkalinize the urine and increase salicylate elimination.

C. The efficacy of the different classes of diuretics varies significantly, with the xanthine diuretics being the least effective and the "high-ceiling" diuretics being the most effective. The establishment of a net negative Na^+ balance, particularly with the less efficacious diuretics, can also depend upon limiting the Na^+ intake.

D. The prolonged usage of some diuretics (mercurials, carbonic anhydrase inhibitors) results in refractoriness, or a reduction in their effectiveness. Thus, these agents are "self-limiting" and because of that are not used as frequently as they once were.

E. Reduction in serum potassium (K^+) levels (hypokalemia) is one of the most important untoward effects of most, but not all, diuretics.

F. Although an individual diuretic can act on several areas of the nephron, the **major sites of action** for the diuretics may be summarized as follows:

1. Those acting on the **proximal tubules:**
   - **a.** Osmotic diuretics.
   - **b.** Xanthine diuretics.
   - **c.** Carbonic anhydrase inhibitors.
   - **d.** Acidifying salts.
2. Those acting on the **ascending limb of the loop of Henle:**
   - **a.** High-ceiling diuretics.
   - **b.** Thiazide diuretics.
   - **c.** Mercurial diuretics.
3. Those acting on the **distal tubules:** Potassium-sparing diuretics.

G. Diuretics can be classified by structure and mechanism of action into the eight groups listed below. Agents in the first four groups are seldom or no longer used but are discussed because their mode of action or their role in the history of diuretics is important.

1. Xanthine diuretics.
2. Mercurial diuretics.
3. Carbonic anhydrase inhibitors.
4. Acidifying salts.

5. Thiazide diuretics.
6. High-ceiling diuretics.
7. Osmotic diuretics.
8. Potassium-sparing diuretics.

II. XANTHINE DIURETICS

A. MECHANISM OF ACTION

1. By increasing cardiac output, these drugs increase renal plasma flow, promoting a higher glomerular filtration rate.
2. They also appear to inhibit Na^+ reabsorption at the proximal convoluted tubule.

B. THERAPEUTIC USES. Xanthines are rarely used as diuretics but their presence in some beverages (e.g., tea and coffee) and in bronchodilators (e.g., aminophylline) warrants remembrance.

C. UNTOWARD EFFECTS. Xanthine diuretics may cause

1. Central nervous system stimulation.
2. Gastrointestinal upset, including vomiting and consequent dehydration.
3. Cardiovascular toxicity, including palpitations, hypotension, and circulatory collapse.

III. MERCURIAL DIURETICS

A. MECHANISM OF ACTION

1. The major effect of organomercurials is to inhibit active chloride transport in the ascending limb of the loop of Henle.
2. In an acidic environment, the mercuric ion (Hg^{2+}) dissociates and binds to sulfhydryl enzymes, inactivating them.
3. As a result, reabsorption of Na^+ is diminished and the excretion of Na^+ and Cl^- is increased.
4. More Cl^- than Na^+ is lost; thus, to maintain electrical neutrality, cations such as H^+ and to a lesser degree K^+ are also lost.
5. Because excess Cl^- is excreted, bicarbonate (HCO_3^-) remains to maintain balanced anions, and the resulting metabolic picture is a hypochloremic alkalosis.
6. In an alkalotic environment, Hg^{2+} does not dissociate from the mercurial diuretics to take an active form; thus, the mercurials become refractory in about a week. However, an acidifying agent such as ammonium chloride ($NH_4^+Cl^-$) can be combined with mercurials to create a metabolic acidosis, offsetting the metabolic alkalosis and combating refractoriness.

B. THERAPEUTIC USES. Mercurial diuretics are poorly absorbed by the oral route and, thus, are given parenterally. Once the most effective class of diuretics available, the mercurials are now seldom used because they must be given parenterally and because of their untoward effects. Since the mercurial diuretics do not disrupt K^+ balance as much as many of the other diuretics, they occasionally are used for congestive heart failure, cirrhosis, and portal obstruction.

C. PREPARATION AND ADMINISTRATION. Mercaptomerin is administered daily, intramuscularly or subcutaneously. The major excretory product is a cysteine complex of the intact organic mercurial molecule.

D. UNTOWARD EFFECTS include

1. Cardiac toxicity. Rapid intravenous administration of a mercurial diuretic can result in ventricular fibrillation, possibly caused by the mercurial's binding to sulfhydryl enzymes in cardiac muscle.
2. Hypersensitivity reactions.
3. Systemic mercury poisoning.
4. Aggravation of acute nephritis or renal insufficiency.

IV. CARBONIC ANHYDRASE INHIBITORS

A. MECHANISM OF ACTION

1. This class of diuretics inhibits the enzyme carbonic anhydrase at both the proximal and distal convoluted tubules.
2. Because of the carbonic anhydrase inhibition, the kidney is deprived of its source of hydrogen ions for $H^+ \rightleftharpoons Na^+$ exchange, so that carbon dioxide (CO_2) reabsorption from the glomerular filtrate is suppressed and HCO_3^- excretion is increased.
3. To maintain ionic balance, Cl^- is retained by the kidney, resulting in a hyperchloremic acidosis.
4. Due to a decrease in the reabsorption of Na^+ in exchange for H^+, the Na^+–K^+ exchange in the distal convoluted tubule increases.
5. Increased urinary amounts of Na^+, K^+, and HCO_3^- result in an alkaline urine.
6. Because plasma Cl^- levels increase and HCO_3^- concentration decreases, a metabolic hyperchloremic acidosis develops.
7. The resulting acidosis eventually causes a refractory state.

B. THERAPEUTIC USES

1. Carbonic anhydrase inhibitors are weak diuretics and essentially have been replaced by the thiazide diuretics. Historically, however, they are very important.
2. They are still used with moderate success for the following purposes:
   a. In glaucoma, for reducing the rate of aqueous humor formation.
   b. In petit mal epilepsy, where they act as an anticonvulsant and decrease the rate of spinal fluid formation. (The therapeutic mechanism of action of this effect is unclear.)
   c. To alkalinize the urine
      (1) In the treatment of salicylate poisoning.
      (2) In combination with HCO_3^- to maintain electrolyte balance.

C. PREPARATION AND ADMINISTRATION

1. As a diuretic, **acetazolamide** is given orally once daily or every other day.
2. For use in glaucoma, it is given 2 to 4 times daily.

D. UNTOWARD EFFECTS

1. Few side effects are associated with the use of carbonic anhydrase inhibitors.
2. Because they are aromatic sulfonamides, they can cause blood dyscrasias and allergic skin reactions, but these are rare.
3. Drowsiness and paresthesias can occur but are reversible.

V. ACIDIFYING SALTS, e.g., ammonium chloride ($NH_4^+Cl^-$)

A. MECHANISM OF ACTION

1. Acidifying salts lower the pH in the extracellular fluid and urine.
2. The ammonium in $NH_4^+Cl^-$ is metabolized by the liver to urea, resulting in the net formation of H^+.
3. H^+ then is buffered by HCO_3^-, and CO_2 is formed.
4. Cl^- from the $NH_4^+Cl^-$ replaces HCO_3^-, and this leads to acidosis.
5. An excess of Cl^- also occurs in the tubular lumen and takes Na^+ along with it to maintain electrical neutrality.
6. The glutaminase system becomes activated, producing ammonia (NH_3).
7. The kidney secretes H^+ in exchange for Na^+, and Cl^- is excreted in combination with NH_4^+.
8. Ultimately, the amount of $NH_4^+Cl^-$ ingested is equal to the amount excreted by the kidney and a refractory state is produced.

B. THERAPEUTIC USE

1. As a primary diuretic, $NH_4^+Cl^-$ is effective for only 1 to 2 days and thus is seldom used.
2. The drug is used to augment the effect of mercurial and high-ceiling diuretics by maintaining an available source of Cl^- in the blood to compensate for diuretic-induced alkalosis.

C. PREPARATION AND ADMINISTRATION. $\mathbf{NH_4^+Cl^-}$ is administered as enteric-coated tablets given orally 4 to 6 times a day for 2 days.

D. UNTOWARD EFFECTS include

1. Gastric irritation.
2. Uncompensated acidosis that occurs when renal function is impaired.
3. Exacerbation of hepatic failure.

VI. THIAZIDE DIURETICS (BENZOTHIADIAZIDES)

A. MECHANISM OF ACTION

1. Structurally, these drugs have a sulfonamyl group which accounts for their inhibition of carbonic anhydrase activity at both the proximal and distal convoluted tubules. Their primary mechanism of action does not, however, rely on inhibition of carbonic anhydrase.
2. They inhibit Cl^- reabsorption, particularly in the distal portion of the ascending limb of Henle's loop and the very early portion of the distal tubule.
3. Refractoriness does not occur.
4. There is increased renal excretion of Na^+, Cl^-, HCO_3^-, and K^+.
5. The initial hypotensive effect of the thiazide diuretics is a result of a reduction in blood volume, and a continued hypotensive effect occurs because of direct relaxation of arteriolar smooth muscle.

B. THERAPEUTIC USE

1. Thiazide diuretics are used to treat chronic edema, usually associated with cardiac decompensation. A diuretic response occurs in 2 to 3 hours and lasts for about a day.
2. Thiazides sometimes are effective in the treatment of nephrosis.
3. They occasionally are used for the palliation of nephrogenic and neurohypophyseal diabetes insipidus. By decreasing the urinary volume through their natriuretic action, these drugs may enhance the action of antidiuretic hormone (ADH).
4. They are used in the management of hypercalciuria.
5. They are used in the treatment of essential hypertension.

C. PREPARATIONS AND ADMINISTRATION. There are many analogs but the two most important prototypes are

1. **Chlorothiazide**, given orally 1 or 2 times a day.
2. **Hydrochlorothiazide**, given orally 1 or 2 times a day.

D. UNTOWARD EFFECTS

1. Electrolyte abnormalities such as hypokalemia can occur.
   a. Thus, K^+ supplementation is recommended.
   b. Particular caution is needed when a thiazide is administered in combination with a digitalis preparation for the treatment of congestive heart failure. Digitalis administered in the presence of hypokalemia can result in digitalis intoxication and serious cardiac arrhythmias.
2. Hyperuricemia may result from an inhibition of renal tubular secretion of uric acid.
3. Hyperglycemia can occur, aggravating preexisting diabetes mellitus.
4. Renal and hepatic insufficiency occasionally may be aggravated.
5. Lassitude, weakness, and vertigo can occur with large doses.

VII. HIGH-CEILING DIURETICS

A. MECHANISM OF ACTION

1. These diuretics inhibit active Cl^- reabsorption in the ascending limb of the loop of Henle, and this leads to Na^+ and water loss.
2. Cl^- excretion is greater than Na^+ excretion.
3. Large doses promote uric acid excretion.
4. Alkalosis can occur but it does not produce a refractory state.
5. **Furosemide** is a weak inhibitor of carbonic anhydrase, probably as a result of the diuretic's substituted sulfonamide side chain.
6. **Ethacrynic acid** lacks a sulfonamyl group and does not inhibit carbonic anhydrase.

B. THERAPEUTIC USES

1. The high-ceiling diuretics are the most efficacious diuretic agents available.
2. They are useful for the treatment of acute episodes of pulmonary edema.
3. They are also effective for edema associated with congestive heart failure, cirrhosis, and renal disease.
4. Because of its potent edema-reducing ability, furosemide has been used to treat elevated intracranial pressure.

C. PREPARATIONS AND ADMINISTRATION

1. **Furosemide** is usually administered orally in a single dose. It also can be administered intramuscularly or (more frequently) intravenously.
2. **Ethacrynic acid** is administered orally or intravenously once or twice daily. One of the main differences between furosemide and ethacrynic acid is that the former has a broader dose–response curve.

D. UNTOWARD EFFECTS

1. Electrolyte imbalances can occur. Because the high-ceiling diuretics frequently are administered with digitalis, hypokalemia may be a particular problem.
2. Hyperuricemia results because furosemide and ethacrynic acid are actively secreted by the renal and biliary secretory systems, and thus they block renal uric acid secretion.
3. Transient deafness is a risk if a potentially ototoxic drug (e.g., an aminoglycoside antibiotic) is administered concomitantly. In such circumstances, another class of diuretic should be employed.

VIII. OSMOTIC DIURETICS

A. MECHANISM OF ACTION

1. Osmotic diuretics increase urine volume by increasing the amount of osmotically active solute in the voided urine.
2. They are filtered at the glomerulus but are not well reabsorbed due to their size.
3. They do not markedly influence Na^+ and Cl^- excretion.

B. THERAPEUTIC USES

1. The osmotic diuretics are used to reduce cerebrospinal fluid pressure.
2. They will transiently reduce intraocular fluid pressure.
3. They have also served as an adjunct in the prevention or treatment of oliguria and anuria.
4. The osmotic diuretics, especially mannitol, are employed prophylactically for acute renal failure in conditions such as cardiovascular operations, treatment with nephrotoxic anticancer agents, severe traumatic injury, and management of hemolytic transfusion reactions.

C. PREPARATIONS AND ADMINISTRATION

1. **Mannitol** is a six-carbon sugar alcohol that is administered intravenously because it is not absorbed well from the gastrointestinal tract. It is not metabolized.
2. **Urea** is the least used osmotic diuretic. It can be given orally but because of its bitter taste is generally administered intravenously.
3. **Isosorbide** is used orally for ophthalmologic emergencies such as acute angle-closure glaucoma.

D. UNTOWARD EFFECTS

1. Because they do not penetrate cells and their mode of excretion is by glomerular filtration, osmotic diuretics increase blood volume, which can cause decompensation in patients with congestive heart failure.
2. When osmotic diuretics are used for the treatment of renal failure or cirrhotic disease, hyperosmolality and hyponatremia can occur.

IX. POTASSIUM-SPARING DIURETICS

A. TRIAMTERENE

1. **Mechanism of action**
   a. Triamterene inhibits active Na^+ reabsorption and thus reduces the availability of Na^+ to the Na^+–K^+ exchange pump in the distal nephron, resulting in the decreased secretion of K^+.
   b. It causes a moderate increase in Na^+ and HCO_3^- excretion.
   c. Its action is independent of aldosterone.
2. **Therapeutic uses.** Triamterene is used in combination with other diuretic agents for the treatment of hypertension; this combined therapy augments the natriuretic effect while diminishing kaliuresis.
3. **Administration**. Triamterene is administered twice daily, as a capsule, by the oral route only.
4. **Untoward effects**
   a. Reversible azotemia is relatively common.
   b. Gastrointestinal disturbances, including nausea and vomiting, occur on occasion and are thought to be caused by a central mechanism.
   c. Leg cramps may occur.
   d. Dizziness has been reported.
   e. Triamterene causes a slight increase in serum uric acid and thus should be used with caution in patients with gout.

B. SPIRONOLACTONE

1. **Mechanism of action**
   a. Spironolactone is a competitive antagonist of the mineralocorticoid, aldosterone.
   b. It interferes with the aldosterone-mediated Na^+–K^+ exchange, increasing Na^+ loss at the distal tubular site while decreasing K^+ loss.
   c. It is most effective when circulating aldosterone levels are high.
2. **Therapeutic uses**
   a. Spironolactone is often used as an adjunct to other diuretics to reduce the loss of K^+ in the management of refractory edema, such as that associated with Laennec's cirrhosis.
   b. It also is used when adrenal gland tumors result in increased aldosterone levels.
   c. It can be used for edema due to congestive heart failure, although other diuretic agents are more effective.
3. **Administration**. Spironolactone is usually given orally 4 times a day.
4. **Untoward effects**
   a. Gastrointestinal disturbances include diarrhea.
   b. Androgenic side effects include menstrual irregularities and hirsutism.
   c. Central nervous system disturbances include lethargy and mental confusion.
   d. Exacerbation of hyperkalemia is likely (spironolactone is contraindicated in this condition).

STUDY QUESTIONS

Directions: Each question below contains five suggested answers. Choose the **one best** response to each question.

1. A 67-year-old man with a history of congestive heart failure is found to have tachypnea, pitting edema, and audible S_3 and S_4 heart sounds. A chest x-ray supports the diagnosis of congestive heart failure. The diuretic of choice would be

(A) mannitol
(B) hydrochlorothiazide
(C) furosemide
(D) triamterene
(E) spironolactone

2. Adverse effects resulting from the administration of furosemide can include all of the following EXCEPT

(A) hypokalemia
(B) hyperuricemia
(C) hypercalcemia
(D) dose-related ototoxicity
(E) alkalosis

3. The thiazide diuretics have a useful therapeutic effect in all of the following conditions EXCEPT

(A) chronic edema associated with cardiac decompensation
(B) antidiuretic hormone-secreting pulmonary tumors
(C) hypercalciuria
(D) hypertension
(E) nephrosis

4. All of the following statements about mercurial diuretics are true EXCEPT that

(A) their mercuric ion dissociates in an acidic environment
(B) they can induce a hypochloremic alkalosis
(C) they rarely produce a refractory state
(D) administration of ammonium chloride can mitigate the metabolic alkalosis that they produce
(E) rapid intravenous administration can result in ventricular fibrillation

5. All of the following statements about xanthine diuretics are true EXCEPT that

(A) they promote a high glomerular filtration rate by increasing cardiac output
(B) they are less effective than newer diuretics
(C) they can produce central nervous system stimulation
(D) they rarely produce cardiovascular toxicity
(E) they are closely related to substances in tea and coffee

Directions: The group of questions below consists of lettered choices followed by several numbered items. For each numbered item select the **one** lettered choice with which it is **most** closely associated. Each lettered choice may be used once, more than once, or not at all.

Questions 6–10

For each diuretic agent that follows, select its *major* mechanism of action.

(A) Inhibits carbonic anhydrase
(B) Inhibits Cl^- reabsorption in the distal portion of the ascending limb of the loop of Henle
(C) Competitively antagonizes aldosterone
(D) Binds to sulfhydryl enzymes
(E) Inhibits the Na^+–K^+ exchange pump in the distal nephron

6. Ethacrynic acid
7. Spironolactone
8. Chlorothiazide
9. Acetazolamide
10. Triamterene

ANSWERS AND EXPLANATIONS

1. The answer is C. *(VII B 3)* A rapid-acting, potent "loop" diuretic is needed in a patient presenting with acute congestive heart failure. Furosemide is such a diuretic. The other agents listed would not give the immediate diuretic response that is needed.

2. The answer is C. *(VII A 4, D)* All of the untoward effects listed in the question have occurred with furosemide except hypercalcemia. In fact, furosemide lowers plasma calcium concentrations by increasing the renal excretion of calcium. Hyperuricemia results because furosemide is actively secreted by the renal and biliary secretory systems. Transient deafness has occurred, particularly with large doses. Electrolyte imbalance, especially hypokalemia, can be a particular problem if furosemide is administered with digitalis. Alkalosis can occur but is not refractory.

3. The answer is B. *(VI B)* The thiazide diuretics are useful in all the listed therapeutic situations except for pulmonary tumors which secrete antidiuretic hormone (ADH). By decreasing the urinary volume (due to their natriuretic action), thiazide diuretics may enhance the action of ADH, and have been used for the palliative treatment of diabetes insipidus.

4. The answer is C. *(III A, D 1)* All the statements about mercurial diuretics listed in the question are true except that refractoriness does occur. Mercurial diuretics can produce a clinical metabolic picture of hypochloremic alkalosis. In an alkalotic environment the mercuric ion will not dissociate from the drug into its active form; the result is that the mercurials become refractory. Ventricular fibrillation is probably the result of binding to cardiac sulfhydryl enzymes.

5. The answer is D. *(II A 1, B, C)* Cardiovascular toxicity can occur with xanthine diuretics; all other statements in the question are true. The cardiovascular toxicity can include palpitations, hypotension, and circulatory collapse. Being phosphodiesterase inhibitors, the xanthine diuretics increase cyclic adenosine monophosphate (cyclic AMP) levels, which can cause an increase in cardiac output. If toxicity ensues, the above cardiovascular effects can occur.

6–10. The answers are: 6-B, 7-C, 8-B, 9-A, 10-E. *(IV A; VI A; VII A; IX A, B)* Ethacrynic acid inhibits Cl^- reabsorption in the ascending limb of the loop of Henle, producing an increased urinary excretion of Na^+, Cl^-, and K^+. The molecular mechanism responsible for the inhibition of Cl^- reabsorption is not yet known.

Spironolactone is a competitive antagonist of the mineralocorticoid, aldosterone. It competes for the aldosterone receptor site in the distal convoluted tubule. It interferes with the aldosterone-mediated Na^+–K^+ exchange, increasing Na^+ loss at the distal tubular site while decreasing K^+ loss.

Chlorothiazide inhibits Cl^- reabsorption in the ascending limb of the loop of Henle in addition to inhibiting Cl^- reabsorption in other areas of the nephron. The thiazides also can inhibit carbonic anhydrase but this is not the major mechanism of action.

Acetazolamide is a carbonic anhydrase inhibitor. It inhibits this enzyme at both the proximal and distal convoluted tubule. Carbon dioxide reabsorption from the glomerular filtrate is suppressed and HCO_3^- excretion is increased. Due to a decrease in the reabsorption of Na^+ in exchange for H^+, the Na^+–K^+ exchange in the distal convoluted tubule increases. The result is an alkaline urine.

Triamterene inhibits active Na^+ reabsorption and thus reduces the availability of Na^+ to the Na^+–K^+ exchange pump in the distal nephron, resulting in the decreased secretion of K^+.

7
Drugs Affecting Hematopoiesis and Hemostasis

I. DRUGS FOR IRON-DEFICIENCY ANEMIA: IRON AND IRON SALTS

A. PHYSIOLOGY

1. The major portion of iron in body stores is found in **hemoglobin**.
   a. Molecular oxygen is bound reversibly by the iron of hemoglobin.
   b. The ferric state of iron (Fe^{3+}) in methemoglobin is less able to carry oxygen than the Fe^{2+} in hemoglobin.

2. Inorganic iron in the ferrous (Fe^{2+}) form is most readily absorbed from the gastrointestinal tract.
   a. Men require a nutritional input of about 0.5 to 1 mg iron per day.
   b. Menstruating women require up to 2 mg per day.

3. About 1 mg of iron is lost per day in the feces, sweat, and desquamated skin.
   a. Menstruating women can lose up to 30 mg of iron per menstrual period.
   b. Pregnant women can lose up to 500 mg per full-term pregnancy.

4. About 1 gram of iron is stored as **ferritin** and **hemosiderin** in the bone marrow, liver, and spleen. This stored iron is available for the synthesis of hemoglobin should blood be lost from the body.

B. IRON-DEFICIENCY ANEMIA

1. Depletion of body iron can be associated with fatigability, anorexia, headache, and a characteristic hypochromic, microcytic anemia.

2. A low plasma iron level in iron-deficiency anemia is associated with an elevated total iron-binding capacity of plasma transferrin, so that the ratio of serum iron to iron-binding capacity is less than 10 percent:

$$\frac{\text{Serum iron level}}{\text{Total iron-binding capacity}} < 10\%$$

   In other words, the serum iron carrier, transferrin, is less than 10 percent saturated with iron. This ratio in normal individuals is $35\% \pm 15\%$.

3. A definitive diagnosis of iron-deficiency anemia is made by confirming reduced bone marrow iron stores.

4. Severe iron deficiency can cause Plummer-Vinson syndrome, which is associated with dysphagia, hypopharyngeal webs, gastritis, and hypochlorhydria.

5. Iron-deficiency anemia is often caused by significant blood loss. Underlying disorders should be sought where appropriate.

C. ORAL IRON

1. The different salt forms used in oral iron preparations have about the same bioavailability.
   a. **Ferrous sulfate,** containing about 20 percent elemental iron, is the drug of first choice for iron-deficiency anemia.

b. **Ferrous fumarate** contains 33 percent elemental iron. It is principally used as the iron in multivitamin–mineral mixtures.
c. **Ferrous choline citrate** contains 12 percent elemental iron.
d. **Ferrous gluconate** contains 12 percent elemental iron.

2. **Untoward effects** are related to the amount of soluble iron in the upper gastrointestinal tract.
   a. Nausea, heartburn, diarrhea, and constipation can all occur.
   b. Hemochromatosis is rare and is usually the result of an underlying disorder that augments the absorption of iron.

D. **PARENTERAL IRON** is used in patients unable to take iron orally and in patients with malabsorption syndromes.

1. **Iron dextran** is the preparation used parenterally.
   a. Iron dextran is a complex of ferric hydroxide and low-molecular-weight dextran.
   b. Each ml of iron dextran preparation contains 50 mg of elemental iron.
   c. Iron dextran delivered intramuscularly may become fixed (up to 50 percent) locally.
   d. Reticuloendothelial cells phagocytize the iron dextran, splitting off the iron from the dextran molecule.
   e. Due to serious local reactions, the intravenous route is preferred. A test dose is first given over a 5-minute period to test for anaphylaxis.

2. **Untoward effects**
   a. If given intramuscularly, iron dextran may cause local discomfort, discoloration, and potentially malignant skin changes. This route is therefore inappropriate unless the intravenous route is inaccessible.
   b. Headache, fever, arthralgias, and lymphadenopathy can occur.
   c. Anaphylactic reactions, though rare, can be fatal.

II. DRUGS USED IN MEGALOBLASTIC ANEMIAS

A. ETIOLOGY OF MEGALOBLASTIC ANEMIA

1. More than 95 percent of megaloblastic anemias are caused by deficiencies of vitamin B_{12} or folic acid.

2. The most helpful diagnostic tests are serum folate and vitamin B_{12} levels, the Schilling test for urinary vitamin B_{12} excretion, and analysis of gastric function.

B. FOLIC ACID

1. Folic acid is found in a wide variety of foods, with its highest content being found in yeast, liver, and green vegetables.

2. The minimum daily adult intake requirement is 50 μg.

3. **Physiology**
   a. Folic acid is completely absorbed in the proximal third of the small intestine.
   b. Folates present in food are in the reduced polyglutamate form. The mucosa of the duodenum and the upper jejunum contains dihydrofolate reductase, which methylates the reduced folate.
   c. Once absorbed, folate is transported to tissues where it is stored within cells as polyglutamates.
   d. Supplies are maintained by food intake and by the enterohepatic cycle.
   e. The urine is the major route of excretion for folates and their cleavage products.
   f. Folic acid is a precursor of several coenzymes, and several derivatives of tetrahydrofolic acid are important in single carbon atom transfers; for example, the synthesis of thymidylate from deoxyuridylate.

4. **Folate deficiency** can result from
   a. Inadequate dietary supply.
   b. Disease involving the small intestine.
   c. Defects in the folate enterohepatic cycle (e.g., hepatic toxicity from alcoholism).
   d. A low concentration of folate-binding proteins in plasma.

5. Normal pregnancy can also produce an increased requirement for folate intake.

6. Folate deficiency can result in megaloblastic anemia.
   a. The onset is more rapid than with a vitamin B_{12} deficiency.

b. There is *no* neurologic abnormality associated with folate deficiency.

7. Therapeutic uses

a. The major therapeutic use for folic acid is in the therapy of folic acid deficiency.

b. Leucovorin calcium injection (folinic acid) is used to circumvent the action of dihydrofolate reductase inhibitors such as methotrexate. It should *not* be used as a treatment for ordinary folate deficiency.

8. Preparation and administration

a. Folic acid can be given orally and will usually cure an uncomplicated megaloblastic anemia resulting from folate deficiency.

b. Folic acid injection contains the sodium salt, and is principally used in acute illness. It is given by intramuscular, intravenous, or deep subcutaneous injection.

c. Leucovorin calcium injection (folinic acid) is administered intramuscularly.

9. Untoward effects

a. The oral form is nontoxic at therapeutic doses.

b. Large amounts may counteract the antiepileptic action of phenobarbital, phenytoin, and primidone.

c. There have been rare allergic reactions to parenteral administration.

C. VITAMIN B_{12}

1. Physiology

a. Vitamin B_{12} (cyanocobalamin) is a cobalt-containing compound that is synthesized by the bacterial flora in the colon. However, it cannot be absorbed there, and humans must obtain the vitamin from the dietary intake of animal products.

b. Intrinsic factor, a glycoprotein produced by the gastric parietal cells, is necessary for the gastrointestinal absorption of vitamin B_{12}.

(1) Gastric acid releases the vitamin from proteins, allowing it to become complexed to intrinsic factor.

(2) The vitamin B_{12}–intrinsic factor complex binds to ileal mucosal cell receptors whence it is transported into the circulation.

c. Once in the circulation, vitamin B_{12} is transported to the tissues by a plasma β-globulin, transcobalamin II.

d. The liver preferentially stores vitamin B_{12}. A portion of the stored vitamin is secreted into the bile each day and is normally reabsorbed in the ileum.

e. Vitamin B_{12} is essential for cell growth and for maintenance of normal myelin. It is also important for the normal metabolic functions of folate.

2. Vitamin B_{12} deficiency can result from

a. An insufficient dietary supply.

b. Inadequate secretion of intrinsic factor.

c. Ileal disease.

d. Congenital absence of transcobalamin II.

e. Interference with the reabsorption of vitamin B_{12} excreted in the bile.

3. Vitamin B_{12} deficiency can result in

a. Megaloblastic anemia. Although this is most common, all blood cell lines can be affected, resulting in panycytopenia.

b. Demyelination and cell death. This can produce irreversible damage to the central nervous system.

4. Therapeutic uses

a. The most common justified therapeutic use for vitamin vitamin B_{12} is the treatment of pernicious anemia (addisonian anemia). This condition is usually caused by atrophy of the gastric mucosa with achlorhydria and failure to secrete intrinsic factor; maintenance therapy with vitamin B_{12} is required for life.

b. Vitamin B_{12} should not be used as a placebo.

5. Preparation and administration

a. If the patient lacks intrinsic factor or has ileal disease, vitamin B_{12} must be administered parenterally. Cyanocobalamin injection, a bright red solution, is administered by the intramuscular or deep subcutaneous route but never intravenously.

b. Combinations of oral vitamin B_{12} with intrinsic factor usually produce unreliable absorption, and therefore this approach is not recommended.

6. Untoward effects from vitamin B_{12} administration are rare.

III. HEMOSTASIS AND ANTICOAGULANTS

A. HEPARIN

1. Pharmacologic properties
- **a.** Heparin prolongs the clotting time of blood, both in vivo and in vitro.
- **b.** This highly negatively charged mucopolysaccharide is prepared commercially from bovine lung and porcine intestinal mucosa.
- **c.** Heparin prevents fibrin formation in the process of coagulation.
  - **(1)** It increases the activity of antithrombin III.
  - **(2)** Antithrombin III then inhibits the conversion of prothrombin to thrombin by thromboplastin.
  - **(3)** Antithrombin III also directly inactivates thrombin.
- **d.** Injected heparin causes the release of tissue-bound lipoprotein lipase, which hydrolyzes the triglycerides of chylomicrons and low-density lipoproteins bound to capillary endothelial cells. This produces a clearing effect on postprandial turbid lipemic plasma.
- **e.** Heparin suppresses the rate of aldosterone secretion and increases the concentration of free thyroxine.
- **f.** Heparin slows wound healing and probably also depresses cell-mediated immunity.

2. Pharmacokinetics
- **a.** Because of its highly negative charge and large molecular size, heparin is administered parenterally.
- **b.** It displays dose-dependent half-life kinetics.
- **c.** Heparin is metabolized in the liver by heparinase. The inactive products are excreted in the urine.
- **d.** Intramuscular injections are contraindicated because they cause painful hematomas.

3. Preparation and therapeutic uses
- **a.** Since the anticoagulants reduce the rate of fibrin formation, they are primarily used in the prophylaxis of venous thrombosis. Venous (red) thrombi consist of a fibrin network enmeshed with red blood cells and platelets.
- **b.** The anticoagulants are generally ineffective in the treatment of arterial (white) thrombi, made up of adhering platelets. Arterial thrombi are treated with the antithrombotics and thrombolytics (see III, C, below).
- **c.** The prophylactic treatment of venous thrombotic disease usually involves continuous infusion of **heparin sodium injection**, as well as intravenous bolus administration.
- **d.** In the preoperative use of heparin to prevent postoperative venous thrombosis and embolism, a low dose is given by subcutaneous injection. This is followed by additional intermittent subcutaneous injections.

4. Heparin therapy is monitored by the partial thromboplastin time (PTT).
- **a.** The test is done at any time during continuous infusion therapy; if the heparin is given intermittently, the PTT is measured prior to an injection.
- **b.** During therapy, the PTT should be twice the control value.
- **c.** Once the PTT is stable, daily monitoring is performed.

5. Untoward effects and contraindications
- **a.** Hypersensitivity reactions can occur. A test dose should be given to patients with a prior allergic history.
- **b.** Hemorrhage due to excessive blockade of fibrin formation and interference with normal hemostasis accounts for the primary toxicity of heparin. Bleeding should be reduced by careful control of dosage.
- **c.** Osteoporosis may complicate prolonged heparin therapy.
- **d.** Transient alopecia can occur.
- **e.** Transient thrombocytopenia can occur in up to 25 percent of patients receiving heparin therapy. This can result from heparin-induced platelet aggregation; more severe cases result from the formation of heparin-dependent antiplatelet antibodies.
- **f.** Heparin is contraindicated in patients who are hypersensitive to the drug. Bacterial endocarditis, active tuberculosis, and certain types of surgery are also contraindications for heparin administration.

6. Reversal of the anticoagulant actions
- **a.** Often, discontinuation of heparin therapy is sufficient to correct excessive anticoagulant effects.
- **b.** If rapid reversal is indicated, the strongly basic protamine sulfate is given by slow intravenous injection.
  - **(1)** About 1 to 1.5 mg of protamine sulfate will usually antagonize 100 units of heparin.

(2) Protamine inhibits the anticoagulant effect of heparin but not necessarily the effect of heparin on platelet aggregation.

B. ORAL ANTICOAGULANTS

1. Warfarin sodium is the drug of choice and is considered the prototype of the **coumarin-derived anticoagulants.**

2. Pharmacologic properties

a. The coumarin-derived anticoagulants interfere with vitamin K–dependent synthesis of active coagulation factors II (prothrombin) VII, IX, and X.

b. They are effective only in vivo. Their therapeutic effect is dependent on the half-lives of factors II, VII, IX, and X, and thus 8 to 12 hours are required for action.

3. Factors affecting activity

a. Anything that can cause vitamin K deficiency, such as disease of the small bowel, can increase the response to these anticoagulants.

b. Impaired hepatic synthesis of clotting factors can lead to an increased hypoprothrombinemic response to oral anticoagulants during hepatic disease or in alcoholic individuals. Excessively reduced levels of prothrombin will result in hemorrhage.

c. Hypermetabolic states such as hyperthyroidism increase the response to oral anticoagulants.

d. The older the patient, the greater the response to these anticoagulants.

e. During pregnancy, vitamin K–dependent factors are increased, resulting in a decreased responsiveness to oral anticoagulants. Since heparin does not cross the placenta, it is considered safe for the fetus.

f. Drug interactions. Table 7-1 lists the drugs which increase or decrease the response to oral anticoagulants.

Table 7-1. Drug Interactions with Oral Anticoagulants

Drugs	**Effect on Reponse to Anticoagulant**	**Mechanism**
Acetylsalicylic acid	↑	↓ADP release by platelets, impairing platelet aggregation
Phenylbutazone, oxyphenbutazone	↑	Impair platelet aggregation; displace warfarin from albumin
Disulfiram, metronidazole, trimethoprim-sulfamethoxazole	↑	↑hypoprothrombinemia by prolonging levowarfarin half-life
Cimetidine	↑	Unknown
Clofibrate	↑	↓platelet adhesiveness and ↑ turnover of vitamin K–dependent factors
Barbiturates, glutethimide	↓	Induce drug microsomal metabolizing system
Rifampin	↓	↓blood concentration of drug
Cholestyramine	↓	↓hypoprothrombinemia; ↑plasma clearance of drug

4. Pharmacokinetics

a. Racemic warfarin (i.e., the mixture of the dextro- and levo- forms) is well absorbed orally and reaches peak plasma concentrations in one hour.

b. It is 99 percent bound to plasma albumin, which prevents its diffusion into red blood cells, cerebrospinal fluid, urine, and breast milk.

c. It is metabolized in the liver and undergoes enterohepatic circulation, and then is excreted in the urine and feces.

5. Preparations and therapeutic uses

a. For warfarin sodium and warfarin potassium the maintenance dose is determined by one-stage prothrombin activity, which should be about 1½ to 2½ times the control value. Once the prothrombin activity is stable, bimonthly checks are sufficient.

b. Warfarin sodium is available in injectable form, but parenteral administration is seldom needed.

c. These agents are widely used in the secondary prophylactic treatment of venous thrombosis and pulmonary embolism, to prevent the recurrence or extension of venous thrombus formation.

d. Since oral anticoagulants have no effect on platelets, they are not used in the treatment of thrombotic disease in the arterial system.

6. Untoward effects

a. Hemorrhage is the most important complication, as in the case of heparin administration.

b. Anorexia, urticaria, purpura, and alopecia have occurred.

7. Reversal of anticoagulant effects

a. Following discontinuation of oral anticoagulants, the one-stage prothrombin time gradually returns to normal. Oral administration of vitamin K_1 (phytonadione) will enhance recovery.

b. For severe hemorrhage, phytonadione is given intravenously. The one-stage prothrombin activity will return to normal within 6 to 12 hours, whatever the amount of coumarin anticoagulant ingested. The phytonadione is administered slowly to avoid precipitating a hypotensive episode. Fresh frozen plasma or coagulation-factor concentrate may be needed when bleeding is severe.

C. ANTITHROMBOTIC AND THROMBOLYTIC DRUGS

1. The term **antithrombotic** is reserved for those agents that prevent or reduce the formation of platelet thrombi in the arterial system.

2. The antithrombotic actions of **aspirin** and **sulfinpyrazone** are discussed in Chapter 9 (II B 6 and X C 5, respectively) and those of **dipyridamole** in chapter 5 (IV D 3).

3. Thrombolytic drugs are used in acute, extensive thromboembolic disease because of their ability to dissolve thrombi by bringing about the conversion of endogenous plasminogen to plasmin, a protease. The newly formed plasmin hydrolyzes fibrin in hemostatic plugs and degrades fibrinogen and factors V and VII.

a. **Streptokinase** is obtained from group C β-hemolytic streptococci.

(1) Intravenous streptokinase has been used to treat acute pulmonary embolism and deep vein thrombosis.

(2) Thrombin time is monitored during therapy and should be 2 to 5 times the control value.

(3) Heparin and oral anticoagulants are given once streptokinase therapy is terminated.

(4) Because streptokinase therapy results in degradation of fibrinogen and factors V and VII, the incidence of bleeding can be high.

(5) Fever and allergic reactions are common.

b. **Urokinase** was originally isolated from human urine. It is given by intravenous injection.

(1) Thrombin time is evaluated before subsequent heparin therapy is started.

(2) Excessive bleeding results twice as often in urokinase-treated patients as in patients treated with heparin.

(3) Since urokinase therapy is very expensive, it is limited to those patients allergic to streptokinase.

4. **Antagonists. Aminocaproic acid** is a specific fibrinolysis antagonist that is given intravenously until bleeding caused by a thrombolytic drug is under control. Too rapid intravenous administration can lead to cardiac irregularities.

STUDY QUESTIONS

Directions: Each question below contains five suggested answers. Choose the **one best** response to each question.

1. All of the following statements about iron-deficiency anemia are true EXCEPT

(A) menstruating females require about twice as much dietary iron as men do
(B) iron deficiency can lead to the Plummer-Vinson syndrome
(C) ferrous sulfate is the drug of first choice for iron-deficiency anemia
(D) ferrous sulfate contains more than 90 percent elemental iron
(E) diarrhea or constipation can occur with ferrous sulfate use

2. Which of the following drug and drug effect pairs is INCORRECTLY matched?

(A) Urokinase—converts plasminogen to plasmin
(B) Heparin—prevents fibrin formation
(C) Heparin—antagonized by zinc sulfate
(D) Warfarin sodium—interferes with vitamin K-dependent reactions
(E) Warfarin sodium—interferes with the synthesis of clotting factors

3. All of the following statements about therapeutic iron preparations are true EXCEPT that

(A) ferrous sulfate is the drug of first choice for iron-deficiency anemia
(B) ferrous sulfate contains about 20 percent elemental iron
(C) untoward effects of ferrous sulfate are often inversely related to the amount of soluble iron in the upper gastrointestinal tract
(D) iron dextran is useful in treating patients with malabsorption syndromes
(E) reticuloendothelial cells phagocytize iron dextran

Directions: Each question below contains four suggested answers of which **one or more** is correct. Choose the answer

A if **1, 2, and 3** are correct
B if **1 and 3** are correct
C if **2 and 4** are correct
D if **4** is correct
E if **1, 2, 3, and 4** are correct

4. Vitamin B_{12} deficiency can result from

(1) an insufficient dietary supply
(2) inadequate secretion of intrinsic factor
(3) ileal disease
(4) excessive transcobalamin II

5. The thrombolytic agent streptokinase has which of the following properties?

(1) It is obtained from group C β-hemolytic streptococci
(2) It stimulates the conversion of endogenous plasminogen to plasmin
(3) It has been used to treat acute pulmonary embolism
(4) It produces fever and allergic reactions infrequently

6. Correct statements about the anticoagulant heparin include which of the following?

(1) It is effective in vivo and in vitro
(2) It is antagonized by vitamin K
(3) It prolongs the partial thromboplastin time (PTT)
(4) Approximately 25 percent is orally absorbed

7. Correct statements about folic acid include which of the following?

(1) It is completely absorbed in the proximal third of the small intestine
(2) The urine is the major route of excretion
(3) Deficiency can be a result of inadequate dietary intake
(4) A deficiency of folic acid is usually associated with neurologic complications

SUMMARY OF DIRECTIONS

A	B	C	D	E
1, 2, 3 only	1, 3 only	2, 4 only	4 only	All are correct

8. In which of the following pairs is the anticoagulant drug correctly matched with its characteristic?

(1) Heparin—is a strongly positively charged molecule
(2) Warfarin sodium—overdose is treated with vitamin K
(3) Warfarin sodium—overdose results in a shortened prothrombin time (PT)
(4) Heparin—prevents the conversion of prothrombin to thrombin

9. Correct statements concerning vitamin B_{12} deficiency include which of the following?

(1) It is capable of producing demyelination and irreversible neurologic damage
(2) It is associated with a defect in folate-binding proteins
(3) It is one of two major causes of megaloblastic anemia
(4) It is treated by leucovorin administration

10. Which of the following drugs, if given concomitantly with warfarin, would probably require a reduction in warfarin dosage?

(1) Disulfiram
(2) Aspirin
(3) Phenylbutazone
(4) Barbiturates

11. Which of the following substances help to prevent or reduce arterial thrombi?

(1) Warfarin
(2) Urokinase
(3) Heparin
(4) Aspirin

12. Heparin administration would be contraindicated in which of the following situations?

(1) Known hypersensitivity
(2) Bacterial endocarditis
(3) Active tuberculosis
(4) Diffuse intravascular coagulopathy

13. The therapeutic effect of sodium warfarin is dependent on the half-lives of which of the following coagulation factors?

(1) IX
(2) X
(3) II
(4) VII

14. The response to a dose of an anticoagulant is often changed by concomitant administration of other drugs, which affect the dose-response by different mechanisms. Which of the following drugs and mechanisms are CORRECTLY matched?

(1) Phenylbutazone—impairs platelet aggregation
(2) Phenobarbital—induces drug microsomal metabolism system
(3) Acetylsalicylic acid—impairs platelet aggregation
(4) Glutethimide—inhibits drug microsomal metabolizing system

15. Folate deficiency can result from

(1) an inadequate dietary supply
(2) disease involving the small intestine
(3) a low concentration of folate-binding proteins in plasma
(4) defects in the folate enterohepatic cycle

ANSWERS AND EXPLANATIONS

1. The answer is D. *(I A 2, B 4, C 1 a, 2)* Ferrous sulfate contains about 20 percent elemental iron. All of the other statements are true. Men require about 0.5–1 mg of iron daily, while menstruating females require up to 2 mg/day. The Plummer-Vinson syndrome is associated with severe iron deficiency and is characterized by dysphagia, hypopharyngeal webs, gastritis, and hypochlorhydria. Diarrhea or constipation, nausea, and heartburn can all occur with oral iron preparations.

2. The answer is C. *(III A 1 c, 6 b, B 2 a, C 3)* The antidote for heparin is protamine sulfate. It is strongly basic, and 1 to 1.5 mg of protamine sulfate will antagonize 100 units of heparin. All of the other drugs listed in the question are correctly matched with their effects.

3. The answer is C. *(I C; D)* Ferrous sulfate, which contains 20 percent elemental iron, is the drug of first choice for iron-deficiency anemia. The untoward effects seen with ferrous sulfate are directly, not inversely, related to the amount of soluble iron in the upper gastrointestinal tract. Iron dextran, which is parenterally administered, is useful in patients with malabsorption syndromes. The iron is split off from the sugar molecule of iron dextran by phagocytization in the reticuloendothelial cells.

4. The answer is A (1, 2, 3). *(II C 2)* Because vitamin B_{12} is available in many dietary animal products, and because only minute amounts are required, vitamin B_{12} deficiency is highly unlikely to occur, except in strict vegetarians or in those with ileal disease or with inadequate secretion of intrinsic factor. Congenital absence of transcobalamin II, the plasma β-globulin that transports vitamin B_{12}, can also result in vitamin B_{12} deficiency.

5. The answer is A (1, 2, 3). *(III C 3)* Fever and allergic reactions are fairly common side effects of streptokinase. All of the other statements about this thrombolytic agent are correct. Streptokinase is a protein without known enzymatic activity that is obtained from group C β-hemolytic streptococci. Its interaction with a proactivator of plasminogen results in a proteolytic activity that converts plasminogen to plasmin, which is then capable of hydrolyzing fibrin clots. This property is the basis for the use of streptokinase in treating acute pulmonary embolism.

6. The answer is B (1, 3). *(III A 1 a, 2, 4, 6 b)* Heparin is effective in vivo and in vitro. It is antagonized by protamine sulfate, not by vitamin K. The partial thromboplastin time (PTT) is the only laboratory test that is used to monitor the action of heparin; during therapy, the PTT should be twice the control value. Due to its large molecular size and polarity, heparin is only administered parenterally.

7. The answer is A (1, 2, 3). *(7, II B 3, 4, 6)* Folate deficiency can result in megaloblastic anemia. There is *no* neurologic abnormality associated with folate deficiency. This is in contrast to vitamin B_{12} deficiency, which produces both effects. The remaining statements listed in the question are true.

8. The answer is C (2, 4). *(III A 1, B 5 a, 7)* Heparin is a negatively charged mucopolysaccharide which does interfere with the conversion of prothrombin to thrombin. An overdose of warfarin sodium is effectively treated with vitamin K; however, an overdose will result in a lengthened prothrombin time (PT).

9. The answer is B (1, 3). *(II C)* Vitamin B_{12} is essential for the maintenance of myelin and for normal cell growth. Neurologic abnormalities are associated with vitamin B_{12} deficiency. A deficiency of either folate or vitamin B_{12}, or of both, accounts for 95 percent of megaloblastic anemias. Folate-binding proteins are important for folic acid transport but are not involved in vitamin B_{12} transport. Leucovorin (folinic acid) is an antidote for the antimetabolite methotrexate but is not used to treat vitamin B_{12} deficiency, nor is it usually used for ordinary folate deficiency.

10. The answer is A (1, 2, 3). *(III B 3; Table 7-1)* Warfarin, a coumarin-derived anticoagulant, acts by interfering with the vitamin K–dependent synthesis of active coagulation factors II, VII, IX, and X. Disulfiram, aspirin, and phenylbutazone increase the response to warfarin and other oral anticoagulants, and thus their use would probably require a reduction in warfarin dosage. Disulfiram affects warfarin activity by prolonging the half-life of levowarfarin, and this effect increases hypoprothrombinemia. Aspirin and phenylbutazone both impair platelet aggregation. Barbiturates and glutethimide have the reverse effects on anticoagulation. These drugs reduce the response to warfarin, and thus would probably require an increase in warfarin dosage, because they induce the hepatic enzyme system that increases drug metabolism.

11. The answer is C (2, 4). *(III A 3 b, B 5 d, C 2, 3; Chapter 9, II B 6)* Heparin and warfarin are anticoagulants, and thus are ineffective in the treatment of arterial (white cell) thrombi, which are made up of adhering platelets. Heparin reduces the rate of fibrin formation, and thus is primarily used in the prophylaxis of venous thrombosis, which consists of a fibrin network of red cells and platelets. Warfarin is used in the secondary prophylactic treatment of venous thrombosis and pulmonary embolism. Aspirin and urokinase are both antithrombotic drugs, that is, agents that prevent or reduce the formation of platelet thrombi in the arterial system.

12. The answer is A (1, 2, 3). *(III A 5 f)* Hypersensitivity reactions to heparin can occur, and patients with a known hypersensitivity should not be given the drug. Bacterial endocarditis and active tuberculosis are also contraindications to heparin use. Heparin is an acceptable form of therapy for diffuse intravascular coagulation.

13. The answer is E (all). *(III B 2 b)* Sodium warfarin is the prototype of the coumarin-derived anticoagulants. The therapeutic effect of this class of anticoagulants is dependent on the half-lives of factors II, VII, IX, and X and thus 8 to 12 hours are required for action.

14. The answer is A (1, 2, 3). *(III, Table 7-1)* Both phenylbutazone and aspirin affect platelet aggregation; phenylbutazone is also capable of displacing warfarin from albumin. These two drugs, therefore, *increase* the response to oral anticoagulants, which can cause severe hemorrhage. Phenylbutazone, in addition, can displace warfarin from albumin, which increases the warfarin blood level. Glutethimide, like phenobarbital and other barbiturates, induces the drug microsomal metabolizing system. This *decreases* the response to oral anticoagulants, so that higher doses are required to produce the desired anticoagulant effect.

15. The answer is E (all). *(II B 4 a, d)* Folate deficiency can result from an inadequate dietary supply or disease which would affect its absorption in the small intestine. Low concentrations of folate binding proteins in plasma can result in folate deficiency. Hepatic toxicity from alcoholism can result in defects in the folate enterohepatic cycle.

8
Autacoids and Their Antagonists

I. INTRODUCTION

A. DEFINITIONS

1. **Autacoids** are circulating or locally acting hormone-like substances which originate from diffuse tissues.
2. **Autacoid antagonists** are agents that inhibit the synthesis or the receptor interactions of certain autacoids.

B. PHYSIOLOGIC ROLES

1. Two main functions of the autacoids are to modulate local circulation and to influence the process of inflammation.
2. Other physiologic—and pathologic—functions of many autacoids remain obscure.
3. Some autacoid antagonists have important therapeutic value.

C. MAJOR CLASSES. Autacoids can be divided into three categories on the basis of their structure:

1. **Decarboxylated amino acids:** Histamine, serotonin.
2. **Polypeptides:** Angiotensins, kinins, vasoactive intestinal polypeptide, substance P.
3. **Eicosanoids:** Prostaglandins, leukotrienes, thromboxanes.

II. AUTACOIDS

A. HISTAMINE

1. Structure

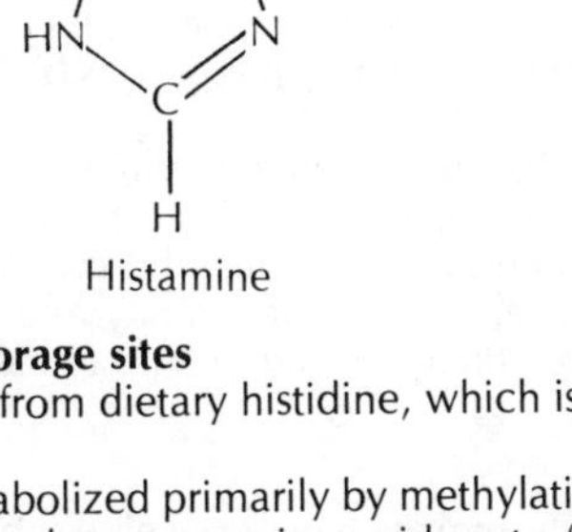

H, $CH_2CH_2NH_2$, C=C, HN, N, C, H

Histamine

2. Synthesis, metabolism, and storage sites

a. Histamine is derived chiefly from dietary histidine, which is decarboxylated by L-histidine decarboxylase.

b. In humans, histamine is metabolized primarily by methylation to form 1-methylhistamine, which can undergo oxidation by monoamine oxidase to form 1-methylimidazole-acetic acid.

c. Histamine is stored in almost all mammalian tissues, although its concentration varies greatly.

(1) Mast cells are the primary storage sites, although some nonmast cells can store the autacoid.

(2) In most nonmast cells, histamine is synthesized but not stored.

(a) Histamine that is stored in the mucosal cells of the stomach can be released by mechanical stimuli, such as food and vagal stimulation. The released gastric histamine regulates intestinal contraction and gastric secretion.

(b) In skin and lung tissue, histamine is thought to be important in tissue growth and repair as well as in allergic responses.

(c) In the central nervous system, a high concentration of histamine can be found in the hypothalamus, where it is thought to be released as a neurotransmitter.

3. Mechanism of action

a. Histamine acts via specific cell surface receptors.

b. It is currently believed that stimulation by cyclic adenosine monophosphate (cyclic AMP) or increased calcium influx may be important mediators of certain histamine actions.

4. Receptor classification. Two classes of receptors mediate the action of histamine.

a. H_1 receptors are responsible for the bronchoconstriction and intestinal contraction produced by histamine. 2-Methylhistamine is the prototypic H_1 receptor agonist, and pyrilamine is the prototypic antagonist.

b. H_2 receptors are responsible for gastric secretion caused by histamine. 4-Methylhistamine is the prototypic H_2 receptor agonist, and cimetidine is the prototypic antagonist.

5. Pharmacologic effects. Considerable species differences exist; human pharmacology is listed below.

a. Extravascular smooth muscles

(1) The activation of H_1 receptors in bronchial smooth muscle results in bronchoconstriction and decreased lung capacity.

(2) The activation of H_1 receptors on gastrointestinal smooth muscle produces spasmodic contractions.

b. Cardiovascular system

(1) Histamine dilates the fine vessels of the microcirculation and causes increased permeability. This results in local edema.

(2) A decrease in blood pressure reflects the capillary and arteriolar dilation.

(3) Histamine produces a positive inotropic and chronotropic effect that is mediated by both H_1 and H_2 receptors.

(4) An intradermal injection of histamine results in the classic **triple response:**

(a) A **reddening** at the site of injection due to local vasodilation.

(b) A **wheal,** or disk of edema, due to increased capillary permeability, seen within 1 or 2 minutes after the histamine injection.

(c) A bright crimson **flare** or halo surrounding the wheal, which may be as large as 5 cm and may last for 10 minutes.

c. Exocrine glands

(1) Histamine is a potent gastric secretagogue, causing the release of large quantities of highly acidic gastric juices, pepsin, and the intrinsic factor of Castle.

(2) Histamine also can stimulate pancreatic and bronchiolar secretion, as well as lacrimation and salivation.

6. Physiologic and pathologic roles

a. Gastric secretion: Histamine is a mediator of normal gastric secretion.

b. Allergic reactions and anaphylactic shock: Histamine is one of several autacoids that participate in hypersensitivity reactions. Antigenic substances cause the release of histamine when they bind to immunoglobulin E (IgE) molecules located on a mast cell membrane.

c. Inflammation: Histamine may be responsible for the delayed vasodilation seen in inflammatory responses.

d. Tissue repair and growth: A high histamine-synthesizing capacity is found in rapidly proliferating tissues; for example, in liver, bone marrow, and a variety of malignancies.

e. Neurotransmission: Histamine may be involved in the initiation of sensory impulses for pain and itching; also, high concentrations are found in the hypothalamus.

f. Regulation of the microcirculation: Histamine plays a role through its vasoactive properties.

7. Clinical uses

a. Histamine and its analogs have no well established therapeutic uses.

b. However, they can be used diagnostically to distinguish between pernicious anemia and other forms of anemia. The loss of the gastric parietal cells in pernicious anemia results in an inability to secrete gastric acid in response to histamine.

8. **Preparations**
   a. Histamine phosphate is injected intravenously. It has been used as a diagnostic agent for testing gastric acid secretion, but side effects (see II A 9, below) have limited its use.
   b. **Betazole hydrochloride** is an isomer of histamine with preferential effects on gastric secretion: it is ten times more potent as a stimulator of gastric secretion than as a vasodilator. It is used as an alternative for histamine phosphate in tests of gastric function because it does not require premedication with a H_1 or H_2 receptor blocker.
   c. **Pentagastrin** is a pentapeptide that also stimulates the secretion of gastric acid, pepsin, and the intrinsic factor of Castle. The gastric secretory responses are similar to those induced by histamine or betazole. It has become popular because it is short-acting and has minimal untoward effects.

9. **Untoward effects of histamine**
   a. Cardiovascular effects include vasodilation, which produces a decrease in blood pressure; flushing; and tachycardia.
   b. Skin temperature increases, and headache and visual disturbances occur.
   c. Bronchoconstriction, dyspnea, and diarrhea are caused by smooth muscle stimulation.

B. SEROTONIN (5-HYDROXYTRYPTAMINE)

1. **Synthesis and structure.** 5-Hydroxytryptamine is primarily derived from dietary tryptophan, which is first hydroxylated and then decarboxylated to form serotonin.

Serotonin

2. **Metabolism, distribution, and function**
   a. Serotonin is initially deaminated by monoamine oxidase to form 5-hydroxyindoleacetaldehyde and is then rapidly oxidized to the major metabolite, 5-hydroxyindoleacetic acid.
   b. Ninety percent of the body's serotonin is found in the enterochromaffin and enterochromaffin-like cells of the gastrointestinal tract. The function of this serotonin is uncertain.
   c. Serotonin is also found in platelets, where its function is not established, and in the central nervous system, where it is believed to be involved with the regulation of temperature, sleep, aggression, pain, and mood. As a component of the pineal gland, serotonin functions as a precursor of melatonin, a hormone that may influence endocrine function.
   d. Carcinoid tumors synthesize large quantities of serotonin.

3. **Pharmacologic effects.** Serotonin, like histamine, shows wide species variations; human pharmacology is listed below.
   a. Serotonin constricts most arteries and veins, especially in the renal and splanchnic beds.
   b. It is notable that serotonin dilates the blood vessels in skeletal muscle.
   c. Serotonin produces a positive inotropic and chronotropic effect on the heart, but these effects may be masked by reflex responses.
   d. The effects of a serotonin injection are complex.
      (1) Initially, a brief depressor phase is seen, which is the result of a transient reflex response to serotonin and vagus nerve stimulation.
      (2) This phase is followed by an increase in blood pressure, which is due to an increase in cardiac output and a reduction in peripheral resistance.
      (3) Finally, a prolonged depressor action results from the dilation of blood vessels in skeletal muscles.

4. Serotonin currently has no **therapeutic use.**

C. ANGIOTENSINS. The angiotensins are a group of polypeptide autacoids.

1. **Synthesis**
   a. The precursor for all angiotensins is **angiotensinogen,** a plasma α-globulin.
   b. Angiotensinogen is metabolized by renin to form the decapeptide **angiotensin I.**
   c. Angiotensin I is hydrolyzed by a peptidyl dipeptidase, called **angiotensin-converting enzyme.** This enzyme is found in large amounts on capillary endothelial cells in the lung. Its product is the pharmacologically active octapeptide, **angiotensin II.**

d. Angiotensin II is metabolized by an aminopeptidase to form a less active autacoid, angiotensin III.
e. Other routes of metabolism have been observed but appear not to be as important as those listed above.

2. Pharmacologic effects

a. One of the major functions of the **renin–angiotensin system** is to regulate blood pressure.
  (1) Renin, a juxtaglomerular enzyme, controls the formation of angiotensin II, which causes vasoconstriction.
  (2) Angiotensin II is one of the most potent vasoconstrictors known, being 40 times more potent than norepinephrine.
  (3) Angiotensin II has a positive inotropic and chronotropic effect, which is due to central and peripheral sympathetic stimulation.
b. In addition to its centrally mediated hypertensive effect, blood-borne angiotensin II has a centrally mediated dipsogenic action.
c. Angiotensin II also stimulates sympathetic ganglion cells and enhances ganglionic transmission. This may be mediated by increased biosynthesis of norepinephrine, decreased reuptake of norepinephrine, or increased release of the neurotransmitter.
d. Angiotensin II stimulates the synthesis and secretion of aldosterone, but this has very little effect on blood pressure.
e. Angiotensin II can stimulate the secretion of antidiuretic hormone when injected intraventricularly.

3. Mechanism of action

a. Angiotensin II acts through specific cell surface receptors located on target tissues.
b. The precise mechanism responsible for the ultimate pharmacologic effects of angiotensin II remains unknown, but both prostaglandins and cyclic nucleotides have been implicated.

4. Therapeutic uses

a. There are no approved therapeutic uses for angiotensin.
b. Angiotensin II amide, given as an infusion, has produced a sustained pressor response, but its value in the treatment of shock is controversial because the vasoconstriction that angiotensin produces can lead to decreased tissue and organ perfusion.

D. KININS

1. Synthesis and degradation

a. Like angiotensin, the kinins are vasodilating polypeptides.
b. Two enzymes, called **kallikreins,** catalyze the formation of the plasma kinins kallidin, a decapeptide, and bradykinin, a nonapeptide.
  (1) A high-molecular-weight complex in the plasma made of prekallikrein and an α_2-globulin called kininogen, is the precursor.
  (2) The prekallikrein, which is activated by the Hageman factor (coagulation factor XII) and plasmin, rapidly hydrolyzes high-molecular weight kininogen to form **bradykinin.**
  (3) In the tissues low-molecular-weight kininogens are hydrolyzed by tissue and glandular kallikrein to form **kallidin** (lysyl-bradykinin), which is further converted to bradykinin by plasma and tissue aminopeptidases.
c. Extensive biochemical control mechanisms exist to regulate the formation and degradation of the kinins.
d. Bradykinin is inactivated by the same peptidyl dipeptidase that converts angiotensin I to angiotensin II (see II C 1 c, above).

2. Pharmacologic effects

a. Kinins are potent vasodilators. They act directly on smooth muscles of fine resistance vessels and will also cause the classic triple response seen with histamine (see II A 5 b (4), above).
b. Kinins are powerful algesic agents, an action mediated by a direct stimulation of nerve endings.
c. In contrast to their actions on the fine resistance vessels, plasma kinins cause constriction of large arteries and most large and small veins.
d. Kinins affect the neonatal circulation, causing constriction of the ductus arteriosus, ductus venosus, and umbilical vessels, and dilation of the pulmonary vessels.
e. Kinins are capable of constricting most nonvascular smooth muscle (e.g., bronchiolar, gastrointestinal).

3. Although the **mechanism of action** of kinins is not well understood, some responses may be

mediated by prostaglandins resulting from the stimulation of phospholipase A_2 (see II G 1 d, below).

4. No **therapeutic use** currently exists for kinins.

E. VASOACTIVE INTESTINAL POLYPEPTIDE (VIP)

1. This autacoid derives its name from the original site of isolation, but it is prevalent in both central and peripheral nerves, including those serving the pancreas.

2. It is a potent vasodilator and a pancreatic secretagogue.

F. SUBSTANCE P

1. An undecapeptide, substance P produces vasodilation; contraction of various smooth muscles, including intestinal muscle; salivary secretion; and diuresis.

2. Substance P causes depolarization of central and peripheral nervous system neurons, an action which is believed to be responsible for many of its effects.

3. Substance P is thought to be a neurotransmitter and, in addition, is found in enterochromaffin cells. It is secreted by enterochromaffin tumors and thus plays a role in the carcinoid syndrome.

G. PROSTAGLANDINS, THROMBOXANES, AND LEUKOTRIENES

1. **Synthesis**
   a. The prostaglandins and related autacoids are ubiquitous substances, and are derived from unsaturated 20-carbon essential fatty acids, primarily **arachidonic acid**, which is a component of membrane phospholipids.
   b. These autacoids are synthesized de novo by a complex biochemical pathway and generally are not stored. The major synthetic steps are shown in Figure 8-1.
   c. The numeric subscripts used with the prostaglandins (PGs), thromboxanes (TXs), and leukotrienes denote the number of double bonds in the alkyl side chain.
   d. The essential fatty acid precursors are released from lipid storage sites by a group of enzymes called acylhydrolases; the most notable enzyme is **phospholipase A_2.**
      (1) The activity of the acylhydrolases is stimulated by a wide variety of physical, chemical, hormonal, and neurochemical influences.
      (2) The result of acylhydrolase activation is the release of **arachidonic acid.**
   e. Once released, arachidonic acid can be rapidly metabolized by two distinct enzyme activities, cyclooxygenase and lipoxygenase.
      (1) The **cyclooxygenases** oxygenate and cyclize arachidonic acid to form the cyclic endoperoxides PGG_2 and PGH_2, which are the precursors for other prostaglandins, including prostacyclin (PGI_2), and for the thromboxanes.
      (2) The **lipoxygenases** form the leukotrienes.
   f. Most of these autacoids are rapidly inactivated and thus have short-lived biologic activities.

2. **Physiologic effects**
   a. The physiologic role and pharmacologic actions of the prostaglandins, thromboxanes, and leukotrienes are extensive and still being discovered.
   b. It appears that these autacoids act frequently as **modulators** of neural and hormonal activities. Often two autacoids of this class have opposing effects in a given tissue.
   c. Some important functions are as follows:
      (1) In the **central nervous system**, both stimulation and depression have been observed with specific prostaglandins.
         (a) Prostaglandins of the E series are pyrogens when injected into the cerebral ventricles.
         (b) Prostaglandins may be involved in regulating food and water consumption.
         (c) Prostaglandins modulate the actions of peptide neurotransmitters and hormones.
      (2) Prostaglandins sensitize pain receptors to chemical and mechanical stimuli during the inflammatory process.
      (3) In the **cardiovascular system**, these autacoids have varying effects.
         (a) Prostaglandins of the E and A series and prostacyclin (PGI_2) **dilate** blood vessels, block hormone-mediated vasoconstriction, and, thus, cause decreased blood pressure.
         (b) PGF_2 principally causes **vasodilation**, although it constricts the superficial veins of the heart.
         (c) TXA_2 has local **vasoconstrictor** effects.

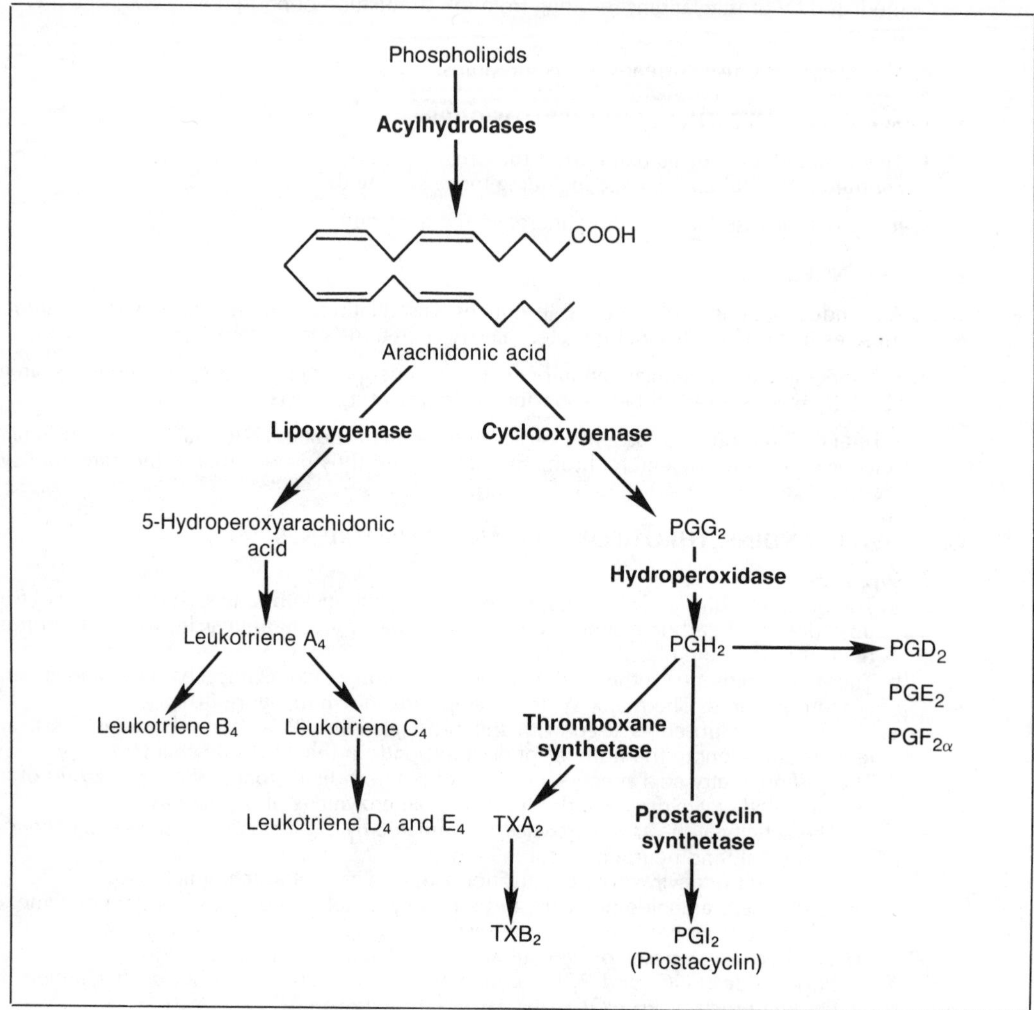

Figure 8-1. Major steps in the synthesis of prostaglandins and related structures.

(4) PGI_2 is a potent **inhibitor** of platelet aggregation, while TXA_2 is a potent **stimulator** of aggregation. PGD_2 and PGE_1 also **inhibit** platelet aggregation but are much less potent than PGI_2.

(5) The prostaglandins and thromboxanes can contract and relax smooth muscles in a variety of tissues. For example:

(a) Prostaglandins of the E series **relax** bronchial smooth muscle, while those of the F series and TXA_2 **constrict** it.

(b) The prostaglandins of the E and F series **contract** uterine smooth muscle. Sensitivity to this effect is increased during the final phase of pregnancy.

(c) The prostaglandins of the E and F series **contract** the longitudinal muscles of the gastrointestinal tract.

(6) PGE_2 and PGI_2 are cytoprotective and prevent mucosal injury induced by noxious agents.

(7) PGI_2 is capable of inhibiting gastric acid secretion induced by gastrin, histamine, or feeding.

(8) Prostaglandins are involved in luteinizing hormone (LH) release, in ovulation, and in the termination of corpus luteum function. They may also have a role in the endometrial changes associated with menstruation.

(9) Prostaglandins may modulate the release of trophic hormones from the anterior pituitary gland, and may play a role in steroidogenesis, insulin release, and thyroid response to thyroid-stimulating hormone.

3. Mechanism of action

a. Receptors for prostaglandins of the E and F series have been identified.

b. In many cells and tissues, prostaglandins activate adenylate cyclase and thus increase the level of cyclic AMP, which mediates their pharmacologic actions.

c. In other tissues, prostaglandins appear to act via mechanisms that are not dependent upon cyclic AMP.

d. The cyclic AMP–dependent and –independent actions of prostaglandins and thromboxanes may be related, in some tissues and cells, to the mobilization of intracellular calcium.

e. The mechanism of action of the leukotrienes is being investigated.

4. Therapeutic uses

a. $PGF_{2\alpha}$ and PGE_2 are used for inducing abortion.

b. Prostacyclin derivatives are currently being developed for the treatment of gastrointestinal ucleration by virtue of their cytoprotective effects on the gastric mucosa. Also being investigated are therapeutic uses for the vasodilating effects of PGI_2 and for its ability to inhibit platelet aggregation.

III. AUTACOID ANTAGONISTS

A. HISTAMINE ANTAGONISTS fall into two classes, depending on whether they block H_1 or H_2 receptors.

1. H_1 receptor antagonists are the classic antihistamine agents.

a. H_1 receptor antagonists block the histamine effect on:

(1) Bronchial smooth muscle.

(2) Intestinal smooth muscle.

(3) Small blood vessels.

(4) Sensory impulses for itching.

b. Structure and classification

(1) H_1 receptor antagonists are substituted ethylamines.

(2) The nucleus of H_1 antagonists has the following structure:

$$\begin{matrix} R_1 \diagdown & & \diagup CH_3 \\ & X{-}CH_2{-}CH_2{-}N & \\ R_2 \diagup & & \diagdown CH_3 \end{matrix}$$

(a) X can be nitrogen, carbon, or an ether moiety.

(b) R_1 and R_2 are cyclic structures.

(3) The major classes, their substituents at X, and typical drugs of each class are shown in Table 8-1.

c. Pharmacokinetics

(1) H_1 antagonists are rapidly and almost completely absorbed from the gastrointestinal tract, allowing effective oral administration.

(2) The onset of action is usually within 30 minutes, and the duration is between 4 and 6 hours.

Table 8-1. Classes of Antihistamine Agents (H_1 Blockers) and Typical Members

Class	Substituent at X	Typical Members*
Ethylenediamines	N	Tripelennamine (Pryribenzamine, etc.) Pyrilamine (Neo-Antergan, etc.)
Phenothiazines	N	Promethazine (Phenergan, etc.)
Alkylamines	C	Chlorpheniramine (Chlor-Trimeton, etc.)
Piperazines	C—N	Cylizine (Marezine) Meclizine (Antivert, Bonine)
Ethanolamines	C—O	Diphenhydramine (Benadryl, etc.) Dimenhydrinate (Dramamine, etc.) Carbinoxamine (Clistin)

Note.—C = carbon; N = nitrogen; O = oxygen.

*Names in parentheses are trade names.

(3) Most H_1 antagonists are metabolized by hydroxylation and are capable of inducing the hepatic microsomal enzyme system.

d. Pharmacologic effects

(1) **Sedation** is a common effect and may be desirable in some clinical settings. There is little correlation between antihistamine potency and degree of sedation. Alcohol consumption will greatly increase sedation.

(2) The **anticholinergic properties** of H_1 receptor antagonists are useful in the treatment of motion sickness.

(3) The **local anesthetic and antipruritic effects** of the H_1 receptor antagonists are due to their ability to prevent histamine-induced itching and pain in the skin and mucous membranes.

e. Therapeutic uses

(1) H_1 receptor antagonists are useful in the symptomatic treatment of allergic conditions.

(a) Disorders that respond include urticaria and seasonal rhinitis and conjunctivitis.

(b) H_1 receptor antagonists are also effective for drug reactions caused by allergic phenomena.

(c) They are ineffectual in bronchial asthma but have an adjuvant role in systemic anaphylaxis.

(2) Prophylaxis of asthma is accomplished with **cromolyn sodium**, which is neither an antihistamine nor a bronchodilator agent. Cromolyn sodium inhibits the release of histamine and other autacoids from mast cells in the lung.

(3) H_1 receptor antagonists are used in cough preparations.

(4) H_1 receptor antagonists are used prophylactically for motion sickness as well as for vestibular disturbances such as Meniere's disease. The ethanolamines and piperazines are especially useful in the treatment of motion sickness.

(5) H_1 blockers are also used as somnifacients.

(6) H_1 receptor antagonists are effective for urticaria and pruritus. Topical application, as well as oral administration, has been used for this purpose.

f. Untoward effects

(1) Acute poisoning due to overdosage with these agents does occur, especially in children, and the principal symptoms reflect CNS stimulation:

(a) Hallucinations.

(b) Excitement.

(c) Ataxia.

(d) Convulsions, which precede death.

(2) With therapeutic doses, sedation is the most frequently seen untoward effect, and it can interfere with the patient's daily activities. If it occurs, the dose is simply reduced or the antihistaminic agent changed.

(3) Other CNS effects include tinnitus, nervousness, and lassitude.

(4) Nausea, vomiting, or gastric distress can occur, and the agent should be given with meals.

(5) Atropine-like untoward effects can be generated.

(6) Allergic manifestations can occur when the drug is topically administered.

(7) The piperazine compounds are rarely teratogenic.

g. Preparations (see Table 8-1).

2. H_2 receptor antagonists block the histamine effect on gastric acid secretion.

a. Cimetidine

(1) The prototype of the H_2 receptor blockers, cimetidine, is a substituted imidazole compound which acts as a competitive antagonist at H_2 receptors.

(2) **Pharmacologic effects**

(a) The principal effect of cimetidine is to inhibit histamine-stimulated gastric acid secretion.

(b) In addition, it inhibits gastric acid secretion induced by gastrin and acetylcholine.

(c) Cimetidine thus inhibits all phases of physiologic secretion of gastric acid.

(3) Cimetidine is well absorbed when administered orally and is rapidly excreted by the kidney.

(4) Its major **therapeutic use** is in the treatment of duodenal ulcer and gastric hypersecretory states such as the Zollinger-Ellison syndrome.

(5) **Untoward effects**

(a) Generally, cimetidine is well tolerated.

(b) High doses in elderly patients, especially those with some degree of renal dysfunction, have resulted in CNS disturbances such as confusion.

(c) Rarely, a weak antiandrogenic effect has been observed with very high doses, resulting in gynecomastia in men and galactorrhea in women.

(d) Cimetidine reduces liver blood flow and thus can markedly decrease the hepatic clearance of drugs whose metabolism is dependent on liver blood flow; for example, propranolol.

(e) Because cimetidine inhibits the cytochrome P-450 hepatic enzyme system, a number of drug interactions have been observed.

b. Ranitidine

(1) Ranitidine is a new H_2 receptor antagonist which is 4 to 12 times more potent than cimetidine.

(2) Ranitidine is not metabolized to a significant extent by the cytochrome P-450 enzyme system.

(3) Adverse CNS effects and drug interactions have recently been reported.

(4) The risk of untoward antiandrogenic effects from ranitidine use appears to be minimal.

B. SEROTONIN ANTAGONISTS are of two general classes: ergot alkaloid derivatives and phenothiazine derivatives.

1. Methysergide

a. Methysergide is a semisynthetic ergot alkaloid congener which lacks any intrinsic vasoconstrictor or oxytocic activity.

b. It is a competitive antagonist of serotonin, inhibiting its vasoconstrictor and pressor effects.

c. Methysergide is useful for the prophylactic treatment of migraine and other vascular headaches, but the mechanism for this action is unknown.

d. The major adverse effects seen with methysergide are gastrointestinal irritation; CNS effects such as insomnia, restlessness, nervousness, and unsteadiness; and retroperitoneal fibrosis.

2. Cyproheptadine

a. Cyproheptadine is a phenothiazine which also blocks H_1 receptors.

b. It also has weak anticholinergic activity and possesses mild central depressant properties.

c. It is a competitive antagonist of serotonin, blocking the vascular effects of serotonin.

d. Cyproheptadine is used mainly to treat pruritic dermatoses.

e. Adverse effects are usually mild, with dry mouth and drowsiness being the most common.

C. ANTAGONISTS OF THE RENIN–ANGIOTENSIN SYSTEM. There are two major classes of substances that can inhibit the renin–angiotensin system: angiotensin II receptor antagonists and inhibitors of the enzyme peptidyl dipeptidase.

1. Angiotensin II receptor antagonists

a. The prototype agent is **saralasin**, a competitive inhibitor of angiotensin II receptors.

b. In normal individuals, the angiotensin II receptor antagonists have partial agonist activity, resulting in both mild pressor response and increased secretion of aldosterone.

c. In patients with malignant hypertension, who are sodium-depleted, saralasin and congeners produce profound hypotension and decreased secretion of aldosterone.

d. For clinical usage, see Chapter 5, V G 2.

2. Inhibitors of peptidyl dipeptidase

a. Captopril, the prototype, blocks the enzymatic conversion of angiotensin I to angiotensin II.

(1) Captopril and others of this class are not angiotensin II antagonists, nor do they possess agonist activity.

(2) They reduce systemic blood pressure in patients with increased angiotensin I levels but not in normal individuals who are in sodium balance. (See Chapter 5, V G, for further discussion).

(3) Captopril, when administered orally, will reduce blood pressure in hypertensive patients with high, normal, and low plasma renin levels.

(4) The fact that many hypertensive patients with normal renin levels respond to captopril suggests that other factors affecting the renin–angiotensin system, e.g., sodium depletion, may have a role in hypertension.

b. These agents also increase the actions of bradykinin, since it is inactivated by peptidyl dipeptidase.

c. They are also able to depress the secretion of aldosterone by lowering angiotensin II production.

D. INHIBITORS OF PROSTAGLANDINS AND THROMBOXANES are effective nonsteroidal anti-inflammatory agents, discussed in Chapter 9.

STUDY QUESTIONS

Directions: Each question below contains five suggested answers. Choose the **one best** response to each question.

1. Which of the following effects might be observed in a patient who is accidentally given a large overdose of histamine while being tested for achlorhydria?

(A) Severe localized blanching of the skin
(B) Decreased capillary permeability
(C) Bronchoconstriction
(D) Relaxation of gastrointestinal smooth muscle
(E) Gastric acid suppression

2. Classic antihistamines (H_1 receptor blockers) are *indicated* for the treatment of

(A) peptic ulcer
(B) an acute asthma attack
(C) motion sickness
(D) the common cold
(E) oversedation

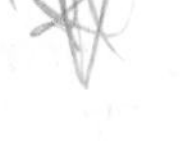

Directions: Each question below contains four suggested answers of which **one or more** is correct. Choose the answer

A if **1, 2, and 3** are correct
B if **1 and 3** are correct
C if **2 and 4** are correct
D if **4** is correct
E if **1, 2, 3, and 4** are correct

3. Drugs effective for the prevention of motion sickness include

(1) chlorpromazine
(2) scopolamine
(3) pyridoxine
(4) meclizine

4. True statements concerning the classic antihistamines include which of the following?

(1) They block histamine receptors on bronchial and intestinal smooth muscle
(2) They are substituted ethylamines
(3) They may induce hepatic microsomal enzymes
(4) Overdosage may cause death in children following generalized convulsions

5. Which of the following statements characterize the autacoids?

(1) They are enzymes
(2) They all have a decarboxylated amino acid structure
(3) They are found only in circulating blood
(4) They originate from diffuse tissues

6. H_2 receptor blockers have which of the following effects?

(1) They inhibit gastric acid secretion
(2) They decrease the liver blood flow
(3) They cause gynecomastia
(4) They are highly toxic

7. True statements concerning the autacoids include which of the following?

(1) Histamine and serotonin are decarboxylated amino acids
(2) Antiserotonins have not been found
(3) Angiotensin II is formed from angiotensin I by an enzyme in lung tissue
(4) Prostaglandins are found only in reproductive organs

8. Which of the following histamine antagonists will successfully inhibit gastric acid secretion?

(1) Diphenhydramine
(2) Ranitidine
(3) Tripelennamine
(4) Cimetidine

9. Which of the following autacoids are correctly matched with a recognized clinical use?

(1) Angiotensin II—diagnosis of gout
(2) Histamine—diagnosis of pernicious anemia
(3) Serotonin—peripheral vascular disease
(4) Prostaglandin $F_{2\alpha}$—therapeutic abortion

10. Which of the following statements characterize cimetidine?

(1) It is a competitive H_2 receptor antagonist
(2) It is useful for the treatment of duodenal ulcers
(3) It is approved for use in the treatment Zollinger-Ellison syndrome
(4) It is useful for the treatment of allergic reactions

ANSWERS AND EXPLANATIONS

1. The answer is C. *(II A 9)* Bronchoconstriction would be the most prominent untoward effect. The overdose of histamine would increase capillary permeability, stimulate gastrointestinal smooth muscle, and stimulate gastric acid secretion. Vasodilation and increased skin temperature would also occur.

2. The answer is C. *(III A 1 e)* Antihistamines, or H_1 receptor blockers, by virtue of their anticholinergic activity, are used in the treatment of motion sickness. Although H_1 blockers are *used* for the common cold, they are not *indicated* for this condition. Antihistamines are not indicated in asthma; epinephrine is the drug of first choice for the acute treatment of asthma. H_2 receptor blockers, not H_1 blockers, are used for the treatment of peptic ulcer disease. Antihistamines are sedating, and thus would not be used to treat oversedation.

3. The answer is C (2, 4). *(III A 1 e (4); Chapter 2, VI B 2; Chapter 3, V B 5)* Chlorpromazine is principally an antipsychotic agent. Pyridoxine (vitamin B_6) is not used in the treatment of motion sickness. Scopolamine is a muscarinic blocker which is useful in the treatment of motion sickness. Meclizine is a piperazine antihistamine which, because of its antichlolinergic properties, is also useful for the treatment of motion sickness.

4. The answer is E (all). *(III A 1 a, b, c (3), f (1))* The classic antihistamines block receptors on bronchial and intestinal smooth muscle. They may induce hepatic microsomal enzymes. Therapeutic doses produce CNS depression, but convulsions can occur with toxic doses. The basic structure of the classic antihistamines is a substituted ethylamine.

5. The answer is D (4). *(I A, B, C)* Autacoids are hormone-like substances, and generally not enzymes. However, they originate from diffuse tissues, and generally not from discrete glands. Not all autacoids are decarboxylated amino acids; some are polypeptides and some are eicosanoids. Autacoids can be found in the circulation and within tissues, and they are thought to modulate local circulation and to influence the processes of inflammation.

6. The answer is A (1, 2, 3). *(III A 2)* H_2 receptor blockers inhibit gastric acid secretion, can decrease the liver blood flow, and have a weak antiandrogenic effect that produces gynecomastia in men. These agents are well tolerated and have a low incidence of untoward effects.

7. The answer is B (1, 3). *(I C 1; II C 1, G 1; III B)* Histamine and serotonin are decarboxylated amino acids. Antagonists of serotonin include methysergide and cyproheptadine. Angiotensin II is formed from angiotensin I by angiotensin-converting enzyme in lung tissue. Prostaglandins are found in almost every tissue.

8. The answer is C (2, 4). *(III A 2)* Ranitidine and cimetidine are H_2 receptor blockers and therefore are capable of inhibiting gastric acid secretion. Both diphenhydramine and tripelennamine are H_1 receptor antagonists and thus are not capable of inhibiting gastric acid secretion.

9. The answer is C (2, 4). *(II A 7, B 4, C 4, G 4)* Histamine, betazole, and pentagastrin are capable of stimulating gastric acid secretion and are useful diagnostically to distinguish between pernicious anemia, in which parietal cells are nonfunctioning, and other forms of anemia. Serotonin and angiotensin II have no current clinical use. Prostaglandin $F_{2\alpha}$ is used to achieve therapeutic abortion because of its ability to cause contraction of uterine smooth muscle.

10. The answer is A (1, 2, 3). *(III A 1 e, 2 a)* Cimetidine is the prototype H_2 receptor antagonist. It is used in the treatment of duodenal ulcers and hypersecretory states such as the Zollinger-Ellison syndrome. The H_2 blockers are not effective in the treatment of allergic reactions, which usually respond to H_1 blockers.

9

Non-Narcotic Analgesics, Nonsteroidal Anti-Inflammatory Drugs, and Drugs Used in the Treatment of Gout

I. INTRODUCTION

A. The commonly used non-narcotic analgesics (aspirin, acetaminophen) are effective as both analgesic and antipyretic agents.

B. In addition, the salicylates (e.g., aspirin) and the newer nonsteroidal anti-inflammatory drugs (NSAIDs) also possess excellent anti-inflammatory activity due to their inhibition of prostaglandin biosynthesis.

1. For example, aspirin acetylates and irreversibly inactivates cyclooxygenase.
2. This blocks the synthesis of the prostaglandins PGE_2, PGI_2, and $PGF_{2\alpha}$, which are believed to be involved in inflammation-associated vasodilation, pain, and edema (see Chapter 8, II G).
3. Additionally, the inhibition of thromboxane (TXA_2) synthesis due to blockade of platelet cyclooxygenase results in increased bleeding time (see II B 6).

C. In contrast, acetaminophen, although an excellent analgesic and antipyretic, does not possess anti-inflammatory activity.

D. Besides their use in rheumatoid arthritis, many of the nonsteroidal anti-inflammatory agents are also useful in the treatment of acute gout.

E. Unlike narcotics, the agents discussed in this chapter have no tolerance or addiction liability.

F. In the treatment of rheumatoid arthritis, the **NSAIDs** and the **salicylates,** as discussed in this chapter, are the drugs of first choice. Several other agents, which are not primarily used for their anti-inflammatory activity, can be of variable therapeutic benefit in rheumatoid arthritis. The **glucocorticoids** have obvious anti-inflammatory actions, but hazards with long-term therapy preclude their use as a treatment of choice. The **antimalarials, chloroquine,** and the **hydroxychloroquines,** also exhibit some antirheumatic activity. The cytotoxic agents such as **azathioprine** and **cyclophosphamide,** primarily used in cancer chemotherapy, can also reduce arthritic symptoms. The immunopotentiating action of the anthelmintic, **levamisole,** is believed to underlie the improvement in rheumatoid arthritis sometimes seen with this agent. Finally, **penicillamine** can also reduce arthritic symptoms in some cases. The mechanism of action is unknown.

II. ASPIRIN (ACETYLSALICYLIC ACID) AND OTHER SALICYLATES

A. CHEMISTRY. A white crystalline substance, acetylsalicylic acid is stable in dry air but hydrolyzes to salicylic and acetic acids in moist air. Its chemical structure is shown below.

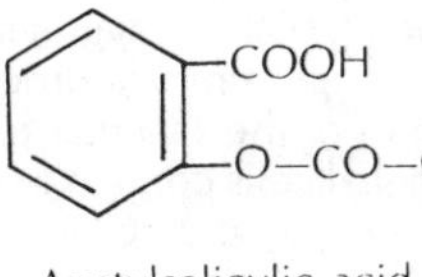

[benzene ring with –COOH and –O–CO–CH_3]

Acetylsalicylic acid

B. PHARMACOLOGIC EFFECTS

1. Antipyretic action

a. Aspirin is rapidly effective in febrile patients, yet has little effect on normal body temperature.

b. The antipyretic effect of aspirin appears to occur in the central nervous system (CNS).

(1) Aspirin, by inactivating cyclooxygenase, inhibits the synthesis of PGE_2.

(2) During fever, PGE_2 is thought to be released from the hypothalamus via the mediation of an endogenous pyrogen.

c. *Hyperpyrexia occurs with toxic doses of aspirin* and the other salicylates (e.g., sodium salicylate); it is, in part, the result of an increase in oxygen consumption and in metabolic rate.

2. Analgesic action

a. Low-intensity pain arising from integumental structures is relieved better than pain from visceral areas.

b. The salicylates have a lower maximal analgesic effect as compared to narcotic analgesics.

c. Aspirin is widely used because chronic administration does not lead to tolerance or addiction and because its toxicity is lower than that of more potent analgesics.

d. Relief of pain occurs through both peripheral and central mechanisms.

(1) The salicylates inhibit the synthesis of prostaglandins in inflamed tissues, thus preventing the sensitization of pain receptors to both mechanical and chemical stimuli.

(2) Centrally, the analgesic site exists in close proximity to the antipyretic region in the hypothalamus. The analgesia produced by the salicylates is not associated with mental alterations such as hypnosis or changes in sensation other than pain.

3. Effects on respiration

a. Full therapeutic doses of the salicylates increase oxygen consumption and carbon dioxide production in skeletal muscle. The resulting increase in alveolar ventilation is characterized by an increase in the depth as opposed to the rate of respiration.

b. Higher doses result in medullary stimulation, leading to hyperventilation and a respiratory alkalosis. Compensation rapidly occurs because the kidney is able to increase the excretion of bicarbonate, producing a compensated respiratory alkalosis.

c. Toxic doses or very prolonged administration can depress the medulla, resulting in an uncompensated respiratory acidosis. Since renal bicarbonate excretion is elevated and since the salicylates cause the accumulation of organic acids, a metabolic acidosis also results.

4. Cardiovascular effects

a. No untoward effects occur at therapeutic doses.

b. Large doses tend to dilate peripheral vessels.

c. Vasomotor paralysis occurs at toxic doses, producing circulatory depression.

5. Gastrointestinal effects

a. The salicylates can cause epigastric distress and can stimulate the chemoreceptor trigger zone in the CNS.

b. They produce a dose-related gastric ulceration and hemorrhage, due in part to exfoliation of gastric mucosal cells.

c. The secretion of protective gastric mucus is inhibited, and gastric acid secretion increases because salicylates suppress the formation of PGI_2, which is known to inhibit gastric acid secretion.

6. Effects on blood

a. Aspirin has no effect on leukocyte count, hemoglobin, or hematocrit at therapeutic doses.

b. There is, however, a prolongation of bleeding time with doses as small as 300 mg of aspirin.

c. Because it can acetylate and inactivate cylooxygenase, aspirin has important effects on the delicate balance that exists between the initiation and the inhibition of **platelet aggregation.**

(1) Platelets are ordinarily nonadherent. However, vascular injury and exposure to subendothelial structures result in activation of the platelet cylooxygenase enzyme system, leading to the production of thromboxane A_2 (TXA_2), via thromboxane synthetase. TXA_2 is capable of inducing platelet aggregation.

(2) Concurrently opposing this physiologic process is the cylooxygenase and prostacyclin synthetase enzyme system of the vascular endothelium. Instead of thromboxane synthetase, vascular endothelial cells contain a prostacyclin synthetase which converts the cyclooxygenase products PGG_2 and PGH_2 to prostacyclin, a potent inhibitor of platelet clumping.

(3) It is thought that aspirin in appropriate doses can preferentially inhibit the platelet cyclooxygenase system, blocking the formation of TXA_2 and thereby suppressing platelet clumping.

(4) By inhibiting initial platelet aggregation to subendothelial structures, aspirin also prevents the secondary release of adenosine diphosphate (ADP) from platelet granules, a process that normally occurs when platelets clump. ADP release ordinarily brings about additional waves of platelet aggregation, leading to thrombus formation.

d. In doses greater than 6 g/day aspirin may reduce plasma prothrombin levels.

e. Because of its effects on the blood, aspirin should be avoided in patients with severe hepatic disease, hypoprothrombinemia, vitamin K deficiency, or hemophilia.

7. Effects on the kidney

a. High doses of the salicylates (above 5 g) will promote the renal excretion of sodium urate.

b. Low doses of the salicylates (below 2 g) will decrease the renal excretion of sodium urate, producing an elevation of serum uric acid levels. The salicylates appear to negate the action of many uricosurics and thus should not be administered in conjunction with these agents during therapy for gout (see X F 3, below).

8. Metabolic effects

a. The salicylates uncouple oxidative phosphorylation.

b. Large doses of the salicylates can produce hyperglycemia and glycosuria.

c. Aspirin, like other salicylates, can reduce lipogenesis by blocking the incorporation of acetate into fatty acids.

9. Endocrine effects

a. The salicylates, in very large doses, can cause stimulation of steroid secretion by the adrenal cortex. This effect is mediated through action on the hypothalamus.

b. The competitive displacement of thyroxine and triiodothyronine from prealbumin by aspirin and other salicylates leads to their enhanced rate of disappearance.

c. The salicylates may prolong the gestational period during pregnancy. This may be due to a delay in the onset of labor caused by the inhibition of prostaglandin synthesis in the uterus, since prostaglandins are believed to be involved in eliciting uterine contractions.

C. PHARMACOKINETICS

1. Upon oral administration of the salicylates, a portion is rapidly absorbed from the stomach. The majority of an orally ingested salicylate dose, however, is absorbed from the upper portion of the small intestine.

2. Once absorbed, the salicylates are distributed throughout the body by a pH-dependent passive diffusion process.

3. Most of the salicylates bind avidly to serum proteins. Aspirin as such binds to a lesser extent.

4. Biotransformation occurs in the microsomal drug-metabolizing system, and the following metabolic products are seen in the urine: salicyluric acid (75 percent), phenolic glucuronide (10 percent), acylglucuronide (5 percent), and free salicylic acid (10 percent).

5. Alkalinization of the urine (pH 8) significantly increases the excretion of salicylates because of increased ionization and decreased reabsorption through the kidney tubules.

6. Rectal absorption of the salicylates is slow and unpredictable.

D. SALICYLATE INTOXICATION

1. Mild intoxication from aspirin or other salicylates is referred to as **salicylism** and usually occurs with repeated administration of large doses. Characteristic findings include:

a. Headache, mental confusion, lassitude, drowsiness.

b. Tinnitus, difficulty in hearing.

c. Hyperthermia, sweating, thirst, hyperventilation, vomiting, diarrhea.

2. More severe salicylate intoxication can result in more severe CNS disturbances, including hallucinations, vertigo, or convulsions. In addition, skin eruptions and, more important, marked alterations in acid–base balance are observed.

3. Ingestion of as little as 10 g of aspirin by a child can result in death.

4. Fatal intoxication can be produced in children by ingestion of as little as 5 g of methyl salicylate, which is widely used as a counterirritant in liniments and has the characteristic odor and taste of wintergreen.

5. Treatment of salicylate poisoning includes:
   a. Inducing emesis with syrup of ipecac and/or administering gastric lavage.
   b. Appropriate infusion measures to correct abnormal electrolyte balance and dehydration.
   c. Alkalinization of the urine.

6. Dialysis may be required in severe intoxication.

E. THERAPEUTIC USES

1. The salicylates are used in restricted situations for the symptomatic relief of fever.
   a. They have no effect on the underlying cause of a fever, and since the hyperthermic response in an illness may be a normal protective physiologic mechanism, they should not be used routinely or trivially for this purpose.
   b. Because of an increased incidence of Reye's syndrome in children who have been given aspirin for the relief of fever, it is now recommended that acetaminophen be given instead, if medication is required.

2. The salicylates are useful as analgesics for certain categories of pain (e.g., headache, arthritis, dysmenorrhea).

3. The salicylates, by way of their anti-inflammatory action, provide symptomatic relief in acute rheumatic fever.

4. The salicylates remain the standard, first-line drug in the therapy of **rheumatoid arthritis.**
   a. Both the analgesic and the anti-inflammatory actions provide symptomatic relief in this disorder.
   b. Relatively large doses are required, however, and these may not be well tolerated in some individuals, necessitating the use of other agents either alone or in combination with the salicylates.

F. PREPARATIONS

1. Aspirin is available as tablets, capsules, and suppositories in a wide range of dosages. Rectal administration may be required in infants or if oral administration is impossible.

2. Sodium salicylate is available as tablets.

3. Buffered or enteric-coated preparations of aspirin may be better tolerated but the slightly enhanced absorption rate of buffered aspirin may not be significant.

III. ACETAMINOPHEN AND PHENACETIN

A. CHEMISTRY. A para-aminophenol derivative, acetaminophen is the major active metabolite of phenacetin. Its chemical structure is shown below.

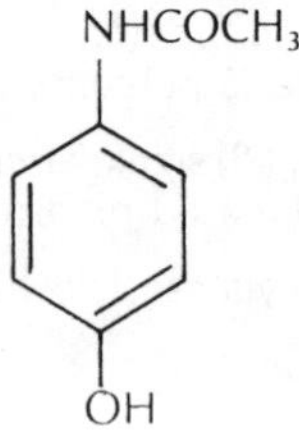

Acetaminophen

B. PHARMACOLOGIC EFFECTS

1. Both phenacetin and acetaminophen are effective analgesic and antipyretic agents, but they have no anti-inflammatory activity for reasons that are not completely understood.

2. Acetaminophen appears to be an inhibitor of prostaglandin synthesis in the brain, thus explaining its analgesic and antipyretic activity, but it is much less effective than aspirin as an inhibitor of the peripherally located prostaglandin biosynthetic enzyme system that plays such an important role in inflammation.

3. Acetaminophen and phenacetin exert little or no pharmacologic effect on the cardiovascular, respiratory, or gastrointestinal system, on acid–base regulation, or on platelet function.

C. PHARMACOKINETICS

1. Acetaminophen is completely and rapidly absorbed from the gastrointestinal tract.
2. About 3 percent is excreted unchanged in the urine, while 80 to 90 percent is conjugated with glucuronic or sulfuric acid in the liver and then excreted in the urine.
   - a. Small amounts of hydroxylated metabolites are ordinarily excreted.
   - b. At high doses, one of these metabolites undergoes spontaneous dehydration to form *N*-acetyl-*p*-benzoquinone, the metabolite thought to be responsible for hepatotoxicity (see D 3 below).
3. About 70 to 80 percent of administered phenacetin is rapidly metabolized to acetaminophen. The remaining 20 percent is metabolized to several other metabolites.

D. UNTOWARD EFFECTS

1. At therapeutic doses both acetaminophen and phenacetin are well tolerated.
2. Untoward effects include:
   - a. Skin rash and drug fever (hyperpyrexia caused by an allergic reaction to the drug).
   - b. Rare instances of blood dyscrasias; in addition, with prolonged use phenacetin can produce a hemolytic anemia.
   - c. Renal tubular necrosis and renal failure.
   - d. Hypoglycemic coma.
3. An overdose of acetaminophen (about 15 g in an adult; about 4 g in a child) can result in severe hepatotoxicity.
   - a. The toxic metabolite of acetaminophen appears to be inactivated in the liver via glutathione.
   - b. It is thought that when glutathione stores are consumed, the *N*-acetyl-*p*-benzoquinone metabolite binds covalently to cellular constituents, producing hepatocellular damage.
   - c. Although clinical symptoms such as nausea and vomiting occur during the first 24 hours after toxic ingestion, signs of hepatic damage (e.g., enzyme abnormalities) may not occur for 2 to 6 days.
   - d. Treatment consists of:
     - (1) Emptying the stomach and administering activated charcoal.
     - (2) Hemodialysis, if begun within the first 12 hours after ingestion.
     - (3) Administration of sulfhydryl compounds (e.g., acetylcysteine), which probably replenish hepatic stores of glutathione.
4. High doses of phenacetin can produce cyanosis, respiratory depression, and cardiac arrest.
5. Hepatic damage is *not* associated with phenacetin overdosage, but overall toxic liability is greater than with acetaminophen.

E. THERAPEUTIC USES. Acetaminophen and phenacetin provide an effective alternative for aspirin in individuals for whom aspirin is contraindicated (e.g., because of peptic ulcer) and who do not require the anti-inflammatory action of aspirin.

F. PREPARATIONS AND ADMINISTRATION

1. Acetaminophen is available in tablet and liquid form and is administered orally.
2. Phenacetin, also given orally, is principally used in analgesic mixtures.

IV. PHENYLBUTAZONE

A. CHEMISTRY AND PHARMACOLOGIC EFFECTS

1. A congener of antipyrene, phenylbutazone is an effective anti-inflammatory agent but toxicity prohibits its long-term use.
2. Phenylbutazone possesses anti-inflammatory and analgesic activity that is qualitatively similar to that of aspirin. Its analgesic effect against nonrheumatic pain, however, is less than that produced by aspirin.

B. MAJOR UNTOWARD EFFECTS

1. Significant sodium and chloride retention occurs through a direct effect on renal tubules; this can cause cardiac decompensation and acute pulmonary edema.

2. As many as 10 to 50 percent of patients experience nausea, vomiting, or skin rashes.
3. Phenylbutazone can cause agranulocytosis or aplastic anemia.
4. Peptic ulceration has been reported.
5. Because phenylbutazone binds to plasma proteins and displaces other drugs (e.g., warfarin), a number of undesirable drug interactions may occur.
6. Phenylbutazone also has a direct effect in reducing platelet function.

C. **THERAPEUTIC USES**

1. Because it is poorly tolerated by many patients, phenylbutazone is not used as an antipyretic or general analgesic agent.
2. Phenylbutazone is chiefly used in the short-term therapy of acute gout and in acute exacerbations of rheumatoid arthritis, and only after other agents have failed.
3. Brief courses of the drug may be of benefit in the treatment of osteoarthritis and ankylosing spondylitis, with the same reservations described above.

D. Phenylbutazone is administered orally. It should be taken with meals to lessen gastric irritation.

V. INDOMETHACIN

A. **CHEMISTRY.** Indomethacin is a methylated indole derivative.

B. **PHARMACOLOGIC EFFECTS**

1. Indomethacin has prominent anti-inflammatory, antipyretic, and analgesic activity.
2. Although, in vitro, indomethacin is one of the most potent inhibitors of prostaglandin synthesis, in vivo, indomethacin does not prolong bleeding time, as does aspirin. Thus, indomethacin apparently does not gain access to the platelet cylooxygenase.
3. Although indomethacin is a more potent anti-inflammatory agent than aspirin, the doses of indomethacin that are well tolerated by rheumatoid arthritis patients do not show superior results compared to the salicylates.

C. **UNTOWARD EFFECTS.** These occur in up to 30 percent of patients, and include:

1. Gastrointestinal disturbances, including peptic ulceration.
2. CNS complaints, including severe frontal headache, dizziness, vertigo, and mental confusion.
3. Blood dyscrasias, including neutropenia and thrombocytopenia.

D. **THERAPEUTIC USES**

1. The major uses of indomethacin are in the treatment of rheumatoid arthritis, ankylosing spondylitis, osteoarthritis, and acute gout.
2. It has also been used in the treatment of patent ductus arteriosis in neonates.
3. Because of its toxicity and side effects, it is not routinely used for analgesia or antipyresis.

E. **PREPARATION AND ADMINISTRATION.** Indomethacin is administered orally. It should be taken with meals to lessen gastric irritation.

VI. SULINDAC

A. Structurally, sulindac is closely related to indomethacin.

B. It is half as potent as indomethacin and has a lower incidence of untoward effects. Gastrointestinal disturbances are the most common adverse effect.

C. Its long half-life of 16 hours is due to an active sulfide metabolite and its assumed enterohepatic circulation.

D. The major **therapeutic uses** of sulindac are in the treatment of osteoarthritis, rheumatoid arthritis, ankylosing spondylitis, and acute gout.

Hypersens. Rxns. in SLE

E. Sulindac is administered orally.

VII. IBUPROFEN AND NAPROXEN

A. CHEMISTRY AND PHARMACOLOGIC EFFECTS

1. Both ibuprofen and naproxen are propionic acid derivatives possessing anti-inflammatory, analgesic, and antipyretic activity.
2. Ibuprofen is equipotent to aspirin in its anti-inflammatory effect.
3. Both are potent inhibitors of cyclooxygenase and prolong bleeding time.
4. Both are firmly bound to serum proteins (over 98 percent).

B. THERAPEUTIC USES AND UNTOWARD EFFECTS

1. Naproxen and ibuprofen are used as nonsteroidal anti-inflammatory agents and as non-narcotic analgesic agents.
2. Gastrointestinal and CNS untoward effects occur with both, although these are significantly less severe than those seen with indomethacin.
3. Ibuprofen appears to be better tolerated than aspirin with regard to gastrointestinal complaints.

C. Ibuprofen and naproxen are administered orally.

VIII. TOLMETIN

A. Tolmetin is a nonsteroidal anti-inflammatory agent more potent than aspirin but less potent than indomethacin.

B. Tolmetin also produces analgesic and antipyretic effects.

C. It is rapidly and completely absorbed from the gastrointestinal tract. Tolmetin has a short half-life in plasma (about 1 hour).

D. Untoward effects are those common to most of the other nonsteroidal anti-inflammatory agents, i.e., gastrointestinal and CNS symptoms.

E. The major therapeutic indication for tolmetin is the treatment of juvenile and adult rheumatoid arthritis.

IX. GOLD

A. CHEMISTRY AND MECHANISM OF ACTION

1. Most gold preparations used in the treatment of rheumatoid arthritis are aurous salts in which gold is attached to sulfur.
2. It is hypothesized that gold is taken up by macrophages, resulting in inhibition of phagocytosis and lysosomal enzyme activity. In addition, gold probably suppresses cellular immunity.

B. PHARMACOKINETICS

1. Water-soluble gold salts are rapidly absorbed after intramuscular administration.
2. More recently, an orally active gold preparation has come under investigation.

C. UNTOWARD EFFECTS occur in 25 to 50 percent of patients receiving parenteral gold therapy.

1. Cutaneous reactions, ranging from erythema to exfoliative dermatitis, and lesions of the mucous membranes, are often observed.
2. Eosinophilia is quite common.
3. Proteinuria occurs frequently, although this nephrosis is reversible.
4. Blood dyscrasias, including thrombocytopenia, leukopenia, agranulocytosis, and aplastic anemia, have occurred.

5. Other untoward effects include encephalitis, hepatitis, and peripheral neuritis.

D. **THERAPEUTIC USES.** The major therapeutic use for gold is in the treatment of rheumatoid arthritis that is resistant to salicylate or to other nonsteroidal anti-inflammatory therapy.

1. Gold is commonly used in early, progressive arthritis that is unresponsive to other regimens of therapy.

2. Gold therapy is of little use in advanced arthritis.

X. DRUGS USED IN THE TREATMENT OF GOUT

A. **GENERAL CONSIDERATIONS.** Because the drugs used in gout act by various mechanisms, a brief review of some aspects of this condition is in order.

1. Gout is the most readily treated of all the rheumatic disorders.

2. Hyperuricemia is not always accompanied or followed by gout, but when gout occurs it is preceded by hyperuricemia.

3. Causes of hyperuricemia include the following:
   a. Excessive uric acid synthesis associated with myeloproliferative disorders and malignancies especially after antineoplastic or radiation therapy. Conditions that lead to high rates of cell formation and destruction will lead to increased serum levels of purines, derived from cellular nucleic acids, and will thus result in hyperuricemia.
   b. A primary defect in the rate of purine synthesis.
   c. Decreased renal excretion of uric acid caused by certain drugs (e.g., thiazides) or due to genetic deficiency.
   d. Sex-linked uricaciduria (e.g., in Lesch-Nyhan syndrome) due to a lack of the enzyme hypoxanthine–guanine phosphoribosyltransferase.

4. Acute gouty arthritic episodes can be precipitated by excessive alcohol consumption, kidney disease, and possibly by high-purine diets or external stresses. If the gout is a secondary phenomenon unrelated to a genetic defect, the underlying cause of the hyperuricemia must be determined.

5. Twenty-five percent of the body's uric acid is degraded in the gastrointestinal tract by bacterial enzymes. Seventy-five percent is renally excreted. Ninety-eight percent of the filtered uric acid is reabsorbed in the proximal tubule and then secreted in the distal portion of the proximal tubule.

6. **Mechanism of gouty inflammation**
   a. When the plasma is supersaturated with urate, needle-shaped crystals of monosodium urate precipitate in joint tissue.
   b. An acute inflammatory reaction occurs, resulting in the ingestion of monosodium urate crystals by polymorphonuclear leukocytes.
   c. Lysosomal enzymes are released by the granulocytes, producing a decrease in the local pH in the joint tissue.
   d. With a decreased pH, further urate precipitation occurs in joints and cartilage.

B. **PROBENECID**

1. In low doses probenecid blocks the tubular secretion of uric acid, while at therapeutic doses probenecid is uricosuric.
   a. Therapy with probenecid (or with sulfinpyrazone—see C, below) should not be initiated during an acute attack of gout because of this biphasic action.
   b. As a general inhibitor of the tubular secretion of organic acids, probenecid will also increase serum levels of other organic acids, such as penicillin.

2. Because probenecid lowers serum levels of uric acid by inhibiting the proximal tubular reabsorption of uric acid at therapeutic doses, it is useful for the treatment of chronic gout. It has no analgesic activity.

3. It is rapidly absorbed from the gastrointestinal tract, and its metabolic products are also uricosuric.

4. When approximately 1 g of probenecid is administered daily, urinary excretion of uric acid increases by 50 percent, resulting in a corresponding fall in serum urate.

5. Probenecid is administered orally. Its action is blocked by the administration of aspirin.

6. Probenecid is well tolerated, the most common untoward effects being gastrointestinal disturbances and hypersensitivity reactions such as skin rash and drug fever.

C. SULFINPYRAZONE

1. Another uricosuric agent, this sulfoxide derivative of phenylbutazone also inhibits the proximal tubular reabsorption of uric acid.
2. After oral administration, sulfinpyrazone is well absorbed from the gastrointestinal tract and most is excreted unchanged in the urine. A hydroxy metabolite also is a potent uricosuric substance.
3. Untoward effects are similar to those seen with probenecid.
4. Sulfinpyrazone is used for the treatment of chronic gout. Administration with meals is recommended.
5. Sulfinpyrazone also inhibits prostaglandin synthesis and interferes with a number of platelet functions, including adherence to subendothelial cells. Because of these effects it is being examined as an antithrombotic agent.

D. COLCHICINE

1. This alkaloid derivative is effective in the treatment of acute attacks of gout and, in addition, is effective if given prophylactically to prevent such attacks.
2. Colchicine inhibits the migration of polymorphonuclear leukocytes to the inflammatory area. It is proposed that colchicine produces ultrastructural alterations in leukocytes by attaching to the microtubular protein (tubulin) that is involved in cell motility and thus prevents the migration of granulocytes and inhibits phagocytotic activity.
3. Colchicine also blocks cell division by binding to mitotic spindles (mitotic blockade).
4. Colchicine is rapidly absorbed from the gastrointestinal tract.
   a. Large amounts of the drug and its metabolites re-enter the intestinal tract in the bile and intestinal secretions.
   b. This high local concentration of drug, together with the rapid turnover of intestinal epithelial cells, which makes the cells particularly susceptible to mitotic blockade by colchicine, leads to altered function of the intestinal mucosa and produces one of the drug's major untoward effects, diarrhea.
5. Nausea, vomiting, and abdominal pain with diarrhea are cardinal signs that more serious toxicity could result, and could call for discontinuation of colchicine therapy.
6. The most serious untoward effects that occur with chronic administration are agranulocytosis, aplastic anemia, myopathy, and alopecia.
7. In an acute attack of gout colchicine is usually administered orally in intermittent doses until pain disappears or gastrointestinal symptoms occur.
   a. The patient usually experiences a marked improvement in joint symptoms within 12 hours.
   b. A total of no more than 10 mg should be administered in one such course of therapy.
8. Colchicine is excreted unchanged by the liver and kidney; therefore, the dosage may have to be reduced if renal or liver disease is present.
9. A fatal dose of colchicine can be as little as 8 mg in 24 hours.

E. ALLOPURINOL

1. Allopurinol is an isomer of hypoxanthine, a purine.
2. Allopurinol, together with its primary metabolite alloxanthine, prevents the terminal steps in uric acid synthesis by inhibiting the enzyme xanthine oxidase, which converts xanthine or hypoxanthine to uric acid. Hyperuricemia is thus reversed by the blockade of uric acid production.
3. Allopurinol acts as a competitive inhibitor, while alloxanthine acts noncompetitively.
4. The inhibition of xanthine oxidase causes serum levels of the catabolic intermediates xanthine and hypoxanthine to increase. Renal clearance of these substances, however, is rapid and their increased plasma concentrations do not exceed their solubility. Thus, crystallization within joint tissue does not occur as it would with comparable levels of uric acid.

5. Allopurinol is well tolerated. The most common untoward effects are hypersensitivity reactions, including cutaneous reactions.

6. Acute attacks of gout occur more frequently during initial therapy with allopurinol.
   a. This may be due in part to the active dissolution of microcrystalline deposits of sodium urate (tophi) within subcutaneous tissue, resulting in transient periods of hyperuricemia and crystal deposition in joint tissue.
   b. To reduce this complication, simultaneous prophylactic therapy with colchicine is indicated.

7. Allopurinol is administered orally. Starting with a low dose may lessen the probability of precipitating recurrent acute gouty attacks.

F. NONSTEROIDAL ANTI-INFLAMMATORY AGENTS USED IN THE TREATMENT OF GOUT

1. **Indomethacin** may provide symptomatic relief in acute attacks. The dosage of indomethacin must be reduced for patients who are also taking probenecid, since the latter increases the plasma levels of indomethacin.

2. **Phenylbutazone** is an alternative drug to indomethacin in the treatment of acute gouty arthritis.

3. Aspirin and other salicylates, although they may provide symptomatic relief, actually antagonize the action of the uricosurics probenecid and sulfinpyrazone. Therefore, the salicylates are contraindicated when probenecid or sulfinpyrazone is being administered.

STUDY QUESTIONS

Directions: Each question below contains five suggested answers. Choose the **one best** response to each question.

1. Which of the following drugs used in the treatment of gout has as its primary effect the reduction of uric acid synthesis?

(A) Allopurinol
(B) Sulfinpyrazone
(C) Colchicine
(D) Aspirin
(E) Indomethacin

2. A patient has rheumatoid arthritis and is taking medication which is causing headaches, nausea, and vomiting. Which agent is the patient most likely to be taking?

(A) Indomethacin
(B) Aspirin
(C) Acetaminophen
(D) Phenylbutazone
(E) Phenacetin

3. Which of the following drugs or procedures would probably be *least effective* in the treatment of gout?

(A) Restriction of the diet, with avoidance of foods having a high purine content
(B) Allopurinol
(C) Uricosuric agents such as probenecid or sulfinpyrazone
(D) Colchicine
(E) Small doses of steroids given chronically

4. A hemophiliac patient has rheumatoid arthritis. Which drug might be prescribed to relieve the pain?

(A) Acetaminophen
(B) Acetylsalicylic acid
(C) Phenylbutazone
(D) Ibuprofen
(E) Naproxen

5. All of the following are undesirable effects of the salicylates EXCEPT for

(A) exfoliation of gastric mucosal cells
(B) inhibition of peripheral PGE_2 and $PGF_{2\alpha}$ synthesis
(C) stimulation of the chemoreceptor trigger zone
(D) salicylism
(E) decreased gastric mucus secretion

Directions: Each question below contains four suggested answers of which **one or more** is correct. Choose the answer

A if **1, 2, and 3** are correct
B if **1 and 3** are correct
C if **2 and 4** are correct
D if **4** is correct
E if **1, 2, 3, and 4** are correct

6. Allopurinol has which of the following characteristics?

(1) It is a uricosuric agent
(2) It blocks the conversion of hypoxanthine to uric acid
(3) It is a pyrimidine derivative
(4) It lowers blood uric acid

7. Characteristics of probenecid include which of the following?

(1) It inhibits the renal tubular secretion of penicillin
(2) It is useful in the treatment of gout
(3) At appropriate doses, it promotes the excretion of uric acid
(4) It has a mechanism of action similar to sulfinpyrazone

SUMMARY OF DIRECTIONS

A	B	C	D	E
1, 2, 3 only	1, 3 only	2, 4 only	4 only	All are correct

8. Drugs and their characteristics are *incorrectly* matched in which of the following?

(1) Aspirin—is uricosuric in high doses
(2) Sulindac—has a long half-life
(3) Indomethacin—causes frontal headaches
(4) Ibuprofen—has more potent anti-inflammatory effects than aspirin

9. Major therapeutic uses for gold include the treatment of

(1) infectious hepatitis
(2) acute gout
(3) ankylosing spondylitis
(4) rheumatoid arthritis

Directions: The group of questions below consists of lettered choices followed by several numbered items. For each numbered item select the **one** lettered choice with which it is **most** closely associated. Each lettered choice may be used once, more than once, or not at all.

Questions 10–13

For each of the characteristics listed below, choose the drug that is most likely to show that characteristic.

(A) Aspirin
(B) Acetaminophen
(C) Phenylbutazone
(D) Probenecid
(E) Ibuprofen

10. Produces significant fluid retention
11. Possesses no analgesic activity
12. Is a uricosuric whose action is antagonized by salicylates
13. Possesses no anti-inflammatory activity but is a central prostaglandin inhibitor

ANSWERS AND EXPLANATIONS

1. The answer is A. *(X C 1, D 2, E 2, F)* The only agent listed in the question that interferes with the synthesis of uric acid is allopurinol. It does this by inhibiting xanthine oxidase, which converts xanthine and hypoxanthine to uric acid. Sulfinpyrazone is a uricosuric agent, while colchicine acts by preventing the migration of granulocytes. Indomethacin is useful for symptomatic relief in acute attacks of gout. Aspirin is also anti-inflammatory and analgesic; in high dosages it can be uricosuric.

2. The answer is A. *(V C)* Although all of the agents listed in the question can produce nausea and vomiting, indomethacin is the only one associated with a significant incidence of frontal headaches. Aspirin, phenacetin, and acetaminophen are effective analgesics and do not cause frontal headaches. Phenylbutazone also has the analgesic potency of aspirin.

3. The answer is E. *(X A–F)* Diet, uricosuric agents, colchicine, and allopurinol are the mainstay of therapy for the treatment of gout. Small doses of steroids are not used in treating this condition.

4. The answer is A. *(II B 6 e; III B 3; IV B 6; VII A 3)* All of the agents listed in the question except acetaminophen are capable of reducing platelet aggregation and thus prolonging bleeding times. Acetaminophen might be useful, therefore, in relieving the pain of arthritis in the hemophiliac patient, who is already at risk for deficient hemostasis.

5. The answer is B. *(I B 2; II B 1 b, 5, D 1)* Salicylates (e.g., aspirin) inhibit prostaglandin synthesis and thus have excellent anti-inflammatory properties. For example, the enzyme cyclooxygenase is irreversibly inactivated by aspirin and this blocks the synthesis of PGE_2 and $PGF_{2\alpha}$. Both of these prostaglandins are thought to be involved in inflammation-associated vasodilation, pain, and edema. The salicylates can cause epigastric distress and stimulate the chemoreceptor trigger zone in the CNS. Dose-related gastric ulceration and hemorrhage can occur, caused in part by exfoliation of gastric mucosal cells. Because the formation of PGI_2 (prostacyclin), which is known to inhibit gastric acid secretion, is suppressed, protective gastric mucus secretion is suppressed and gastric secretion increases. Salicylism is a mild salicylate intoxication and usually occurs with repeated ingestion of moderately large doses of salicylates.

6. The answer is C (2, 4). *(X E 1, 2)* Allopurinol is a purine derivative and a xanthine oxidase inhibitor, not a uricosuric agent. It blocks the conversion of hypoxanthine and xanthine to uric acid and by this mechanism lowers blood uric acid.

7. The answer is E (all). *(X B)* Probenecid prolongs penicillin blood levels by inhibiting its secretion. Probenecid is a uricosuric agent which is useful in the treatment of gout because it blocks the reabsorption of uric acid in the kidney. Sulfinpyrazone has a similar mechanism of action, namely, inhibiting the renal tubular reabsorption of uric acid.

8. The answer is D (4). *(II B 7; V C 2; VI C; VII A 2)* High doses of aspirin are uricosuric and sulindac has a long half-life. CNS complaints, including frontal headache, frequently occur with indomethacin. Ibuprofen is not a more potent anti-inflammatory agent than aspirin, it is equipotent.

9. The answer is D (4). *(IX D; X)* The major therapeutic use of gold is in the treatment of rheumatoid arthritis (RA), particularly RA that is unresponsive to salicylates and other types of nonsteroidal anti-inflammatory therapy. Gold therapy would be contraindicated in persons who have a history of infectious hepatitis. Gold is not used in the treatment of gout; therapeutic drugs for this condition include probenecid, sulfinpyrazone, colchicine, allopurinol, indomethacin, and phenylbutazone. Drugs used for the treatment of ankylosing spondylitis include sulindac, phenylbutazone, and indomethacin.

10–13. The answers are: 10-C, 11-D, 12-D, 13-B. *(III B 1, 2; IV B 1; X B 2, 5, F 3)* Phenylbutazone, by a direct effect on renal tubules, causes salt and water retention. Probenecid is the only agent listed which has no analgesic activity. Probenecid at therapeutic doses is uricosuric; it acts by inhibiting proximal tubular reabsorption of uric acid. Its action is antagonized by the salicylates. Acetaminophen is a central prostaglandin inhibitor, but exerts no anti-inflammatory activity.

10
Agents Affecting Endocrine Function

I. CORTICOTROPIN AND ADRENAL CORTICOSTEROIDS

A. ADRENAL PHYSIOLOGY

1. The adrenal cortex serves as a homeostatic organ, regulating reactions to stress.
2. The release of adrenal corticosteroids is controlled by a pathway that includes the central nervous system (Fig. 10-1).
3. A number of stimuli, including trauma, chemicals, diurnal rhythms, and emotion, can cause the **hypothalamus** to release corticotropin-releasing factor (CRF).
4. CRF traverses the hypophyseal portal system and stimulates the **anterior pituitary gland.**
5. The anterior pituitary gland in turn is stimulated to release corticotropin (adrenocorticotropic hormone, **ACTH).**
6. ACTH circulates in the bloodstream and acts on the **adrenal cortex.**

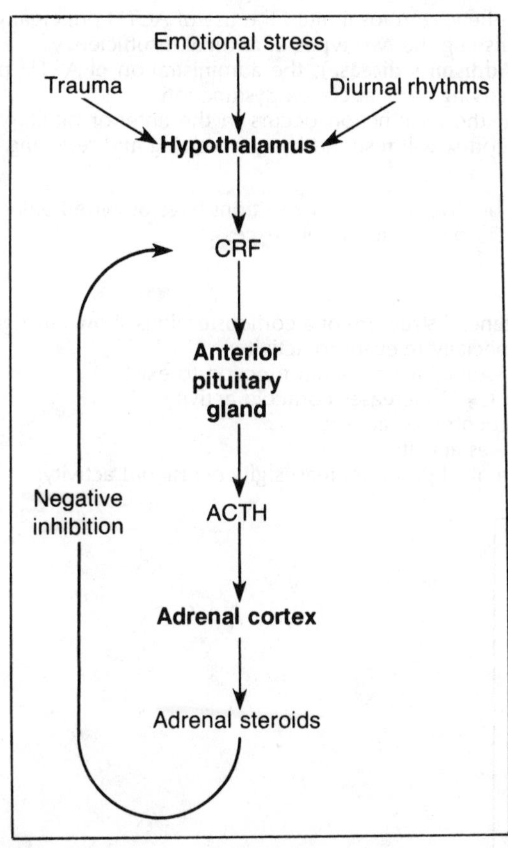

Figure 10-1. The pathway of adrenocorticotropic hormone (ACTH) and adrenal steroid secretion. CRF = corticotropin-releasing factor.

7. The adrenal cortex then releases the following endogenous corticosteroids:
   a. **Glucocorticoids**
      (1) Cortisol.
      (2) Cortisone.
      (3) Corticosterone.
   b. **Mineralocorticoids**
      (1) Aldosterone.
      (2) Desoxycorticosterone.

8. A **negative feedback pathway** maintains homeostasis (see Fig. 10-1). When the levels of endogenous corticosteroids increase, the production of ACTH is reduced, as is that of CRF.

B. ADRENOCORTICOTROPIC HORMONE (ACTH)

1. Human ACTH is a polypeptide hormone consisting of 39 amino acids.

2. Commercial derivatives have only 13 amino acids but still possess the action of endogenous ACTH.

3. **Mechanism of action**
   a. ACTH is thought to stimulate specific protein receptor sites on the adrenal cortical cell membrane.
   b. This membrane receptor is believed to be linked with a system for generating cyclic adenosine monophosphate (cyclic AMP). When the receptor is occupied by ACTH, the cyclic AMP system is activated and the synthesis of corticosteroids is initiated.
   c. The binding of ACTH to the receptor stimulates the rate-limiting step in the corticosteroid synthetic pathway (which originates with cholesterol).
   d. Although ACTH is required for the synthesis of mineralocorticoids, it stimulates the synthesis of glucocorticoids more than that of mineralocorticoids.

4. Since ACTH is a polypeptide hormone, it must be administered parenterally, and is most often given intramuscularly. It is rapidly hydrolyzed in the tissues, with a half-life of 15 minutes.

5. **Therapeutic uses.** The discovery of synthetic steroids limited the use of ACTH principally to serving as a diagnostic tool for distinguishing the two types of adrenal insufficiency.
   a. In **primary adrenal insufficiency (Addison's disease),** the administration of ACTH produces no effect because of the underlying adrenal cortex dysfunction.
   b. In **secondary adrenal insufficiency,** the dysfunction occurs in the anterior pituitary. If ACTH is administered, the adrenal cortex will respond by synthesizing and releasing the adrenocorticosteroids.

6. **Untoward effects** from ACTH are rare, but hypersensitivity reactions have occurred on occasion. **Toxicity** is dose-related and results from corticosteroid excess.

C. ADRENAL CORTICOSTEROIDS

1. **Structure–activity relationships.** The general structure of a corticosteroid is shown in Figure 10-2. Certain structural features are especially relevant to activity:
   a. Position 11: Oxygen or halogen is essential for corticoid function to exist.
   b. Position 17: The presence of OH or C=O increases corticoid activity.
   c. A double bond at 1,2 increases glucocorticoid activity.
   d. Position 6 or 9: Halogenation increases activity.
   e. Position 6 or 16: The presence of an alkyl group increases glucocorticoid activity.

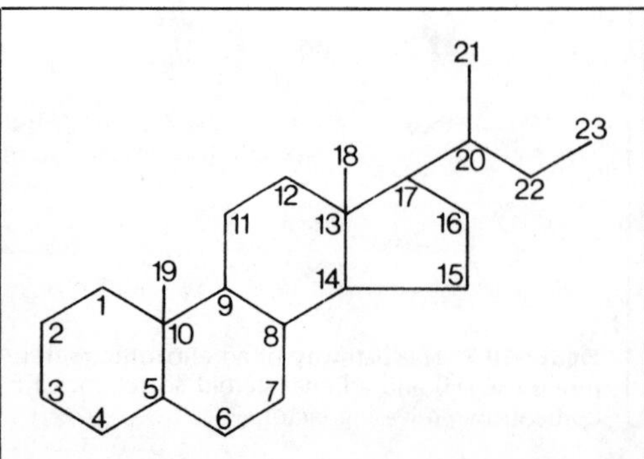

Figure 10-2. Adrenal corticosteroids: general structure.

2. Mechanism of action

a. The steroid receptor is found in the cytoplasm of the cell after the tissue is disrupted.

b. Once the steroid traverses the cell membrane and binds to the receptor, the complex is found in the nucleus of the cell.

c. The drug–receptor–chromatin complex stimulates the formation of messenger ribonucleic acid (mRNA).

d. The mRNA stimulates the synthesis of enzymes that control rate-limiting reactions in the synthetic pathway of the steroids.

3. Glucocorticoid activity

a. Physiologic doses can result in:

(1) Increased liver glycogen stores.

(2) Increased gluconeogenesis.

(3) Increased lipolysis.

(4) CNS effects, at times including euphoria.

(5) Maintenance of cardiovascular function by potentiation of norepinephrine.

(6) Maintenance of skeletal muscle function (in Addison's disease there is wasting of skeletal muscle).

(7) Increased hemoglobin synthesis, resulting in an elevation of the red blood cell count.

b. Pharmacologic doses can result in:

(1) Anti-inflammatory effects, in which steroids:

(a) Suppress leukocyte migration.

(b) Stabilize lysosomal membranes.

(c) Reduce the activity of fibroblasts which are involved in collagen and tissue repair in inflamed areas.

(d) Reverse the capillary permeability that is associated with histamine release.

(e) Suppress the immune response by inhibiting antibody synthesis.

(2) Anti-allergic effects—the mechanism is not well understood, but these effects are thought to be associated with the anti-inflammatory effects.

(3) Inhibition of growth and cell division.

4. Mineralocorticoid activity

a. Unlike the case with glucocorticoids, physiologic and pharmacologic doses of mineralocorticoids produce similar effects; it is the intensity of the effects that differs.

b. Mineralocorticoids increase blood sodium and decrease blood potassium.

c. Control of serum Na^+ depends primarily upon the juxtaglomerular apparatus, where a low Na^+ level in the blood causes the release of renin from the kidney. Renin cleaves angiotensinogen to form angiotensin, which triggers aldosterone release.

d. Aldosterone alters Na^+–K^+ in the distal tubule of the kidney to enhance sodium reabsorption.

5. Pharmacokinetics

a. Adrenal corticosteroids are readily absorbed in the gastrointestinal tract.

b. Some 90 percent of a dose becomes bound to plasma proteins.

c. Steroids are metabolized in the liver and are often bioactivated by reduction reactions. The final or phase II metabolic reaction results in the conjugation of the steroid with sulfate or glucuronide, and the conjugate then is excreted by the kidney.

6. Preparations

a. Mineralocorticoids

(1) Aldosterone is an endogenous mineralocorticoid but is not available as a medicinal agent.

(2) Desoxycorticosterone and **fludrocortisone** are the agents used as replacements for aldosterone in Addison's disease.

b. Glucocorticoids with some mineralocorticoid activity

(1) Hydrocortisone and **cortisone** are examples.

(2) Though they possess primarily glucocorticoid activity, they do cause some sodium retention. This becomes significant only in patients who are not able to tolerate the additional sodium load.

c. Glucocorticoids without mineralocorticoid activity

(1) These are semisynthetic analogs of the natural substances and are very important since an anti-inflammatory dose can be given without the untoward effect of sodium retention.

(2) Examples include **prednisone, prednisolone, methylprednisolone, triamcinolone, betamethasone**, and **beclomethasone.**

(3) Beclomethasone was the first corticosteroid available in the inhalation form; it is used to treat acute bronchial asthma.

d. The commonly used corticosteroids, with their anti-inflammatory potency, equivalent milligram potency, and sodium retention potential, are listed in Table 10-1. In Table 10-2, these preparations are divided on the basis of their duration of action into short-, intermediate-, and long-acting steroids.

7. **Principles of administration.** Corticosteroid dosing varies greatly, depending on the condition of the patient.
   a. The major endogenous glucocorticoid is hydrocortisone, with 10 to 25 mg secreted daily. About 0.5 to 2 mg of corticosterone and 30 to 150 μg of aldosterone are secreted daily. Secretion shows a diurnal rhythm; the peak of secretion occurs between 4 a.m. and 8 a.m.
   b. In stressful situations, these values can increase tenfold.
   c. It is best if oral steroids are taken around 8 a.m. to mimic the natural secretion of the adrenal cortex.
   d. Less than 25 mg of prednisone per day (or equivalent—see Table 10-1) taken at 8 a.m. for fewer than 5 to 10 days usually will not suppress the pituitary–adrenal axis.
      (1) If the axis is suppressed, the adrenal cortex will not respond to stress by releasing steroids; the consequences can be fatal.
      (2) Once this axis is suppressed it may take over a year for normal function to return.
   e. To minimize the effects of pituitary–adrenal axis suppression, when steroid treatment ceases, doses should be tapered off rather than stopped abruptly.
   f. When steroids are used in children, alternate-day therapy is recommended. With this regimen, normal growth patterns can be maintained and suppression of the pituitary–adrenal axis by negative feedback is less likely.

8. **Therapeutic uses**
   a. **Replacement therapy for adrenal insufficiency**
      (1) For acute adrenal insufficiency, cortisol hemisuccinate is given by intravenous injection; it is then given in intravenous fluids.
      (2) For chronic adrenal insufficiency cortisone acetate is taken on arising and in the late afternoon. The mineralocorticoid fludrocortisone acetate is taken daily also.
   b. **Management of arthritis**
      (1) All other therapy must have failed before steroids are used. The patient also should be exhibiting progressive disability.
      (2) Steroids are administered by intra-articular injection for the treatment of affected joints.
   c. Corticosteroids are also widely used in the treatment of:
      (1) Rheumatic carditis.
      (2) Renal diseases, including the nephrotic syndrome.
      (3) Most collagen vascular diseases.
      (4) Severe allergic reactions.
      (5) Ocular disorders involving inflammation.
      (6) Various skin diseases, usually by topical administration.
      (7) Chronic ulcerative colitis.
      (8) Cerebral edema.
   d. The use of corticosteroids in cancer patients is discussed in Chapter 11, V D.

9. **Untoward effects**
   a. Prolonged therapy with corticosteroids can result in the following:
      (1) Suppression of pituitary–adrenal function.
      (2) Increased susceptibility to infection.
      (3) Peptic ulceration, which may be the result of altered mucosal defense mechanisms.

Table 10-1. Glucocorticoids: Anti-Inflammatory Potency, Relative Potency (Oral), and Potential for Sodium Retention

Glucocorticoid	Anti-Inflammatory Potency	Equivalent Oral Potency (mg)	Sodium Retention
Hydrocortisone	1.0	20	2+
Cortisone	0.8	25	2+
Prednisolone	5.0	5	1+
Prednisone	4.0	5	1+
Methylprednisolone	5.0	4	0
Triamcinolone	5.0	4	0
Betamethasone	40.0	0.6	0
Dexamethasone	30.0	0.75	0

Table 10-2. Duration of Action of Some Commonly Used Corticosteroids

Short-Acting (12 hr or less)	Intermediate-Acting (12 to 24 hr)	Long-Acting (over 24 hr)
Hydrocortisone Cortisone	Prednisone Prednisolone Methylprednisolone Triamcinolone	Dexamethasone Betamethasone

(4) Myopathy characterized by proximal arm and leg weakness.
(5) Psychological disturbances, including suicidal tendencies or "steroid psychosis."
(6) Posterior subcapsular cataracts, especially in children.
(7) Osteoporosis, which can lead to vertebral fractures. Glucocorticoids directly inhibit osteoblast formation as well as intestinal calcium absorption. They also increase secretion of parathyroid hormone.
(8) Hyperglycemia

b. Glucocorticoids can arrest growth in small children receiving small doses. Both DNA synthesis and cell division are inhibited.

D. ADRENAL STEROID INHIBITORS

1. Metyrapone reduces cortisol production by inhibiting the 11-β-hydroxylation reaction.
2. It is used in diagnosing primary and secondary adrenal insufficiency. When cortisol production is blocked, negative feedback should increase ACTH and the production of precursors of cortisol if the pituitary and adrenal glands are functional.
3. Metyrapone has also been used to treat hypercortisolism that results from adrenal neoplasms.

II. ORAL CONTRACEPTIVES

A. THE FEMALE MENSTRUAL CYCLE

1. The hypothalamus releases periodic pulses of LHRH (luteinizing-hormone-releasing hormone) which affect the anterior pituitary gland. The gonadotropic hormones FSH (follicle-stimulating hormone) and LH (luteinizing hormone), released from the pituitary gland, influence ovarian secretion.
2. At about day 5 of the menstrual cycle, the level of estrogen in the bloodstream begins to rise as follicles in the ovary develop, stimulated by FSH. Estrogen secretion decreases when one of the follicles ruptures at ovulation on day 14, and the corpus luteum is formed. After day 14, the corpus luteum secretes progesterone and estrogen, and the levels of these steroids remain elevated until the corpus luteum regresses.
3. Estrogen stimulates the midcycle surge of LH and FSH that triggers luteinization. At other times, estrogen exerts a negative feedback, especially on FSH.

B. TYPES OF ORAL CONTRACEPTIVES

1. The "**combination pill**" contains both estrogen and a progestin.
   a. Commonly used components
      (1) Ethinyl estradiol or mestranol is used for estrogen activity.
      (2) Norethindrone, ethynodiol, or norethynodrel is used for progesterone activity.
   b. The main **mechanism of action** appears to be suppression of the midcycle surge of LH and FSH.
   c. Administration of the combination starts on day 5 and continues through the fertile period (day 12 to 16) and until day 25. The next course is started 7 days after the last dose.
2. The "**minipill**," which contains progestin alone, is taken throughout the menstrual cycle. It is 97 percent effective. Menstrual cycles are more irregular than with the combination pill. The mechanism is not known.

C. UNTOWARD EFFECTS

1. Estrogens increase the blood concentrations of some clotting factors as well as increasing platelet aggregation.
2. The risk of thrombophlebitis and thromboembolism is increased significantly with oral contraceptive use. It appears to be estrogen-dose-dependent.

3. The incidence of cerebral and coronary thrombosis is increased, but age, smoking, and hypertension are important associated risk factors.

4. Reversible hypertension occurs in 5 percent of women taking oral contraceptives. Estrogen increases the circulating concentrations of renin and angiotensin, resulting in sodium and water retention.

5. Vaginal and uterine carcinomas are associated with the use of estrogens, but what role oral contraceptives play is poorly defined.

6. Irregular vaginal bleeding (''breakthrough'' bleeding) may occur when pills are first begun.

7. Nausea, vomiting, breast tenderness, weight gain, dizziness, and headaches have all been associated with oral contraceptive use.

8. Depression, various ocular disturbances, and an increased incidence of gallbladder disease have also been associated with oral contraceptive use.

D. OTHER USES OF ESTROGENS. Estrogens are used for replacement therapy in conditions such as primary ovarian failure or inadequate pituitary function or after a hysterectomy. Their use in postmenopausal women is controversial because there is an increased risk of endometrial carcinoma.

III. ANDROGENS

A. PHYSIOLOGY

1. The hypothalamus produces luteinizing-hormone–releasing hormone (LHRH), a peptide that stimulates the release of pituitary luteinizing hormone (LH) and follicle-stimulating hormone (FSH).

2. LH and FSH act on the testes to stimulate spermatogenesis and the formation of **testosterone.**

3. Testosterone or an active metabolite, dihydrotestosterone, exerts negative feedback on the hypothalamus or the pituitary gland, or both, to regulate steroid production.

4. The **actions** of androgens include developmental effects on the male reproductive system in utero and at puberty. Androgens maintain libido and cause the development of secondary male characteristics such as growth of facial hair and increased skeletal muscle mass.

B. CLINICAL USES. Androgens are used:

1. As replacement therapy to induce puberty in adolescent males and to maintain secondary sex characteristics in adults with testicular failure or hypogonadism.

2. To prevent osteoporosis in postmenopausal women. An estrogen is given in combination with the androgen to prevent masculinizing side effects; as mentioned above, the postmenopausal use of estrogens is controversial.

3. As replacement therapy, with other hormones (thyroid, adrenal, corticosteroid, growth hormone, and estrogen), in females with hypopituitarism.

C. UNTOWARD EFFECTS include:

1. Masculinization in women.

2. Precocious puberty and premature closing of epiphyseal plates in children.

3. Fluid retention.

4. Jaundice, with 17-methyl substituted androgens.

D. PREPARATIONS include:

1. Testosterone.
2. Methyltestosterone.
3. Fluoxymesterone.
4. Long-acting ester derivatives such as testosterone propionate and testosterone cypionate.

IV. INSULIN

A. GENERAL COMMENTS

1. In 1921, Banting and Best extracted insulin from the pancreas and demonstrated its therapeutic effects in diabetic dogs and human subjects.
2. It is important to remember that diabetes mellitus involves not only a deficiency of insulin but also an excess of certain other hormones, such as growth hormone, glucocorticoids, and glucagon. Thus, not only the pancreas is involved in glucose homeostasis but also the anterior pituitary gland and the adrenal cortex are.

B. ETIOLOGY OF DIABETES MELLITUS

1. It is currently believed that the juvenile-onset (insulin-dependent) form has an autoimmune etiology.
2. Viruses may also play a role in the etiology of diabetes. Coxsackie B, mumps, and rubella viruses all have been shown to produce morphologic changes in the islet-cell structure.
3. The genetic role in the etiology of diabetes is controversial. Possibly a genetic trait makes an individual's pancreas more susceptible to one of the above viruses.

C. CHEMISTRY OF INSULIN

1. Insulin consists of two amino acid chains joined together by disulfide linkages; it has a molecular weight of about 6,000.
2. Pancreatic β cells form insulin from a single-chain precursor, proinsulin, which possesses little biologic activity.
3. Insulin can exist as a monomer, a dimer, or a hexamer consisting of three dimers.
   - **a.** Two molecules of Zn^{2+} are coordinated in the hexamer form, and it is this form that is stored in the granules of the β cell.
   - **b.** The biologically active form is thought to be the monomer.
4. There are species variations in the amino acid sequence of insulin.

D. REGULATION OF INSULIN SECRETION

1. **Proinsulin,** which is synthesized in the rough endoplasmic reticulum, is packaged, through the Golgi apparatus, into secretory granules. Along the way, an enzymatic process converts proinsulin to insulin.
2. Stored granules containing many insulin molecules are released by exocytosis.
3. Oral glucose has a greater ability to stimulate insulin secretion than intravenously administered glucose. Fatty acids, amino acids, and ketone bodies all increase insulin secretion.
4. Gastrointestinal hormones such as secretin, pancreozymin, and gastrin can stimulate insulin secretion.
5. **Autonomic control of insulin secretion**
   - **a.** β-Adrenergic agonists increase insulin secretion by increasing intracellular cyclic AMP.
   - **b.** Cyclic AMP plus calcium may activate a microtubular–microfilament system that promotes the release of the insulin granule.
6. Glucose-induced insulin release appears to occur in two phases:
   - **a.** An initial-burst phase which peaks in minutes and then rapidly declines.
   - **b.** A slow phase which takes an hour to reach a peak.

E. PHARMACOKINETICS

1. The majority of secreted insulin circulates in the blood and lymphatic system as the free hormone.
2. Though small quantities of insulin can be detected in the urine, the kidney normally filters and reabsorbs the hormone.
3. Both the liver and the kidney are of primary importance in the degradation of insulin by a proteolytic enzyme. Each is capable of destroying 40 percent of the insulin produced per day.

F. SYNDROMES OF DIABETES MELLITUS

1. Juvenile-onset (insulin-dependent) diabetes

- **a.** In this type of diabetes there is no circulating insulin in the plasma.
- **b.** There is complete failure of pancreatic β cell function.
- **c.** The patient is prone to both hyperglycemia and ketoacidosis.

2. Maturity-onset (non-insulin-dependent) diabetes

- **a.** This type may be due to a defect in the receptor on the pancreatic β cell membrane.
- **b.** In the earliest forms of the disease, there is a delay in the initial secretion of insulin after stimulation by glucose.
- **c.** Also, less insulin than normal is secreted at any given glucose concentration.
- **d.** The patient is not prone to ketoacidosis.

3. In both types of diabetes mellitus, plasma immunoreactive glucagon concentrations are increased, especially during ketoacidosis. The normal suppression of glucagon by hyperglycemia is also impaired.

4. The pathognomonic finding of capillary basement membrane thickening occurs early in the course of diabetes mellitus. It is this change which is probably responsible for the major complications of diabetes, including premature atherosclerosis, glomerulosclerosis, retinopathy, neuropathy, and ulceration and gangrene of the extremities.

G. METABOLIC EFFECTS OF INSULIN DEFICIENCY

1. When insulin is deficient, there is a reduction in the rate of transport of glucose across the membranes of certain cells, including muscle and adipose cells.

2. Insulin does not significantly influence the rate of glucose transport across liver cells, erythrocytes, or leukocytes, and the rate of entry of glucose into the brain is only affected in ketoacidosis.

3. There is a reduction in the activity of the enzyme systems necessary for catalyzing glucose to glycogen.

4. Hyperlipemia, ketonemia, and acidosis can all occur with insulin deficiency. This lack of insulin allows hormone-sensitive lipase to mobilize fatty acids, which leads to elevated circulating levels of ketones, acetoacetate, and β-hydroxybutyrate.

5. Insulin deficiency combined with glucagon excess results in the conversion of large amounts of protein to glucose, resulting in an increased excretion of urea and ammonia (azoturia).

H. MECHANISM OF INSULIN ACTION

1. The initial action of insulin is at the cell surface, where the hormone interacts with a highly specific receptor.

2. Exactly how insulin facilitates the transport of glucose and amino acids is not known.

I. PREPARATIONS AND ADMINISTRATION.

Various types of insulin are made which differ in their onset and duration of action. The potency of insulin is expressed in USP units.

1. Crystalline zinc insulin (regular insulin)

- **a.** Regular insulin is a short-acting, soluble insulin which is prepared in a phosphate buffer with Zn^{2+} at a pH of 3.5.
- **b.** Its peak action occurs in 2 to 4 hours and its duration is 5 to 7 hours.
- **c.** It can be administered subcutaneously or intravenously and is a good agent for exerting rapid control for diabetic ketoacidosis.
- **d.** The frequency of injections (4 or 5 /day) is not very convenient.

2. Protamine zinc insulin

- **a.** Adding the basic protein protamine to crystalline zinc insulin causes the formation of large crystals. This produces a compound which is less soluble.
- **b.** When injected, this formulation serves as a tissue depot, producing slow absorption into the bloodstream.
- **c.** The action of protamine zinc insulin peaks in 18 to 16 hours and lasts up to 36 hours.
- **d.** Fine control of hyperglycemia is difficult with such a long-acting preparation.

3. Isophane insulin (NPH, neutral protamine Hagedorn)

- **a.** This intermediate-acting insulin is similar to protamine zinc insulin, but it contains only a small amount of protamine (0.5 mg per 100 units of insulin).

b. Therefore, NPH insulin has an earlier onset and earlier peak effects than protamine zinc insulin, but the duration of action is similar for both preparations.
c. The effects of NPH insulin peak in 8 to 12 hours and have a duration of 24 to 28 hours.
d. These effects are clinically equivalent to combining 2 to 3 units of crystalline zinc insulin with 1 unit of protamine zinc insulin.

4. Lente insulins
a. These insulins do not contain protamine; their insolubility results from the addition of excess zinc in an acetate rather than a phosphate buffer.
b. The onset of action for the lente insulins varies greatly and depends upon the physical state, the ambient zinc concentration, and the pH:
(1) A microamorphous crystalline form known as **prompt insulin zinc suspension (semilente insulin),** peaks in 4 to 8 hours and has a duration of action of 12 to 16 hours.
(2) A large crystalline form with a high zinc content, known as **extended insulin zinc suspension (ultralente insulin),** has an onset and duration of action similar to those of protamine zinc insulin.
(3) Combining 7 parts of ultralente with 3 parts of semilente produces **insulin zinc suspension (lente insulin),** which is quite similar to NPH insulin in its onset and duration of action.

5. Human insulins produced by semisynthetic and recombinant DNA techniques have recently been made available.

J. ROUTE OF ADMINISTRATION

1. The usual route of administration for all insulin preparations is subcutaneous.
2. Insulin is administered intravenously only during emergency circumstances. If administration is via this route the crystalline form is given because it acts rapidly.
3. Since insulin is a protein it can not be given orally because it would be digested.

K. UNTOWARD EFFECTS ASSOCIATED WITH INSULIN THERAPY

1. Hypoglycemia
a. The worst sequela is insulin shock, characterized by abnormalities of the CNS, including hypoglycemic convulsions.
b. Early symptoms of hypoglycemia such as sweating, tachycardia, and hunger are thought to be brought about by the compensatory secretion of epinephrine.
c. Hypoglycemia is best treated by administering glucose intravenously, or by giving fruit juice or other soluble carbohydrates. Glucagon may be given as an alternative to glucose, and it is administered parenterally.

2. Local reactions. Irritation at the site of injection can lead to lipodystrophy and hypertrophy. Sites of injection should be rotated.

3. Antigenic response
a. With the development of new, more highly purified insulin, hypersensitivity reactions are less of a problem.
b. Antigenicity increases as the duration of action of the insulin is increased. Thus, protamine zinc insulin is the most antigenic because of its long duration of action, and also because it contains a large amount of the basic protein protamine. The order of antigenic potency, in descending order, is beef > pork > highly purified ("single-peak") pork > human insulin.

4. Other untoward effects. Psychological problems can occur, especially in the adolescent diabetic.

L. FACTORS ALTERING INSULIN REQUIREMENTS

1. **Other drugs.** Salicylates inhibit the enzymes necessary for gluconeogenesis and also accelerate their utilization. Anticoagulants tend to stimulate insulin secretion, thereby decreasing insulin requirements.
2. **Hormones.** Glucagon, epinephrine, and growth hormone all increase insulin requirements.
3. **Exercise** decreases insulin requirements by making muscle more permeable to glucose and releasing muscle-bound insulin.
4. **Stress,** both physiologic (fever, infection, pregnancy) and psychological, increases insulin requirements, possibly secondary to epinephrine release.

5. **Eating patterns.** Alterations in the diet or a change in eating time may increase or decrease insulin requirements.

6. **Obesity** increases insulin requirements. This may be the result of an increase in the number of insulin binding sites on the greater surface area of the adipose tissue.

V. ORAL HYPOGLYCEMIC AGENTS (SULFONYLUREAS)

A. MECHANISM OF ACTION

1. Sulfonylureas stimulate insulin secretion from pancreatic β cells without entering the cell. This occurs in the absence of glucose.

2. Sulfonylureas may also sensitize the pancreatic β cells to glucose.

B. PHARMACOKINETICS

1. **All sulfonylurea agents** are readily absorbed from the small intestine and have an onset of action varying from 30 minutes to 3 hours. The duration of action also varies from agent to agent.

2. **Tolbutamide**
   a. Onset of action occurs in 30 minutes, while duration of action is 6 to 12 hours.
   b. Tolbutamide is the shortest-acting sulfonylurea and is readily metabolized in the liver to inactive products.
   c. Excretion occurs via the kidney.

3. **Acetohexamide**
   a. Onset of action is rapid; effects peak in 3 hours and last for 12 to 24 hours.
   b. The major metabolite, hydroxyhexamide, is thought to possess most of the activity of this agent. It is renally excreted.

4. **Tolazamide**
   a. Tolazamide is slowly absorbed. Effects do not peak for 6 hours, and the drug has a duration of action of 24 hours.
   b. Its metabolic products are weaker hypoglycemics than the parent compound.
   c. Metabolic products are excreted by the kidney.

5. **Chlorpropamide**
   a. Though rapidly absorbed, this agent becomes bound to plasma proteins.
   b. It has a duration of action of 60 hours.
   c. It is not metabolically altered and is excreted very slowly in its unchanged form.

C. UNTOWARD EFFECTS

1. These are seen in 3 percent to 5 percent of patients treated with a sulfonylurea agent.

2. Hypoglycemia can occur in patients with hepatic or renal insufficiency because the agent will have a longer than expected duration of action.

3. Cutaneous reactions include rashes and photosensitivity.

4. Gastrointestinal reactions include nausea and vomiting.

5. Hematologic reactions—leukopenia, agranulocytosis, thrombocytopenia, pancytopenia, and hemolytic anemia—have occurred.

6. Transient cholestatic jaundice occurs rarely.

7. Inappropriate secretion of antidiuretic hormone has been observed.

D. THERAPEUTIC USES

1. The sulfonylureas are used in the treatment of patients who have insulin-independent diabetes and who cannot be treated with diet alone or who are unwilling to take insulin if dietary control fails.

2. The findings of the University Group Diabetes Program, though controversial, support the above statement, and many physicians have had success using the sulfonylurea agents. The UGDP study did suggest that use of these agents was associated with a higher cardiovascular mortality rate than that produced by diet alone or with insulin therapy.

3. No study to date has demonstrated that sulfonylurea agents prevent the long-term complications of diabetes.

VI. AGENTS AFFECTING THE THYROID GLAND

A. THYROID HORMONES

1. Synthesis

a. Thyroglobulin, a large protein of 600,000 molecular weight, is synthesized in the thyroid gland.

b. The tyrosines on the molecule are iodinated and coupled by a peroxidase.

c. The iodinated thyroglobulin is secreted into the lumen of the gland.

d. The hypothalamus releases thyrotropin-releasing hormone (TRH), which stimulates the pituitary gland to release thyrotropin. In the thyroid gland, thyrotropin stimulates the uptake of thyroglobulin from the lumen back into the cell where it is broken down to yield the thyroid hormones.

e. There are two active forms of thyroid hormone: thyroxine (T_4) and triiodothyronine (T_3) (Fig. 10-3).

2. Physiologic role

a. Thyroid hormones regulate growth and development.

b. They exert a calorigenic effect by increasing the basal metabolic rate.

c. Thyroid hormones accelerate carbohydrate utilization and enhance lipolytic reactions.

d. They inhibit pituitary secretion of thyrotropin by negative feedback.

3. Therapeutic uses

a. Thyroid hormone therapy is used for the treatment of hypothyroidism and myxedema, including myxedema coma.

b. If thyroid hormone therapy is instituted early after birth to hypothyroid infants, cretinism is prevented.

c. It is used in patients with simple goiter and some patients with nodular goiter, who are deficient in the secretion of thyroid hormone. In the case of nodular goiter, carcinoma should be ruled out.

4. Preparation and administration

a. Thyroid tablets are made from extracts of the thyroid gland.

b. Thyroglobulin is a purified extract of pig thyroid.

c. Levothyroxine sodium is the sodium salt of L-thyroxine.

d. Liothyronine sodium is the salt of L-triiodothyronine.

e. Equivalent clinical responses are obtained from the daily administration of about 60 mg of thyroid, 60 mg of thyroglobulin, 100 μg of levothyroxine, or 25 μg of liothyronine.

B. THYROID INHIBITORS

1. Types and their mechanisms of action

a. Antithyroid agents hinder the synthesis of thyroid hormones by preventing the incorporation of iodine into tyrosyl residues of thyroglobulin.

b. Ionic inhibitors block the mechanism for the transport of iodide and thus inhibit thyroidal uptake of iodide ion.

c. Iodide in high concentrations can suppress the thyroid by mechanisms that are not clear.

d. Radioactive iodine concentrates in the thyroid gland, and, in sufficient amounts, can damage the gland through the cytotoxic effects of ionizing radiation.

2. Antithyroid agents

a. Pharmacokinetics

(1) The prototype agent, **propylthiouracil,** is rapidly absorbed and has a short half-life (2 hours). It is concentrated in the thyroid, and is renally excreted.

(2) Antithyroid agents cross the placenta and are found in breast milk.

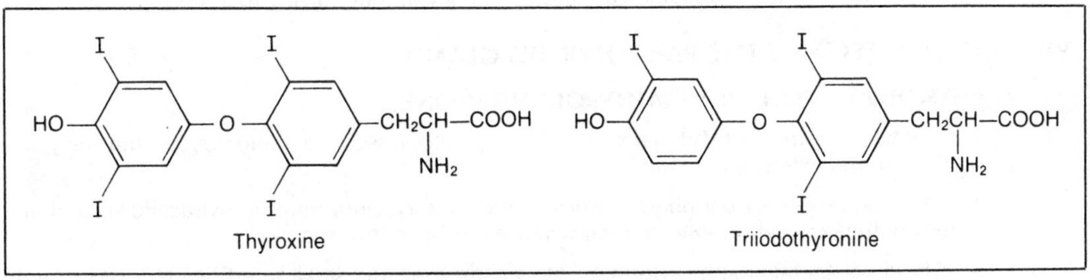

I I I I
HO— —O— —CH_2CH—COOH HO— —O— —CH_2CH—COOH
NH_2 NH_2
I I I
Thyroxine Triiodothyronine

Figure 10-3. Structures of thyroxine (T_4) and triiodothyronine (T_3).

b. **Therapeutic uses.** Antithyroid agents are used in the management of hyperthyroidism. They may be used:
(1) Alone.
(2) With radioiodine, while awaiting the beneficial effects of radiation to appear.
(3) Prior to the surgical treatment of hyperthyroidism (see 3 a (2), below).

c. **Untoward effects**
(1) The most serious untoward effect, though rare, is agranulocytosis.
(2) The most common complaint is a maculopapular rash and fever.

3. **Iodide**

a. **Therapeutic uses in hyperthyroidism**
(1) Iodide is used preoperatively to control hyperthyroidism (i.e., Graves' disease), because it reduces the size of the gland and makes the gland firmer.
(2) It is best to control the hyperthyroidism first with an antithyroid agent such as propylthiouracil. Iodide is then begun 10 days prior to the operative procedure.

b. **Preparations and administration**
(1) **Lugol's solution** contains 5 percent iodine, which is reduced in the intestine to iodide, and 10 percent potassium iodide.
(2) **Potassium iodide** is available for oral use in both solution and solid forms.

c. **Untoward effects**
(1) Preparations containing iodine, as well as iodide, can produce an acute hypersensitivity reaction resulting in angioedema, cutaneous hemorrhages, and symptoms of serum sickness.
(2) Chronic iodide administration can result in iodism.
(a) This is characterized by a brassy taste, increased salivation, and soreness of the teeth and gums. Swelling of the eyelids and symptoms resembling an upper respiratory tract infection can be observed.
(b) Inflammation of the pharynx and larynx can occur, as well as severe frontal headache.
(c) Several types of skin lesions have been observed.
(d) All of the above symptoms usually resolve within a few days after the discontinuation of iodide.

4. **Radioactive iodine**

a. **Pharmacokinetics**
(1) The most commonly used isotope is ^{131}I, which has a half-life of 8 days and emits both β particles and x-rays.
(2) Radioiodine is rapidly incorporated into the colloid of the thyroid follicles.

b. **Therapeutic uses**
(1) Radioiodine is highly effective in the treatment of hyperthyroidism, especially in older patients with heart disease.
(2) It is also a useful diagnostic tool to delineate thyroid disorders.

c. **Preparations and administration**
(1) Sodium iodide I 131 is available both as a solution and as capsules, and can be administered orally or intravenously.
(2) Sodium iodide I 125 is available as capsules for oral administration and as a solution for oral or intravenous use.

d. **Untoward effects**
(1) The treatment of hyperthyroidism with radioiodine is associated with a relatively high incidence of delayed hypothyroidism.
(2) Usually, there is a delayed onset in the control of hyperthyroidism.
(3) There is no conclusive evidence that radioiodine causes cancer in adults, but most physicians are hesitant to use it in patients less than 30 years old, not only because of this possible risk but also because of potential unknown effects on future offspring.
(4) Radioiodine is contraindicated in pregnancy and in nursing mothers.

VII. AGENTS AFFECTING THE PARATHYROID GLAND

A. PHYSIOLOGIC ROLE OF PARATHYROID HORMONE

1. Parathyroid hormone (PTH, parathormone) regulates the concentration of calcium and phosphate in the extracellular fluid.

2. PTH acts on various peripheral tissues to mobilize calcium into the extracellular fluid and restore the concentration to normal when it has been lowered.

3. PTH increases the active absorption of calcium from the small intestine. This is a vitamin D–dependent process.

4. PTH increases the rate of bone resorption of calcium and phosphate.

5. At physiologic doses PTH increases the renal tubular reabsorption of calcium and the excretion of phosphate.

6. The effects on both bone and kidney are probably mediated via cyclic AMP.

B. DISEASES OF THE PARATHYROID GLAND

1. Hypoparathyroidism
  a. Hypoparathyroidism is one of many causes of hypocalcemia.
  b. Symptoms include paresthesias of the extremities, tetany, laryngospasm, and eventually generalized convulsions. Spasms of smooth muscle can also occur. Electrocardiographic changes can include marked tachycardia.
  c. Dietary supplementation of vitamin D and calcium is the principal form of treatment.

2. Hyperparathyroidism
  a. The primary form is due to parathyroid hyperplasia or adenoma, or to tumors at other sites.
  b. The secondary form is a result of conditions producing a negative calcium balance, such as malabsorption or renal disease.
  c. Symptoms and signs include hypercalciuria (which can result in renal calculi), muscle weakness, constipation, nausea, and vomiting.
  d. Treatment is usually by surgical resection, although long-term therapy with neutral phosphate, a low-calcium diet, and plenty of fluids may be given to those patients who are poor surgical candidates.

C. CALCITONIN

1. Parafollicular C cells of the thyroid are the site of production and secretion of calcitonin. Parafollicular C cells are also found in the parathyroid and thymus.

2. The synthesis and secretion of calcitonin are regulated by the plasma calcium concentration. Cyclic AMP, epinephrine, glucagon, gastrin, and cholecystokinin all play a role by stimulating calcitonin release following the ingestion of calcium salts.

3. By altering osteoclastic and osteocytic activity calcitonin can directly inhibit bone resorption.

4. Calcitonin, in part by a cyclic AMP–mediated reaction, increases kidney excretion of calcium, phosphate, and sodium.

5. Preparation and administration
  a. Calcitonin used clinically is salmon calcitonin.
  b. It is administered subcutaneously or intramuscularly.

6. Therapeutic uses
  a. The major uses of calcitonin are to decrease hypercalcemia and hyperphosphatemia in patients with:
    (1) Hyperparathyroidism.
    (2) Idiopathic hypercalcemia of pregnancy.
    (3) Vitamin D intoxication.
    (4) Osteolytic bone metastases.
  b. Though calcitonin is effective for the treatment of Paget's disease of bone, patients may become resistant to therapy in several months.

7. **Untoward effects** include occasional edema and nausea and the stimulation of antibody formation.

D. SODIUM ETIDRONATE

1. Sodium etidronate is used in the treatment of Paget's disease of bone.

2. It is thought to slow the formation and dissolution of hydroxyapatite crystals.

3. Its advantages over calcitonin include:
  a. Oral efficacy.
  b. Lack of antigenicity.

4. Etidronate disodium is given orally. Daily doses, given for not more than 6 months, may produce a long-lasting remission.

STUDY QUESTIONS

Directions: Each question below contains five suggested answers. Choose the **one best** response to each question.

1. All of the following are endogenous corticosteroids released by the adrenal cortex EXCEPT

(A) cortisol
(B) cortisone
(C) beclomethasone
(D) aldosterone
(E) corticosterone

2. Which of the following synthetic steroids shows predominantly mineralocorticoid action?

(A) Hydrocortisone
(B) Spironolactone
(C) Dexamethasone
(D) Fludrocortisone
(E) Cortisol

3. All of the following statements about diabetes are correct EXCEPT

(A) diabetes can be caused by a lack of insulin secretion from the β cells of the pancreas
(B) diabetic patients who are poorly controlled usually have a positive nitrogen balance
(C) In the diabetic patient, lipolysis leads to the accumulation of fatty acids, producing the characteristic acetone breath
(D) insulin allows muscle cells to take up glucose in diabetic and healthy individuals
(E) severe diabetics often have vascular and neurologic complications

4. Edema, thrombophlebitis, and thromboembolism have been associated with the use of oral contraceptives that have an excess of

(A) progestin
(B) estrogen
(C) testosterone
(D) aldosterone
(E) prostaglandins

5. All of the following are short-acting or intermediate-acting antidiabetic agents EXCEPT

(A) chlorpropamide
(B) crystalline zinc insulin
(C) semilente insulin
(D) neutral protamine Hagedorn (NPH) insulin
(E) tolbutamide

6. All of the following statements about adrenocorticotropic hormone (ACTH) are true EXCEPT

(A) release of endogenous ACTH is controlled by corticotropin-releasing factor (CRF)
(B) release of ACTH can be inhibited by cortisol
(C) ACTH is in part responsible for activating the synthesis of corticosteroids
(D) ACTH is most useful clinically as a diagnostic tool to confirm adrenal insufficiency
(E) the oral route is the preferred route of administration

7. All of the following statements about oral contraceptives are true EXCEPT

(A) the "combination pill" contains both estrogen and progestin
(B) ethinyl estradiol and mestranol are commonly used in oral contraceptives
(C) the "minipill" contains estrogen alone
(D) estrogen inhibits the secretion of follicle-stimulating hormone (FSH)
(E) the risk of thromboembolism increases significantly with oral contraceptive use

Directions: Each question below contains four suggested answers of which **one or more** is correct. Choose the answer

A if **1, 2, and 3** are correct
B if **1 and 3** are correct
C if **2 and 4** are correct
D if **4** is correct
E if **1, 2, 3, and 4** are correct

8. Which of the following characteristics would be true for adrenocorticotropic hormone (ACTH)?

(1) It combines with cytoplasmic receptor which then combines with chromatin
(2) It has a steroid structure
(3) It is commonly used to treat arthritis
(4) Cortisol inhibits its release

9. True statements about insulin include which of the following?

(1) It promotes the synthesis of glycogen
(2) It enhances the peripheral utilization of glucose
(3) It enhances the conversion of glucose to fat
(4) It acts on the liver to promote glycogenolysis

10. Which of the following corticosteroids and characteristics are correctly matched?

(1) Desoxycorticosterone—causes hypernatremia (Na^+)
(2) Triamcinolone—is a glucocorticoid
(3) Prednisolone—stabilizes lysosomal membranes
(4) Cortisone—must be bioactivated in the liver

11. True statements about crystalline zinc insulin include which of the following?

(1) It can serve as replacement therapy for juvenile-onset diabetes
(2) Its active precursor is proinsulin
(3) It is a short-acting insulin
(4) It can be administered orally

12. Which of the following are known to be glucocorticoid effects?

(1) A dose-dependent increase in liver glycogen stores
(2) Maintenance of normal cardiovascular function
(3) Changes in mood and behavior
(4) Increased lipogenesis from protein

Directions: The question below consist of lettered choices followed by several numbered items. For each numbered item select the **one** lettered choice with which it is **most** closely associated. Each lettered choice may be used once, more than once, or not at all.

Questions 13–15

For each drug use listed below, select the drug that is most appropriate.

(A) Levothyroxine
(B) Propylthiouracil
(C) Iodide
(D) Parathyroid hormone
(E) Calcitonin

13. Useful in the treatment of hyperparathyroidism

14. Useful in conjunction with radioiodine therapy

15. Useful in the treatment of myxedema

ANSWERS AND EXPLANATIONS

1. The answer is C. *(I A 7)* All of the compounds listed are endogenous corticosteroids released by the adrenal cortex except beclomethasone. Beclomethasone was the first steroid available in a form suitable for inhalation and is used to treat acute bronchial asthma.

2. The answer is D. *(I C 6, 7 a, Table 10-1; Chapter 6, IX B 1)* Hydrocortisone and cortisol are short-acting glucocorticoids with some mineralocorticoid activity. Spironolactone is an aldosterone antagonist. Dexamethasone has no sodium-retaining potency. Fludrocortisone shows predominantly mineralocorticoid action.

3. The answer is B. *(IV F 1, 4, G 1, 4, 5)* Diabetic patients who are poorly controlled usually have a negative nitrogen balance due to gluconeogenesis. Insulin deficiency combined with glucagon excess results in the conversion of large amounts of protein to glucose, resulting in an increased excretion of urea and ammonia. All of the other statements in the question are correct.

4. The answer is B. *(II C)* Estrogen excess can be associated with nausea, monilial infections, chloasma and increased areolar pigmentation, edema, leg cramps, thrombophlebitis, and, in predisposed individuals (smokers, hypertensives), an increased incidence of cerebral and coronary thrombosis.

5. The answer is A. *(IV I 1, 3, 4; V B 2, 5)* Crystalline zinc and semilente insulins are short-acting insulins, while NPH insulin is intermediate-acting. Tolbutamide is a short-acting sulfonylurea, while chlorpropamide has a duration of action of 60 hours.

6. The answer is E. *(I B)* Adrenocorticotropic hormone (ACTH) cannot be administered orally. Since it is a polypeptide hormone, it must be administered parenterally, most often intramuscularly. All of the other statements in the question are true.

7. The answer is C. *(II A, B, C)* The "minipill" contains progestin alone, not estrogen. It is 97 percent effective as a contraceptive agent. All of the other statements in the question are true.

8. The answer is D (4). *(I A 8, B 1, 3, 5, Figure 10-1)* Adrenocorticotropic hormone (ACTH) reacts with a hormone receptor in the adrenal-cell plasma membrane, and this results in the stimulation of adenylate cyclase activity. ACTH does not have a steroid structure and is most commonly used as a diagnostic agent in adrenal insufficiency. It has been used therapeutically for secondary adrenal insufficiency but the patient's response is less predictable than with corticosteroids. Cortisol will inhibit the release of ACTH.

9. The answer is A (1, 2, 3). *(IV G, H)* Insulin promotes the synthesis of glycogen, including synthesis in the liver. This is due, in part at least, to a decrease in the amount of circulating gluconeogenic substrates, such as amino acids and glycerol. In addition it enhances both the peripheral utilization of glucose and the conversion of glucose to fat. How insulin facilitates the transport of glucose and amino acids is not known.

10. The answer is E (all). *(I C 3 b, 4 b, 5 c, 6, Table 10-1)* All of the statements in the question regarding the listed steroids are correctly matched. Since desoxycorticosterone is a mineralocorticoid, sodium retention can occur. Triamcinolone is a glucocorticoid with five times the anti-inflammatory potency of hydrocortisone. Prednisolone can both suppress leukocyte migration and stabilize lysosomal membranes. Cortisone is bioactivated in the liver.

11. The answer is B (1, 3). *(IV I, J)* Crystalline zinc insulin is a short-acting insulin that can serve as replacement therapy in juvenile-onset diabetes. Proinsulin is an inactive precursor of insulin. Crystalline zinc insulin, like any insulin preparation, can only be administered parenterally because it is a protein and would be digested in the gastrointestinal tract.

12. The answer is A (1, 2, 3). *(I C 3 a)* Glucocorticoids will produce a dose-dependent increase in liver glycogen and hyperglycemia. Glucocorticoids participate in blood pressure homeostasis by maintaining normal blood volume and peripheral vascular reactivity. They can affect thought processes and central nervous system metabolism. Glucocorticoids facilitate the conversion of proteins to carbohydrate and facilitate the effect of adipokinetic peptides, causing dipolysis of triglycerides in adipose tissue.

13–15. The answers are 13-E, 14-B, 15-A. *(VI A 3, B 2 a, b; VII C 6)* Calcitonin is chiefly used therapeutically to decrease hypercalcemia and hyperphosphatemia in patients with hyperparathyroidism and other disorders associated with hypercalcemia.

Propylthiouracil may be used with radioiodine, to control the effects of hyperthyroidism until the benefits of radiation take effect. Unlike iodide, which would block thyroidal uptake of the radioiodine, propylthiouracil interferes with the synthesis of thyroid hormone by blocking the incorporation of iodine into tyrosyl residues of thyroglobulin.

Levothyroxine is used for the treatment of hypothyroidism, including myxedema coma. It is also given to infants at birth who have hypothyroidism to avoid cretinism.

11 Cancer Chemotherapy

I. INTRODUCTION

A. Cancer is a disease of uncontrolled cell division, invasion, and metastasis. Most of the current clinical antineoplastic agents act on the proliferating population of cells; none act primarily to influence tumor cell invasion or metastases.

B. There may be as many as 100 different types of cancer, each with its own response rate to a given drug. The sensitivity of a given cancer to a given drug depends upon its location, its degree of differentiation, its size, and, presumably, other biochemical factors that are poorly understood.

C. Cancer is generally considered to be due to the clonal expansion of a single neoplastic cell. However, there may be additional somatic mutations, leading to heterogeneous cell populations in which some individual neoplastic cells become insensitive to a specific drug.

D. Combinations of anticancer agents with different mechanisms of action are therefore often used in an attempt to destroy all the malignant cells. Acronyms for these combinations are frequently employed; for example, **MOPP** for mechlorethamine, vincristine (Oncovin), procarbazine, and prednisone.

E. Antineoplastic agents kill a *constant fraction* of the tumor cells rather than a *fixed number* of cells. In an attempt to eliminate all of the malignant cells, cancer chemotherapeutic agents are often administered as an **adjunct** to surgery or irradiation.

F. THE CELL CYCLE AND ANTICANCER THERAPY

1. The growth of a tumor is a function of
  - **a.** The fraction of the total cell population that is proliferating.
  - **b.** The time required for an individual cell to divide (cell cycle time).
  - **c.** The rate of cell loss.

2. The cell cycle
  - **a.** Both normal and malignant cells that are proliferating pass through four discrete phases (Fig. 11-1):
    - **(1)** Mitosis, or M phase.
    - **(2)** Gap 1, or G_1 phase.
    - **(3)** DNA synthesis, or S phase.
    - **(4)** Gap 2, or G_2 phase.
  - **b.** G_0 is a resting phase in which the cells are not proliferating.
  - **c.** Interphase is any period between episodes of mitosis.

3. Some antitumor therapies, such as irradiation, carmustine, or mechlorethamine, are equally cytotoxic to proliferating and nonproliferating cells. These **proliferation-independent agents** kill both normal and malignant cells.

4. Most antitumor agents are preferentially toxic to proliferating cells.
  - **a.** There are two general classes:
    - **(1) Phase-specific agents** act at specific phases of the cell cycle. For example, hydroxyurea and cytarabine kill only cells in the S phase.

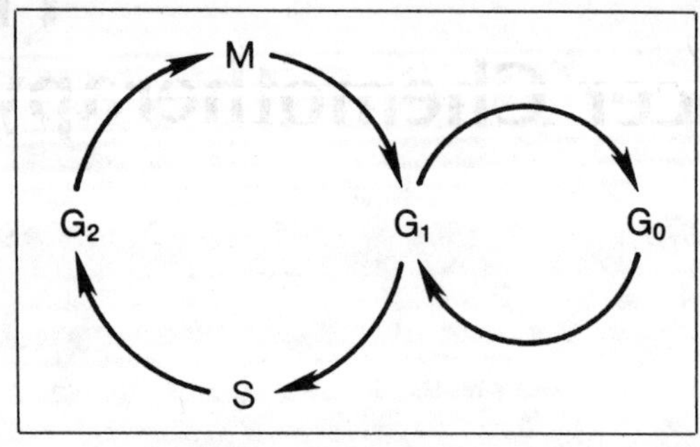

Figure 11-1. The cell cycle. **M,** mitosis; **G_1,** gap 1 phase; **S,** DNA synthesis phase; **G_2,** gap 2 phase; **G_0,** resting phase.

(2) **Phase-nonspecific agents** kill proliferating cells preferentially but do not act on cells at a specific phase in the cell cycle. Examples of these drugs are 5-fluorouracil and cyclophosphamide.

b. Some agents exert their major cytotoxic action in one phase of the cell cycle but also have a more limited activity in other phases.

c. In addition, some agents are **self-limiting** because they are phase-specific but block the cell in another phase of the cell cycle. Thus, methotrexate, which kills cells in the S phase, also can inhibit RNA synthesis in the G_1 and G_2 phases and thereby limits its own cytotoxicity.

G. TOXICITY

1. Anticancer agents frequently show only a moderate selectivity for tumor cells as opposed to normal tissues.

2. Therefore, many of the clinically used antineoplastic agents cause severe toxicity to the patient's normal tissues.

3. Because rapidly proliferating cells are the ones most severely affected, the common side effects are:
a. Bone marrow suppression.
b. Gastrointestinal tract toxicity.
c. Alopecia.

H. DOSAGE CALCULATIONS. Because of their low therapeutic index, the doses of antineoplastic agents are usually calculated on the basis of the patient's body surface area (in square meters) rather than body weight.

I. CLASSIFICATION. The major antineoplastic agents are classified primarily on the basis of their chemical structure, source, or mechanism of action. The five major groups are:

1. Alkylating agents.

2. Antimetabolites.

3. Natural products.

4. Hormones.

5. Miscellaneous agents.

II. ALKYLATING AGENTS

A. INTRODUCTION

1. All of the drugs in this category have or can form an alkyl group that becomes covalently bound to cellular constituents.

2. All alkylating agents are phase-nonspecific. In addition to killing rapidly proliferating cells these drugs also kill nonproliferating cells as a result of alkylation of RNA, DNA, and essential proteins. Thus, some nitrogen mustards are proliferation-independent.

3. Alkylation of DNA is responsible for the cytotoxic antitumor activity of most alkylating agents.
a. The 7-nitrogen and 6-oxygen of guanine are the most favored sites in DNA for alkylation.
b. Once one of these sites has been alkylated, several events may follow:
(1) **Cross-linking.** Bifunctional alkylating agents (those which have two chloroethyl moieties) may form a second covalent bond with an adjacent DNA substituent, a protein, or RNA, resulting in inhibition of DNA replication.

(2) **Mispairing of bases.** Alkylated guanine forms base pairs with thymine rather than cytosine. This leads to miscoding of the gene and the possible production of defective proteins.
(3) **Depurination of DNA.** Alkylation of the 7-nitrogen in guanine causes cleavage of the imidazole ring, which leads to a weakened sugar–phosphate backbone of DNA and strand breakage.

4. Enzymes exist which can repair the DNA damage caused by alkylation, and they may limit the responsiveness of some tumors.

B. NITROGEN MUSTARDS

1. Chemistry
a. The basic structure of the nitrogen mustards is shown in Figure 11-2.
b. The prototype is **mechlorethamine,** in which R = CH_3.

2. Mechanism of action
a. One chloroethyl moiety undergoes cyclization, with the release of a chloride ion.
b. The resulting highly reactive carbonium ion can attack nucleophilic groups on protein, DNA, RNA, and other cellular constituents.
c. As with all alkylating agents, the nitrogen mustards are phase-nonspecific.
d. Acquired resistance to nitrogen mustards can occur and imparts cross-resistance to other alkylating agents.

3. Mechlorethamine

$$R = CH_3$$

a. Pharmacokinetics
(1) Mechlorethamine was the first clinically used nitrogen mustard.
(2) It is highly reactive, with a chemical and biological half-life in plasma of 10 minutes.
(3) It is proliferation-independent.

b. Therapeutic uses
(1) In the treatment of Hodgkin's disease, mechlorethamine is combined with vincristine (Oncovin), procarbazine, and prednisone to form the MOPP regimen.
(2) It has also been used topically for the treatment of mycosis fungoides.

c. Major untoward effects include
(1) Myelosuppression.
(2) Nausea and vomiting.
(3) Alopecia.
(4) Menstrual irregularities.

d. Route of administration
(1) Because it causes severe tissue damage when given by other routes of administration, mechlorethamine must be given intravenously in a rapidly flowing infusion of saline.
(2) Care must be taken to avoid extravasation during administration.

4. Cyclophosphamide (see Fig. 11-3)
a. Pharmacokinetics
(1) Cyclophosphamide is well absorbed orally and must be activated in the liver by the mixed function oxidase system.
(2) The metabolites **phosphoramide mustard** and **acrolein** are believed to be the ultimate cytotoxic species.
(3) Cyclophosphamide and its metabolites are eliminated primarily by the kidneys, and thus renal failure greatly increases their retention.

b. Therapeutic uses
(1) Cyclophosphamide is used alone and in combination in the treatment of a wide variety of neoplastic disorders, including Hodgkin's disease, Burkitt's lymphoma, ovarian and breast carcinomas, oat cell lung cancer, and neuroblastoma.

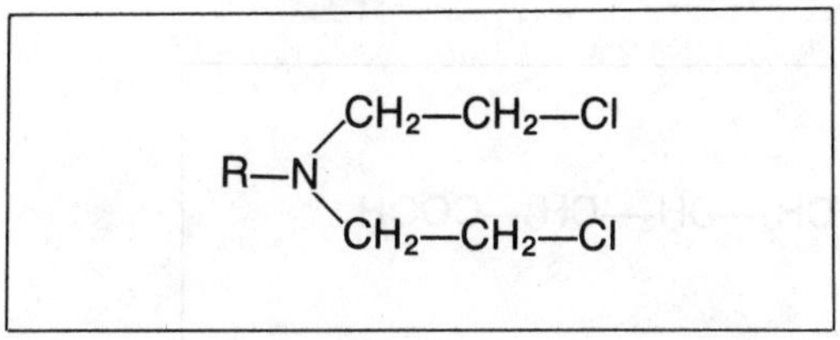

$$R-N(CH_2-CH_2-Cl)_2$$

Figure 11-2. Basic structure of the nitrogen mustards.

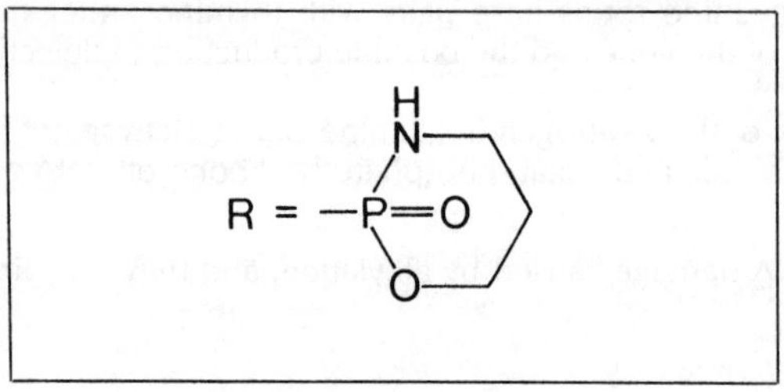

Figure 11-3. R structure of cyclophosphamide.

(2) Cyclophosphamide has also been used as an immunosuppressing agent during organ transplants.

c. Major untoward effects

(1) Unlike other nitrogen mustards, cyclophosphamide rarely induces thrombocytopenia.

(2) Alopecia occurs frequently.

(3) Up to 10 percent of treated patients develop a sterile hemorrhagic cystitis which is probably due to chemical irritation of the bladder mucosa by the metabolite acrolein. A liberal fluid intake dilutes the urinary concentration of acrolein and decreases this side effect.

(4) Prolonged cyclophosphamide treatment can occasionally produce interstitial pulmonary fibrosis.

d. Route of administration

(1) Cyclophosphamide is administered orally or intravenously.

(2) The total leukocyte count is monitored, and the dose is adjusted accordingly.

5. Melphalan (see Fig. 11-4)

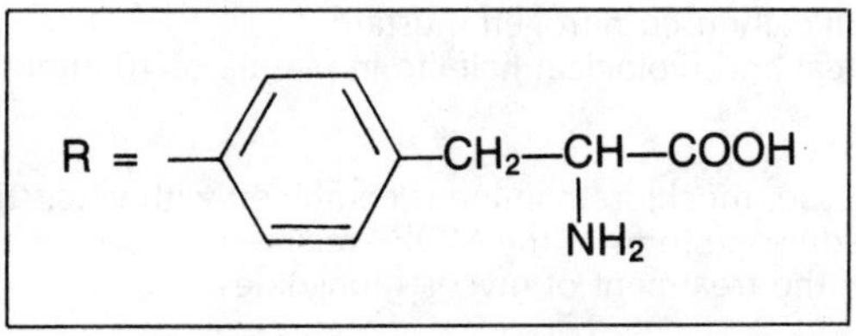

Figure 11-4. R structure of melphalan.

a. Pharmacokinetics and therapeutic uses

(1) Melphalan is well absorbed from the gastrointestinal tract.

(2) Its major use is in the treatment of multiple myeloma.

b. Major untoward effects

(1) Like other alkylating agents, melphalan causes prominent myelosuppression.

(2) Nausea, vomiting, and alopecia are rare.

c. Route of administration

(1) Melphalan is administered orally.

(2) Close hematologic monitoring is essential.

6. Chlorambucil (see Fig. 11-5)

a. Pharmacokinetics

(1) Like melphalan, chlorambucil is well absorbed from the gastrointestinal tract.

(2) It is completely metabolized.

(3) It is the slowest-acting nitrogen mustard.

b. Therapeutic uses include:

(1) Chronic lymphocytic leukemia.

(2) Waldenstrom's macroglobulinemia.

c. Major untoward effects

(1) As with other alkylating agents, myelosuppression is seen.

(2) Nausea and vomiting occur.

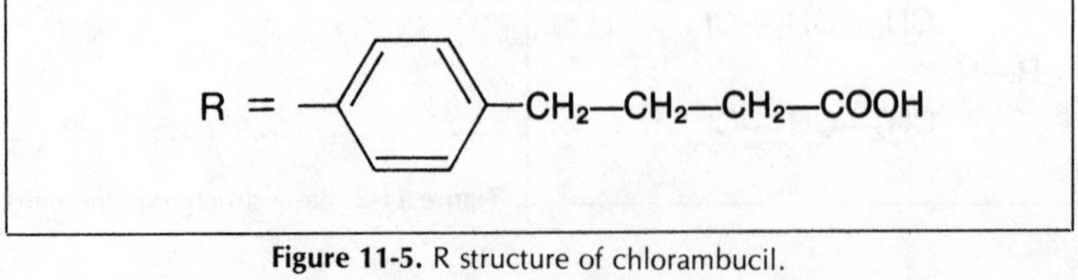

Figure 11-5. R structure of chlorambucil.

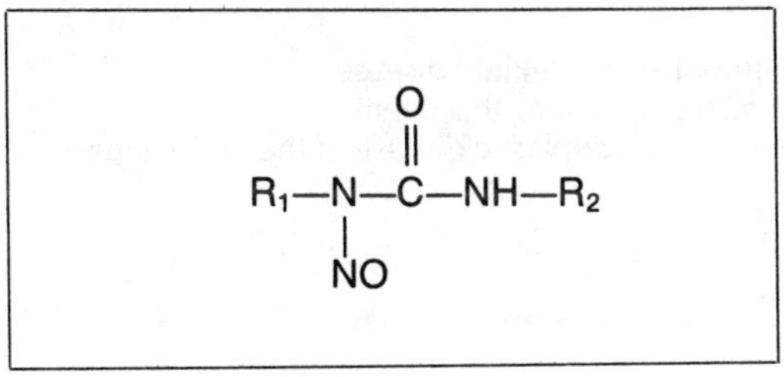

$$\begin{array}{c} \quad\quad\quad O \\ \quad\quad\quad \| \\ R_1—N—C—NH—R_2 \\ | \quad\quad\quad\quad \\ NO \quad\quad\quad\quad \end{array}$$

Figure 11-6. Basic structure of the nitrosoureas.

C. NITROSOUREAS

1. Chemistry

a. The basic structure is shown in Figure 11-6.

b. In general the nitrosoureas are chemically unstable and decompose rapidly.

c. Acronyms derived from their chemical structures are commonly used for the nitrosoureas.

2. Mechanism of action

a. In aqueous environments, the nitrosoureas decompose to alkylating and carbamylating intermediates.

b. The therapeutic and toxic effects of the nitrosoureas are due to both the alkylation of DNA and other nucleophiles and the carbamylation of lysine residues on proteins.

c. The consequences of DNA alkylation by the nitrosoureas are similar to those seen with other alkylating agents (see II A 3, above).

d. The high lipid solubility of some of the nitrosoureas allows these agents to cross the blood–brain barrier. Thus, they are useful in the treatment of malignancies of the central nervous system (CNS).

e. The nitrosoureas are proliferation-independent.

3. Carmustine (BCNU)

a. Chemistry

(1) Carmustine is 1,3-bis(2-chloroethyl) 1-nitrosourea (BCNU).

(2) Both R_1 and R_2 have the same structure.

$$R_1 \text{ and } R_2 = CH_2CH_2Cl$$

b. Pharmacokinetics

(1) Carmustine is administered intravenously due to its rapid tissue uptake and metabolism.

(2) The chemical half-life is less than 10 minutes.

(3) The major degradation and metabolic products are excreted in the urine.

c. Therapeutic uses include:

(1) Hodgkin's disease.

(2) Meningeal leukemia.

(3) Tumors of the brain.

d. Major untoward effects include:

(1) Delayed hematopoietic depression.

(2) Nausea and vomiting.

(3) CNS toxicity.

(4) Pulmonary fibrosis.

4. Lomustine (CCNU)

a. Chemistry

(1) Lomustine is 1-(2-chloroethyl)-3-cyclohexyl-1-nitrosourea (CCNU).

(2) The R structures are:

$$R_1 = CH_2CH_2Cl$$

$$R_2 = \text{(cyclohexyl ring)}$$

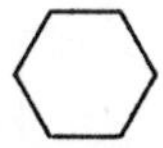

b. Pharmacokinetics

(1) Lomustine, which is given orally, is rapidly absorbed from the gastrointestinal tract and metabolized.

(2) The metabolites, however, have a long half-life (over 16 hours).

(3) The metabolites can enter the cerebrospinal fluid (CSF).

c. **Therapeutic uses**
(1) Lomustine is effective in the treatment of Hodgkin's disease.
(2) Non-Hodgkin's lymphomas can also respond to this agent.
(3) Lomustine has been used to treat primary neoplastic disease of the brain, kidney, stomach, colon, and lung.

d. **Untoward effects** include:
(1) Bone marrow suppression.
(2) Nausea and vomiting.

D. ALKYL SULFONATES

1. The prototype agent is **busulfan.** Its bifunctional structure is shown in Figure 11-7.

2. **Pharmacokinetics**
   a. Busulfan is well absorbed after oral administration.
   b. Almost all of the drug is eliminated in the urine as methanesulfonic acid.

3. **Mechanism of action.** Cleavage of the alkyl–oxygen bond in busulfan produces an electrophile which forms intrastrand DNA cross-links.

4. **Therapeutic uses** of busulfan include:
   a. Chronic lymphocytic leukemia.
   b. Waldenstrom's macroglobulinemia.

5. **Major untoward effects**
   a. Myelosuppression is common.
   b. Endocrine dysfunction, including impotence, sterility, and amenorrhea, can occur.
   c. Hyperuricemia can result from rapid purine catabolism.
   d. Skin pigmentation and pulmonary fibrosis have been noted.

E. TRIAZENES

1. The prototype is **dacarbazine (DTIC).**

2. Its chemical formula is 5-(3,3-dimethyl-1-triazeno) imidazole-4-carboxamide (DTIC); its structure is shown in Figure 11-8.

3. Dacarbazine is *N*-demethylated by liver microsomal enzymes and then functions as an alkylating agent.

4. The active species has a methyl carbonium ion that can methylate DNA and RNA and inhibits the synthesis of DNA, RNA, and protein.

5. Dacarbazine is one of the most active agents against malignant melanoma.

6. Its major untoward effects are nausea, vomiting, myelosuppression, and neurotoxicity.

III. ANTIMETABOLITES

A. INTRODUCTION

1. Antimetabolites are compounds that bear a structural similarity to a naturally occurring substance, such as a vitamin, nucleoside, or amino acid.

2. The antimetabolite competes with the natural substrate for the active site on an essential enzyme or for an important receptor.

3. Some antimetabolites can be incorporated into DNA or RNA, and thus can disrupt cellular function.

4. Most antimetabolites are phase-specific and act during DNA synthesis (the S phase; see Fig. 11-1).

$$H_3C-\overset{\overset{\displaystyle O}{\|}}{\underset{\underset{\displaystyle O}{\|}}{S}}-O-(CH_2)_4-O-\overset{\overset{\displaystyle O}{\|}}{\underset{\underset{\displaystyle O}{\|}}{S}}-CH_3$$

Figure 11-7. Busulfan.

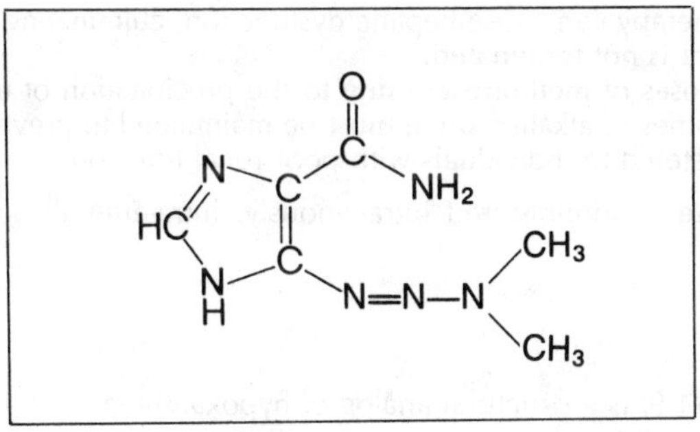

Figure 11-8. Dacarbazine (DTIC).

B. METHOTREXATE

1. Mechanism of action

a. Methotrexate is a folic acid analog that competitively inhibits dihydrofolate reductase, the enzyme that catalyzes the formation of tetrahydrofolate from dihydrofolate.

(1) Normally, tetrahydrofolate is converted to a variety of coenzymes that are necessary for one-carbon transfer reactions involved in the synthesis of purines, thymidylate, methionine, and glycine.

(2) Therefore, methotrexate inhibits the formation of these coenzymes.

b. The primary cause of cell death is the blockade of the biosynthesis of thymidylate and purines required for DNA synthesis.

c. Thus, methotrexate kills cells in S phase.

d. Because methotrexate also inhibits RNA and protein synthesis, the drug slows the rate of entry of cells into S phase, and therefore it is a **self-limiting** S-phase–specific drug.

e. The blockade caused by methotrexate can be circumvented.

(1) Substances such as leucovorin (also called citrovorum factor or folinic acid) can be converted to the tetrahydrofolate coenzymes required for thymidylate and purine biosynthesis even in the presence of methotrexate.

(2) This allows the "rescue" of nonmalignant cells, with a consequent reduction in toxicity from methotrexate.

2. Pharmacokinetics

a. Methotrexate is well absorbed after oral administration.

b. It is eliminated primarily by the kidneys without extensive metabolism and is approximately 50 percent bound to plasma proteins. Weak acids such as salicylates and sulfonamides can increase methotrexate toxicity by inhibiting renal tubular secretion and displacing methotrexate from plasma proteins.

c. Cellular uptake of the drug is by carrier-mediated active transport.

d. After an intravenous injection of methotrexate, plasma decay kinetics are triphasic, with a half-life of 45 minutes for the first (distributional) phase, 3.5 hours for the second (renal clearance) phase, and 27 hours for the third (final excretion) phase.

e. Methotrexate does not penetrate the blood–brain barrier well. However, it is one of the few antitumor agents that can be administered intrathecally for cerebral leukemia.

3. Tumor cell resistance.

Tumor cells may become resistant to methotrexate because:

a. Their cellular transport is impaired.

b. An altered form of dihydrofolate reductase is formed.

c. The tumor cells generate an increased concentration of dihydrofolate reductase.

4. Therapeutic uses

a. Methotrexate is used in combination with other agents to treat acute lymphoblastic leukemia, Burkitt's lymphoma, trophoblastic choriocarcinoma, and carcinomas of the breast, cervix, lung, head, and neck.

b. The drug is also useful in the treatment of mycosis fungoides and psoriasis.

c. High-dose methotrexate therapy combined with leucovorin "rescue" has been used to treat osteogenic sarcoma and lung cancer.

5. Major untoward effects

a. Myelosuppression is significant, with leukopenia and thrombocytopenia occurring 1 to 2 weeks after drug administration.

b. Gastrointestinal toxicity is manifested by ulcerative stomatitis and diarrhea and can disrupt therapy.

c. Nausea and vomiting are common acute untoward effects.

d. Prolonged low-dose methotrexate therapy can cause hepatic dysfunction, culminating in cirrhosis of the liver if drug treatment is not terminated.

e. Renal failure can occur with high doses of methotrexate due to the precipitation of the drug in the renal tubules. Large volumes of alkaline urine must be maintained to prevent this toxicity. The drug is not administered to individuals with poor renal function.

6. Route of administration. Methotrexate is administered intravenously, intra-arterially, intrathecally, or orally.

C. PURINE ANALOGS

1. 6-Mercaptopurine

a. Chemistry. 6-Mercaptopurine (Fig. 11-9) is a structural analog of hypoxanthine.

b. Mechanism of action

(1) 6-Mercaptopurine must be converted intracellularly to the nucleotide 6-mercaptopurine ribose phosphate by hypoxanthine–guanine phosphoribosyl transferase. 6-Mercaptopurine also can be converted to 6-methylmercaptopurine ribonucleotide.

(2) 6-Mercaptopurine ribose phosphate and the methylated nucleotide are cytotoxic primarily because they inhibit de novo purine biosynthesis.

(3) Both block the aminotransferase that is responsible for the first step in purine biosynthesis, namely, the formation of 5-phosphoribosylamine, by feedback inhibition.

(4) In addition, 6-mercaptopurine ribose phosphate inhibits both adenylosuccinate synthetase, the enzyme that converts inosinic acid to adenylosuccinic acid, and inosinate dehydrogenase, the enzyme that converts inosinic acid to xanthylic acid.

c. Pharmacokinetics

(1) 6-Mercaptopurine is well absorbed orally, and 50 percent is recovered in the urine in 24 hours, principally as 6-thiouric acid and inorganic sulfate.

(2) After an intravenous injection, the plasma half-life is approximately 1 hour.

(3) The drug is 20 percent bound to plasma protein and does not cross the blood–brain barrier.

(4) 6-Mercaptopurine can be metabolically inactivated by desulfuration and by oxidation via xanthine oxidase to form 6-thiouric acid.

d. Tumor cell resistance. Tumor cells may become resistant to 6-mercaptopurine due to either a decreased drug activation by hypoxanthine–guanine phosphoribosyl transferase or an increased inactivation by alkaline phosphatase.

e. Therapeutic uses

(1) 6-Mercaptopurine is used in the maintenance therapy of acute lymphoblastic leukemia.

(2) It is also useful in the treatment of acute and chronic myelogenous leukemias.

f. Major untoward effects

(1) 6-Mercaptopurine causes myelosuppression, but this is more gradual in onset than the suppression caused by methotrexate.

(2) 6-Mercaptopurine also causes anorexia and nausea.

(3) One-third of treated patients may develop jaundice associated with bile stasis and hepatic necrosis. Discontinuation of therapy usually reverses this untoward effect.

(4) Hyperuricemia and hyperuricosuria may occur with 6-mercaptopurine therapy.

(a) This is due to the destruction of cells and the release of purines that are metabolized by xanthine oxidase.

(b) Allopurinol, an inhibitor of xanthine oxidase, can block the hyperuricemia and hyperuricosuria (see Chapter 9, X E), but it also prevents the inactivation of 6-mercaptopurine.

(c) Therefore, the dose of 6-mercaptopurine must be reduced when a patient is receiving concurrent allopurinol in order to prevent significant toxicity.

g. Route of administration. 6-Mercaptopurine is administered orally.

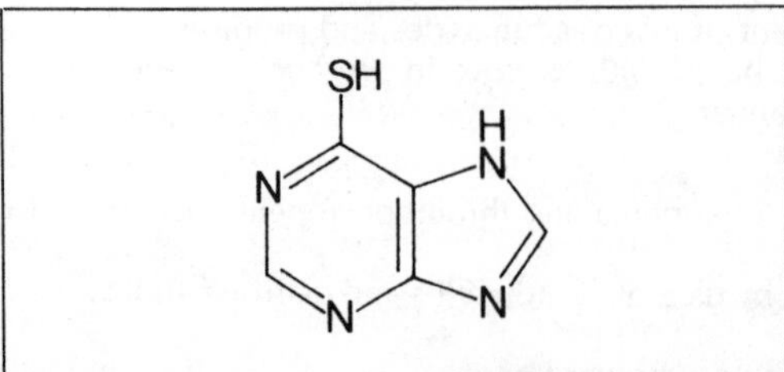

Figure 11-9. 6-Mercaptopurine.

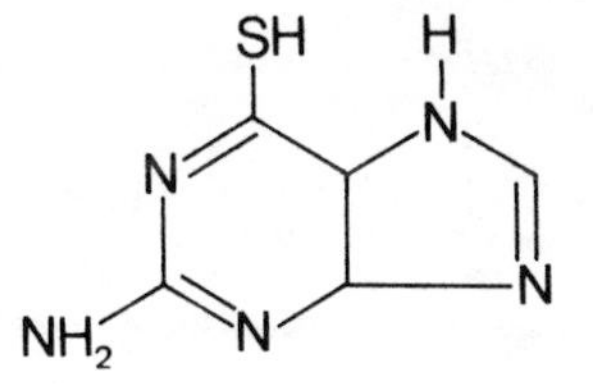

Figure 11-10. 6-Thioguanine

2. **6-Thioguanine**
   a. **Chemistry.** 6-Thioguanine (Fig. 11-10) is a structural analog of guanine in which a sulfhydryl replaces a hydroxyl group in the 6 position.
   b. **Mechanism of action**
      (1) Like 6-mercaptopurine, 6-thioguanine is converted to the nucleotide, in this case 6-thioguanine ribose phosphate, by hypoxanthine–guanine phosphoribosyl transferase.
      (2) The cytotoxicity of 6-thioguanine may be due to feedback inhibition of purine biosynthesis by 6-thioguanine ribose phosphate.
      (3) Alternatively, the cytotoxicity of 6-thioguanine may be due to conversion of 6-thioguanine to the deoxynucleoside triphosphate, which is incorporated into tumor cell DNA and RNA.
   c. **Pharmacokinetics**
      (1) 6-Thioguanine is only slowly absorbed orally, and less than 50 percent of the administered dose is found in the urine in 24 hours, all in the form of metabolites.
      (2) 6-Thioguanine is not a good substrate for xanthine oxidase, in contrast to 6-mercaptopurine, and only small amounts of 6-thiouric acid are detected. Therefore, no dose reduction is required with concurrent allopurinol use.
   d. **Tumor cell resistance.** The proposed mechanisms for tumor cell resistance to 6-thioguanine are the same as those for 6-mercaptopurine.
   e. **Therapeutic uses.** 6-Thioguanine is used primarily in the treatment of acute myelogenous leukemia.
   f. **Major untoward effects**
      (1) Myelosuppression is a common side effect.
      (2) 6-Thioguanine causes mild nausea.
      (3) Hepatotoxicity is less common with 6-thioguanine than with 6-mercaptopurine.
   g. **Route of administration.** 6-Thioguanine is administered orally.

D. PYRIMIDINE ANALOGS

1. **5-Fluorouracil**
   a. **Chemistry.** 5-Fluorouracil is a fluorine-substituted analog of uracil. Its structure is shown in Figure 11-11.
   b. **Mechanism of action**
      (1) Like the purine antimetabolites, 5-fluorouracil must be metabolically activated to a nucleotide, in this case 5-fluoro-2′-deoxyuridine-5′-monophosphate (FdUMP). There are three general pathways for FdUMP formation:
         (a) 5-Fluorouracil can be metabolized to the deoxyribonucleoside, with subsequent phosphorylation by thymidine kinase.
         (b) 5-Fluorouracil can be converted to 5-fluorouridine-5-phosphate by pyrimidine phosphoribosyltransferase and then to the deoxyribonucleoside by ribonucleotide reductase.
         (c) FdUMP can also be formed by the conversion of 5-fluorouracil to fluorouridine, which is subsequently phosphorylated by uridine kinase to form 5-fluorouridine-5′-phosphate and ultimately FdUMP.
      (2) The cytotoxicity of 5-fluorouracil is due primarily to inhibition of DNA synthesis caused by a FdUMP-produced blockage of thymidylate synthetase.
      (3) Thymidylate synthetase normally transfers a methylene group from reduced folic acid to deoxyuridylate monophosphate (dUMP) to form thymidylate, which is essential for DNA synthesis.
      (4) Cytotoxicity may also be due to incorporation of 5-fluorouridine triphosphate into RNA, which leads to "fraudulent" RNA formation.
      (5) 5-Fluorouracil is phase-nonspecific and, thus, kills cells not only in S phase but throughout the cell cycle, perhaps due to its RNA actions.

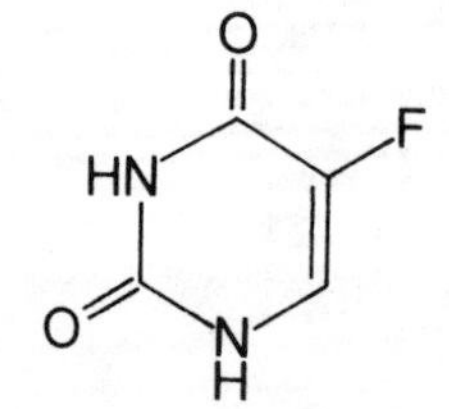

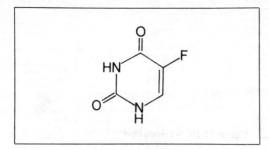

Figure 11-11. 5-Fluorouracil.

c. Pharmacokinetics

(1) 5-Fluorouracil is administered intravenously and is catabolized by the liver.

(2) The first, and rate-limiting, hepatic enzyme involved in 5-fluorouracil catabolism is dihydrouracil dehydrogenase. After cleavage of the pyrimidine ring, the final degradation products are ammonia, urea, 2-fluoro-3-alanine, and CO_2.

(3) 5-Fluorouracil is distributed throughout the body, including the CSF.

d. Tumor cell resistance may result from any of several causes:

(1) An increased synthesis of thymidylate synthetase.

(2) An altered affinity of thymidylate synthetase for FdUMP.

(3) An increased rate of 5-fluorouracil catabolism.

(4) The deletion of enzymes that convert 5-fluorouracil to the active nucleotide.

(5) An increase in the pool of deoxyuridylic acid.

e. Therapeutic uses

(1) 5-Fluorouracil is used in combination with other agents for the treatment of breast cancer.

(2) It has palliative activity in gastrointestinal adenocarcinoma.

(3) It is also used to treat carcinomas of the cervix, bladder, and prostate.

f. Major untoward effects

(1) Myelosuppression, especially leukopenia, frequently occurs.

(2) Oral mucositis, diarrhea, alopecia, and nausea are seen after drug administration.

(3) Neurologic toxicity can be seen in 1 to 2 percent of treated patients.

g. Route of administration

(1) Fluorouracil is usually administered intravenously.

(2) Topical application of the drug has been useful for the treatment of premalignant keratoses of the skin and superficial basal cell carcinoma.

2. Cytarabine (cytosine arabinoside, ara-C, 1-3-D-arabino-furanosylcytosine)

a. Chemistry

(1) Cytarabine is an analog of cytidine in which the ribose moiety has been replaced with an arabinose.

(2) Its structure is shown in Figure 11-12.

b. Mechanism of action

(1) Cytarabine must be activated, by pyrimidine nucleoside kinase, to the nucleotide triphosphate, ara-cytosine triphosphate.

(2) The nucleotide triphosphate competitively inhibits DNA polymerase and thus blocks DNA synthesis and causes cell death.

(3) Cytarabine nucleotides can be incorporated into DNA and RNA, but the biological significance of this remains to be established.

(4) It is an S-phase–specific agent.

c. Pharmacokinetics

(1) Cytarabine is poorly absorbed after oral administration.

(2) It is rapidly metabolized in the liver and other tissues by cytidine deaminase.

(3) It has an extremely short plasma half-life of 10 minutes.

d. Tumor cell resistance may be due to

(1) Depressed levels of the kinase required for activation.

(2) Enhanced levels of the deaminase that inactivates the drug.

e. Therapeutic uses. Cytarabine is used to treat acute myelogenous leukemia in combination with an anthracycline (see IV C) or 6-thioguanine.

f. Major untoward effects

(1) Cytarabine causes severe myelosuppression.

(2) Nausea and mucositis occur.

g. Route of administration

(1) Cytarabine is given by intravenous, intramuscular, or subcutaneous injection.

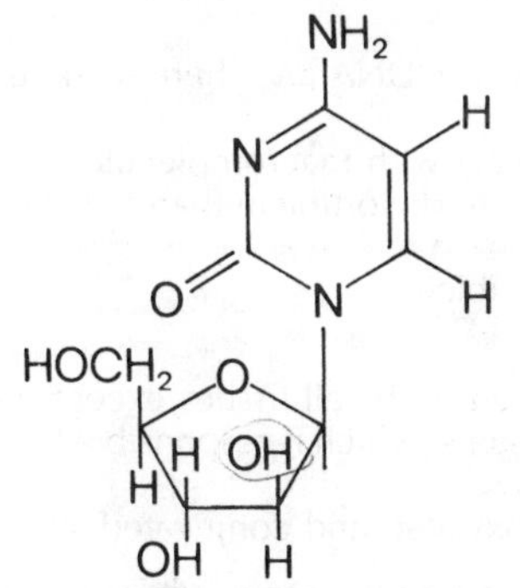

Figure 11-12. Cytarabine.

(2) Because it is a phase-specific agent and rapidly inactivated, continuous infusion is the preferred mode of administration.

IV. NATURAL PRODUCTS

A. INTRODUCTION

1. Unlike the other classes of antitumor agents, membership in this group is determined by the source of the drug.
2. The natural products used in cancer chemotherapy are extracted from a wide variety of plants and lower organisms.
3. Most of the natural products have complex chemical structures and are not illustrated here.

B. DACTINOMYCIN (actinomycin D)

1. **Chemistry**
   a. Dactinomycin is isolated from a *Streptomyces* species.
   b. It contains two cyclic polypeptides that are linked by a chromophore moiety.
2. **Mechanism of action**
   a. Dactinomycin binds noncovalently to double-stranded DNA and inhibits DNA-directed RNA synthesis.
   b. It is a phase-nonspecific agent.
3. **Pharmacokinetics**
   a. Dactinomycin is rapidly cleared from the plasma but is retained in the body for prolonged periods. Only 30 percent of the drug is recovered in the urine and stool after one week.
   b. It does not cross the blood–brain barrier.
4. **Tumor cell resistance** is due to a decreased ability of tumor cells to take up or retain the drug.
5. **Therapeutic uses**
   a. Dactinomycin is used in combination with other agents to treat Wilms' tumor, Ewing's sarcoma, rhabdomyosarcoma, Kaposi's sarcoma, and soft-tissue sarcomas.
   b. Due to its lympholytic effects, it is immunosuppressive and has been used in renal transplantation.
6. **Major untoward effects**
   a. Dactinomycin produces myelosuppression, nausea, and vomiting.
   b. Skin damage can occur in areas of previous irradiation.
7. **Route of administration.** Dactinomycin is administered intravenously.

C. ANTHRACYCLINES

1. **Chemistry**
   a. **Doxorubicin** is the prototype. Isolated from *Streptomyces*, it contains an amino sugar and an anthracycline ring.

b. **Daunorubicin** is structurally almost identical to doxorubicin, lacking only a hydroxyl moiety.

2. **Mechanism of action**
   a. Doxorubicin intercalates between the base pairs in DNA and thereby inhibits both DNA synthesis and DNA-directed RNA synthesis.
   b. Doxorubicin can form free radicals that can react with macromolecules.
   c. Cells traversing the cell cycle are more sensitive to doxorubicin than noncycling cells, and cells in S phase are the most sensitive.
   d. The mechanism of action is similar for daunorubicin.

3. **Pharmacokinetics**
   a. Doxorubicin and daunorubicin are rapidly taken up by all tissues except the brain.
   b. They are extensively bound to cellular components, which is responsible for their long terminal plasma half-life.
   c. Both drugs are metabolized primarily to hydroxylated and conjugated species.

4. **Tumor cell resistance** to doxorubicin or daunorubicin appears to result from reduced cellular uptake of the drug or a more rapid removal of the intracellular drug.

5. **Therapeutic uses**
   a. **Doxorubicin** is one of the most effective agents against solid tumors. It is also effective against acute leukemias and malignant lymphoma.
   b. **Daunorubicin** is most effective against acute lymphocytic and granulocytic leukemia. It has little activity against solid tumors.

6. **Major untoward effects**
   a. Doxorubicin and daunorubicin cause both acute and chronic cardiomyopathy. The depression of cardiac function resulting from repeated doses limits the total amount of drug that can be administered.
   b. Myelosuppression, especially leukopenia, occurs in most patients.
   c. Alopecia is a common side effect.
   d. Both drugs also cause nausea and vomiting.
   e. Dermatitis at the site of previous radiation can occur.

7. **Route of administration**
   a. **Doxorubicin** (Adriamycin) is administered intravenously. Because it causes severe tissue necrosis, doxorubicin *cannot* be injected subcutaneously or intramuscularly, and special care must be taken to avoid extravasation during intravenous infusions or injections.
   b. Cumulative doses of doxorubicin appear to be important in the development of cardiac damage, and a maximum total dose of 550 mg per square meter of body surface area is recommended to avoid cardiotoxicity.
   c. **Daunorubicin** (Cerubidine) is administered similarly.

D. BLEOMYCIN

1. **Chemistry**
   a. Clinically used bleomycin is a group of glycopeptides extracted from a *Streptomyces* species.
   b. The mixture of glycopeptides found in this extract are referred to collectively as bleomycin.

2. **Mechanism of action**
   a. Bleomycin intercalates in DNA and causes both single- and double-strand scissions of DNA.
   b. Bleomycin, which binds to ferrous ion, can transfer an electron to molecular oxygen; this results in superoxide and hydroxyl free radicals that cause DNA strand breaks.
   c. Cells in G_2 and M phase are most sensitive to bleomycin.

3. **Pharmacokinetics**
   a. Bleomycin has a plasma half-life of approximately 1 hour.
   b. More than half of the drug is eliminated unchanged in the urine within 24 hours.
   c. Bleomycin is inactivated in most tissues, except skin and lungs, by an enzyme, bleomycin hydrolase. Toxicity in a specific organ occurs if the organ is lacking in enzyme activity.

4. **Tumor cell resistance**
   a. Tumor cells may fail to respond because of high levels of bleomycin hydrolase activity.
   b. Resistance may also be due to poor cellular accumulation of bleomycin or rapid drug removal.

5. Therapeutic uses

a. Bleomycin is used only in combination with other agents.

b. It is effective with cisplatin and vinblastine for the treatment of testicular carcinoma.

c. It is also used for Hodgkin's and non–Hodgkin's lymphomas and for squamous cell carcinomas of the head and neck, cervix, and skin.

6. Major untoward effects

a. Bleomycin causes an age-related and cumulative-dose–related pulmonary toxicity. This consists of a pneumonitis which can progress to fatal pulmonary fibrosis.

b. Bleomycin does *not* produce significant bone marrow toxicity.

7. Route of administration

a. Bleomycin is administered intravenously or intramuscularly.

b. It is sold in **units of activity**. The units are based upon the toxicity to bacteria; 1 unit equals approximately 1.7 mg.

c. A maximum total cumulative dose of 400 units is recommended to avoid pulmonary toxicity.

E. MITOMYCIN (mitomycin C)

1. Chemistry. Isolated from *Streptomyces,* mitomycin contains an aziridine ring as well as a urethane and a quinone moiety.

2. Mechanism of action

a. Mitomycin is reduced intracellularly by a reduced nicotinamide adenine dinucleotide phosphate (NADPH)–dependent reductase, and then alkylates DNA. Thus, it can also be classified as an alkylating agent.

b. Because oxygen-derived free radicals can be formed, single-strand DNA lesions also can occur.

3. Pharmacokinetics

a. After intravenous administration, mitomycin disappears rapidly from the blood.

b. Mitomycin does not penetrate the CNS.

c. It is extensively metabolized by the liver.

4. Major untoward effects

a. Myelosuppression is a major complication.

b. Dermal, pulmonary, renal, and gastrointestinal toxicity may occur.

c. Extravasation can result in severe local injury.

5. Therapeutic uses and administration

a. Mitomycin has limited use in the treatment of carcinomas of the stomach and cervix.

b. Mitomycin is administered in a rapidly flowing intravenous infusion.

F. VINCA ALKALOIDS

1. Chemistry

a. The two prominent agents in this group, **vincristine** and **vinblastine,** are derived from the periwinkle plant.

b. Both structurally complex compounds, vincristine differs from vinblastine only in having an aldehyde moiety.

c. Despite their similarity in chemical structure, the two alkaloids are quite different in their therapeutic applications and toxicities.

2. Mechanism of action

a. Both alkaloids bind to tubulin and thereby interfere with the assembly of spindle proteins during mitosis.

b. Both agents are M-phase–specific, blocking proliferating cells as they enter metaphase.

3. Pharmacokinetics

a. Both agents are extensively bound to tissue components. Less than 30 percent of a dose of vinblastine or its metabolites, for example, is recovered during a 6-day period after injection.

b. Only a small amount of either of these vinca alkaloids penetrates the brain or enters the CSF.

c. Both agents are metabolized by the liver and excreted in the bile.

4. Tumor cell resistance

a. It is currently believed that resistance to both agents is due to a reduced ability of tumor cells to retain the drugs.

b. Although in experimental murine tumors cross-resistance between vinblastine and vincristine has been observed, in human tumors cross-resistance does *not* appear to occur.

5. Therapeutic uses

a. **Vinblastine** is used in combination with bleomycin and cisplatin for the treatment of testicular carcinoma. It is also effective against lymphomas, neuroblastoma, and Letterer-Siwe disease.

b. **Vincristine**

(1) Vincristine is effective against acute lymphoblastic leukemia, Hodgkin's disease, and non–Hodgkin's lymphomas.

(2) It is also useful in the treatment of solid tumors in children and tumors of the breast, lung, and cervix in adults.

(3) Because vincristine is less likely to cause myelosuppression, it is preferred over vinblastine for use in combination with myelosuppressive agents in the therapy of lymphomas.

(4) Vincristine is used in combination with the corticosteroid prednisone, procarbazine, and an alkylating agent (e.g., mechlorethamine) in the MOPP regimen for treating Hodgkin's disease.

(5) The combination of vincristine with prednisone is considered the treatment of choice for inducing remission in childhood leukemia.

6. Major untoward effects

a. **Vinblastine** causes leukopenia within 4 to 10 days after treatment. Minimal nausea, paresthesias, and jaw pain have been reported.

b. **Vincristine** is significantly neurotoxic, with paresthesias and motor weakness the most prominent effects. These neurologic manifestations are minimized by stopping or reducing the dose at the earliest onset of symptoms.

7. Route of administration

a. **Vinblastine** is administered intravenously, with particular caution being taken not to produce subcutaneous extravasation.

b. **Vincristine** (Oncovin) is also administered intravenously with avoidance of extravasation.

V. HORMONAL THERAPY

A. INTRODUCTION

1. Hormonal therapy relies upon the presence of receptors for endogenous hormones required for cell proliferation.

2. Unlike agents in the other classes of antineoplastic drugs, members of this class generally do not cause severe toxicity.

B. TAMOXIFEN

1. **Chemistry.** Tamoxifen is a nonsteroidal compound containing a triphenylethylene moiety (Fig. 11-13).

2. **Mechanism of action**

a. Some tumors, notably breast carcinomas, require estrogen for cell proliferation.

(1) Estrogen binds to a cytoplasmic protein receptor, and the receptor–hormone complex translocates into the nucleus, inducing RNA synthesis.

Figure 11-13. Tamoxifen.

(2) Estrogen receptors are found in two-thirds of the breast tumors that occur in postmenopausal women.

b. Tamoxifen is useful only in women whose tumors contain estrogen receptors.

(1) Tamoxifen competes with estrogen for the cytoplasmic receptor, although it has little or no estrogenic activity.

(2) Thus, tamoxifen blocks the growth-promoting effects of estrogen in estrogen-dependent tumors.

(3) Tamoxifen is, therefore, an **antiestrogen.**

3. **Pharmacokinetics**

a. The antiestrogen tamoxifen is absorbed when given orally.

b. It is found concentrated in tissues with estrogen receptors such as the ovaries and breast tissue, as well as in tumors that contain these receptors.

c. Tamoxifen undergoes extensive hepatic metabolism.

d. It undergoes enterohepatic recirculation and then is found as metabolites in the stool.

4. **Therapeutic uses.** Tamoxifen is used for palliative treatment of advanced breast carcinoma in the postmenopausal woman.

5. **Major untoward effects**

a. Hot flashes, mild fluid retention, and nausea occur frequently.

b. With high doses corneal and retinal opacities have been observed.

6. **Route of administration.** Tamoxifen is administered orally.

C. ANDROGENS

1. Androgens have been used in the treatment of breast carcinoma in postmenopausal females.

2. The **mechanism of action** is not completely understood.

3. A number of androgens are available, such as fluoxymesterone, dromostanolone, and testosterone. All are equally active and usually produce a response within two months.

4. Common **side effects** are masculinization and fluid retention.

D. ADRENAL CORTICOSTEROIDS

1. Corticosteroids inhibit cellular protein synthesis and also attach to specific corticosteroid-binding proteins associated with leukemia cells. (See Chapter 10, I C for further information about their intracellular mechanism of action.)

2. **Prednisone,** a glucocorticoid (see Chapter 10, I C 6 c), has been used successfully in combination with cytotoxic agents in the treatment of lymphoblastic and chronic lymphocytic leukemia.

3. Prednisone is also active in combination with other cytotoxic agents in the treatment of Hodgkin's disease (e.g., as a component of the MOPP regimen), non–Hodgkin's lymphomas, and multiple myeloma.

4. Because of their ability to suppress estrogen production by the adrenal cortex, adrenal corticosteroids have also been used in the treatment of breast carcinoma.

E. PROGESTINS

1. Progestins bind to cytosolic progesterone receptors and cause maturation of the endometrium to a nonproliferating secretory state. Thus, progestins are sometimes used in the therapy of metastatic endometrial carcinoma that can no longer be treated with irradiation or surgery.

2. The progestins most commonly used as antitumor agents are **medroxyprogesterone,** which is given intramuscularly, and **megestrol,** which is given orally.

3. Progestins also have some limited use in the treatment of metastatic renal cell carcinoma. The mechanism of action in this tumor type is unclear.

4. The progestins cause mild fluid retention and vaginal bleeding.

VI. MISCELLANEOUS AGENTS

A. HYDROXYUREA

1. **Chemistry.** Hydroxyurea is a derivative of urea. Its structure is shown in Figure 11-14.

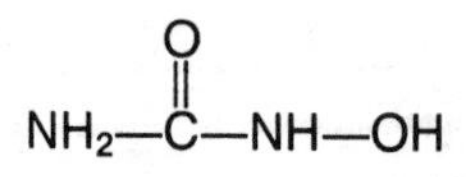

$$NH_2-\overset{O}{\overset{\|}{C}}-NH-OH$$

Figure 11-14. Hydroxyurea.

2. **Mechanism of action**
   a. Hydroxyurea inhibits ribonucleotide reductase. This enzyme is crucial to the biosynthesis of deoxyribonucleotides that are essential for the formation of DNA.
   b. Hydroxyurea is specific for the S phase of the cell cycle.
3. **Pharmacokinetics**
   a. Hydroxyurea is rapidly absorbed from the gastrointestinal tract.
   b. Twenty percent of a dose is metabolized in the liver, while the remainder is excreted via the kidney.
4. **Therapeutic uses**
   a. Hydroxyurea is an alternative to busulfan (see II D, above) in the treatment of chronic myelogenous leukemia.
   b. Hydroxyurea will reduce high white blood cell counts in patients with acute myelogenous leukemia.
5. **Major untoward effects**
   a. Reversible myelosuppression is the major untoward effect.
   b. Gastrointestinal and cutaneous disturbances occasionally occur.
6. **Route of administration**
   a. Hydroxyurea can be administered orally or intravenously.
   b. Because of its renal elimination, administration in patients with impaired renal function must be conducted with caution.

B. PROCARBAZINE

1. **Chemistry.** Procarbazine (Fig. 11-15) is a substituted hydrazine derivative with a structure similar to that of some monoamine oxidase inhibitors.
2. **Mechanism of action**
   a. Procarbazine undergoes auto-oxidation and forms hydrogen peroxide, leading to the degradation of DNA.
   b. It also inhibits DNA, RNA, and protein synthesis.
   c. It also can transmethylate DNA at the 7-nitrogen position of guanine.
3. **Pharmacokinetics**
   a. Procarbazine is rapidly absorbed from the gastrointestinal tract.
   b. It readily equilibrates between the plasma and the CSF.
   c. It is rapidly metabolized, and 40 percent is excreted in the urine.
4. **Therapeutic uses**
   a. The major use of procarbazine is in the treatment of Hodgkin's disease, where it is used in combination with mechlorethamine, vincristine, and prednisone to comprise the MOPP regimen.
   b. Procarbazine also has some activity in the treatment of oat cell carcinomas.
5. **Major untoward effects**
   a. Leukopenia and thrombocytopenia occur commonly.
   b. Gastrointestinal adverse effects as well as potentiation of other CNS-dependent drugs can occur.

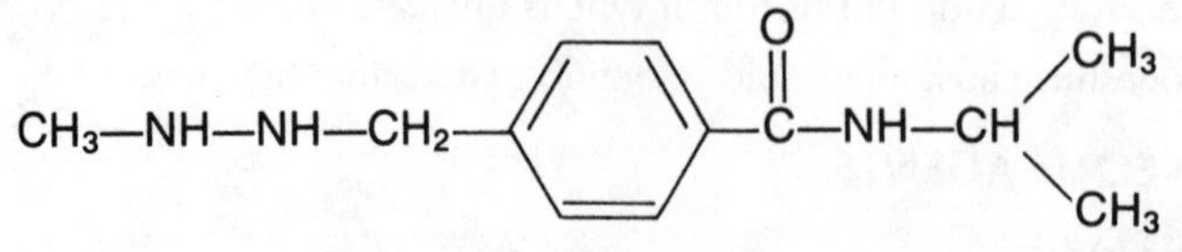

$$CH_3-NH-NH-CH_2-C_6H_4-\overset{O}{\overset{\|}{C}}-NH-CH(CH_3)_2$$

Figure 11-15. Procarbazine.

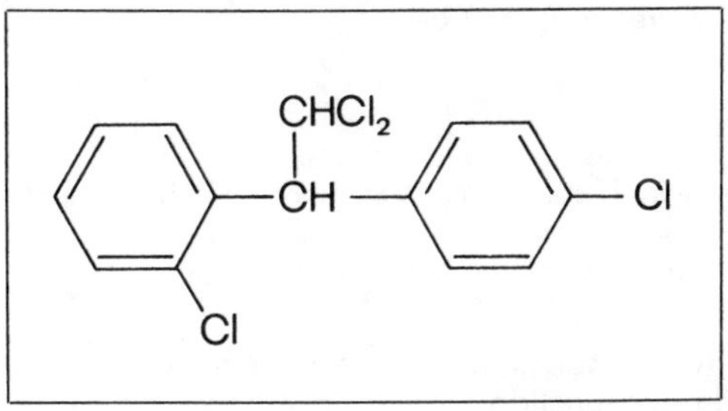

Figure 11-16. Mitotane.

c. Since procarbazine is a weak monoamine oxidase inhibitor, hypertensive reactions can occur when sympathomimetics, tricyclic antidepressants, or foods with a high tyramine content are ingested concomitantly.

6. **Route of administration.** Procarbazine is administered orally until the desired response occurs or limiting toxicity is seen.

C. MITOTANE (o,p′-DDD)

1. **Chemistry**
   a. Mitotane is a derivative of the insecticide DDT.
   b. Its structure is shown in Figure 11-16.

2. **Mechanism of action**
   a. Mitotane selectively destroys normal and neoplastic adrenocortical cells.
   b. It rapidly lowers adrenocorticosteroid levels.

3. **Pharmacokinetics**
   a. Mitotane is partially (40 percent) absorbed from the gastrointestinal tract.
   b. Blood levels persist for up to 9 weeks after cessation of therapy.
   c. Mitotane is widely distributed, with fat being the primary site of storage.

4. **Therapeutic uses.** Mitotane is used as palliative treatment for inoperable adrenocortical carcinomas.

5. **Major untoward effects**
   a. Gastrointestinal disturbances, lethargy, and dermatitis occur.
   b. If patients have Addison's disease, or if shock or trauma occur during mitotane therapy, adrenocorticosteroid replacement is indicated.

6. **Route of administration.** Mitotane is administered orally.

D. CISPLATIN

1. **Chemistry**
   a. Cisplatin (*cis*-diamminedichloroplatinum; Fig. 11-17) is an inorganic coordination complex with a planar configuration.
   b. Only the *cis* isomer is active.

2. **Mechanism of action**
   a. Cisplatin binds to DNA, causing both interstrand and intrastrand cross-linking similar to the actions of the bifunctional alkylating agents.
   b. It also binds extensively to nuclear and cytoplasmic proteins.
   c. Cisplatin is a phase-nonspecific agent.

3. **Pharmacokinetics**
   a. After intravenous administration, 90 percent becomes protein-bound.

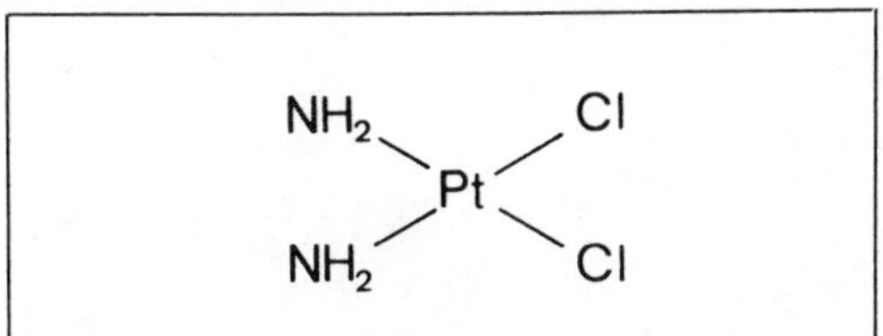

Figure 11-17. Cisplatin.

b. Cisplatin has a long terminal half-life of greater than 2 days.
c. It penetrates the CNS poorly.

4. **Therapeutic uses**
   a. Cisplatin is one of the most effective agents against solid tumors.
   b. It is effective alone and in combination with bleomycin and vinblastine in the treatment of testicular tumors.
   c. Cisplatin is also very useful in the treatment of ovarian carcinoma.

5. **Major untoward effects**

   a. Dose-dependent impairment of renal tubular function can occur, so that cisplatin should not be used in patients with impaired renal function.
   b. High-frequency hearing loss can occur.
   c. Severe nausea and vomiting are almost inevitable.
   d. Anaphylaxis has occurred after intravenous administration.

6. **Route of administration.** Cisplatin is administered intravenously, with vigorous hydration and mannitol diuresis to avoid renal toxicity.

STUDY QUESTIONS

Directions: Each question below contains five suggested answers. Choose the **one best** response to each question.

1. Cyclophosphamide can be used to treat all of the following neoplastic disorders EXCEPT

(A) Hodgkin's disease
(B) Burkitt's lymphoma
(C) choriocarcinoma
(D) ovarian carcinoma
(E) breast carcinoma

2. All of the following have been used as cancer chemotherapeutic agents EXCEPT

(A) alkylating agents
(B) antimetabolites
(C) vitamin D derivatives
(D) plant alkaloids
(E) hormonal agents

Directions: Each question below contains four suggested answers of which **one or more** is correct. Choose the answer

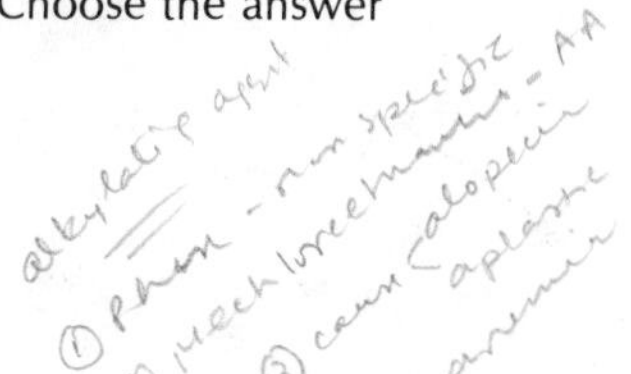

A if **1, 2, and 3** are correct
B if **1 and 3** are correct
C if **2 and 4** are correct
D if **4** is correct
E if **1, 2, 3, and 4** are correct

3. True statements regarding alkylating agents include which of the following?

(1) They are phase-nonspecific
(2) They cause DNA damage that cannot be repaired
(3) Acquired resistance can occur
(4) They are structurally similar to naturally occurring endogenous substances

4. Alkylating nitrogen mustards can produce which of the following side effects?

(1) Aplasia of the bone marrow
(2) Renal toxicity
(3) Alopecia
(4) Cardiac toxicity

5. Proliferation-independent agents include

(1) vincristine
(2) carmustine
(3) hydroxyurea
(4) mechlorethamine

6. Antineoplastic drugs that act only during a specific phase of the cell cycle include

(1) methotrexate
(2) 5-fluorouracil
(3) cytarabine
(4) cyclophosphamide

7. Which of the following drugs are correctly matched with the drug category?

(1) Mechlorethamine—an alkylating agent
(2) Methotrexate—a natural product
(3) 5-Fluorouracil—a pyrimidine analog
(4) Vinblastine—a purine analog

Directions: The group of questions below consists of lettered choices followed by several numbered items. For each numbered item select the **one** lettered choice with which it is **most** closely associated. Each lettered choice may be used once, more than once, or not at all.

Questions 8–10

For each statement about drug action, select the drug that is most likely to be associated with it.

(A) Cyclophosphamide
(B) 5-Fluorouracil
(C) Cytarabine
(D) Vincristine
(E) Mitomycin

8. In addition to being a natural product, it is an alkylating agent because it is reduced intracellularly and alkylates DNA.

9. It inhibits DNA polymerase and can be incorporated into DNA and RNA.

10. It is a phase-specific agent, producing metaphase arrest.

ANSWERS AND EXPLANATIONS

1. The answer is C. *(II B 4 b)* Cyclophosphamide is used alone or in combination for Hodgkin's and Burkitt's lymphomas and for ovarian and breast carcinomas, but not for choriocarcinoma. The latter is most effectively treated with methotrexate. When used for lymphomas, cyclophosphamide is frequently used with vincristine and prednisone. Cyclophosphamide has also been used as an immunosuppressing agent during organ transplants.

2. The answer is C. *(I G; II; III; IV F; V)* Vitamin D derivatives have not been effective as cancer chemotherapeutic agents. A good diet, of course, is always important for the patient. The alkylating agents, antimetabolites, plant alkaloids and hormonal agents are major classes of antineoplastic agents available for clinical use.

3. The answer is B (1, 3). *(II A 2, 4, B 2 d; III A 1)* All alkylating agents are phase-nonspecific. In addition, cell death also occurs during interphase, and, thus, they can be proliferation-independent. Both acquired resistance and cross-resistance can occur. The DNA damage that occurs is subject to repair by enzymes, and repair can be a factor in tumor cell responsiveness. Antimetabolites are substances with structural similarity to endogenous substances.

4. The answer is B (1, 3). *(II B 3 c, 4 c, 5 b, 6 c)* Nitrogen mustards commonly produce nausea, alopecia, myelosuppression, and sometimes diarrhea. Menstrual irregularities have been reported also. Renal and cardiac toxicity are not common problems with the alkylating agents. Renal toxicity is a serious side effect of cisplatin. Doxorubicin causes cardiac damage; this is related to the cumulative dose.

5. The answer is C (2, 4). *(I D 3; IV F 2 b; VI A 2 b)* Proliferation-independent agents are toxic to both proliferating and nonproliferating cells. Examples include carmustine, mechlorethamine, and irradiation. The vinca alkaloids, such as vincristine, bind to tubulin and are M-phase-specific, blocking cells as they enter metaphase. Hydroxyurea inhibits ribonucleotide reductase and blocks cells in S phase.

6. The answer is B (1, 3). *(I D 4 a, c)* Methotrexate acts during the DNA synthetic phase of the cell cycle. Although 5-fluorouracil is proliferation-dependent, it is phase-nonspecific, perhaps due to its RNA actions. Cytarabine is an analog of cytidine which inhibits DNA polymerase and, thus, is an S-phase-specific agent. No alkylating agent is phase-specific.

7. The answer is B (1, 3). *(II B 1, 3; III B, D 1; IV F 1 a)* The administration of mechlorethamine, an alkylating agent, will produce DNA cross-linking, mispairing of bases, and depurination of DNA because of the highly reactive carbonium ion produced from mechlorethamine. This is true of all alkylating agents. Methotrexate is not a natural product but a folic acid antagonist and an antimetabolite. Vinblastine is a plant alkaloid, not a purine analog, while 5-fluorouracil is a fluorine-substituted analog of uracil and, thus, a pyrimidine analog.

8–10. The answers are: 8-E, 9-C, 10-D. *(II A 3, B 2; III D 1 b, 2 b; IV E 2, F 2)* Mitomycin is both a natural product and an alkylating agent. Isolated from a *Streptomyces* species, mitomycin C is reduced by a reduced nicotinamide adenine dinucleotide phosphate (NADPH)–dependent reductase and alkylates DNA.

Cytarabine inhibits DNA polymerase and, thus, kills cells in S phase. Cytarabine nucleotides can be incorporated into DNA and RNA, but the significance is not known.

Vincristine is an M-phase-specific agent, blocking proliferating cells as they enter metaphase. It is useful in the treatment of some lymphomas and leukemias.

12
Anti-Infective Agents

I. INTRODUCTION

A. ANTI-INFECTIVE AGENTS are chemical substances that can kill or suppress the growth of microorganisms.

1. **Antibiotics** are soluble compounds that are derived from certain microorganisms and that inhibit the growth of other microorganisms.
2. The effectiveness of antimicrobial agents usually relies on a biochemical or physiologic difference between the host and the infectious organism.

B. Anti-infective agents can differ from one another in the following ways:

1. Chemical properties.
2. Mechanism of action.
3. Spectrum of activity.
4. Pharmacokinetics.
5. Therapeutic uses.
6. Adverse effects.

C. BACTERIAL INFECTIONS are readily treated in most instances by a wide variety of agents. The major groups of **antibacterial agents** include:

1. Sulfonamides.
2. Penicillins.
3. Cephalosporins.
4. Aminoglycosides.
5. Tetracyclines.
6. Chloramphenicol.
7. Erythromycin, lincomycin, clindamycin, and vancomycin.

D. FUNGAL INFECTIONS, in contrast to bacterial ones, generally are quite resistant to chemotherapy, and thus the number of useful agents for these infections is somewhat restricted. Fungal infections often occur as a result of broad-spectrum antibacterial therapy, which produces a superinfection.

E. INFECTIONS CAUSED BY MYCOBACTERIA, in the past, often required treatment in specialized centers; today such is no longer the case. Tuberculosis is one of the few diseases that requires a combination of antimicrobial drugs, which is used to prevent the appearance of resistant strains of the infecting organism. Leprosy is a disease whose course has been remarkably altered by chemotherapy.

F. HELMINTHIASIS may now affect as many as a billion people a year, and its incidence is increasing with increased agricultural use of land and increased travel. With the advent of several new, highly selective anthelmintic drugs, the older agents used to treat parasitic worm infections have become obsolete.

G. PROTOZOAL INFECTIONS, such as amebiasis and various trypanosomal infections, are treated by a wide variety of agents. Metronidazole is directly trichomonacidal and also is the agent of choice for several other protozoal infections.

H. VIRAL INFECTIONS are difficult to treat because viruses are intracellular parasites, requiring the active participation of a host cell's metabolic processes, and few pharmacologic agents are selective enough to kill a virus without injuring the involved host cell.

II. THE SULFONAMIDES

A. CHEMISTRY

1. The sulfonamides are derivatives of sulfanilamide, which has the following structural formula:

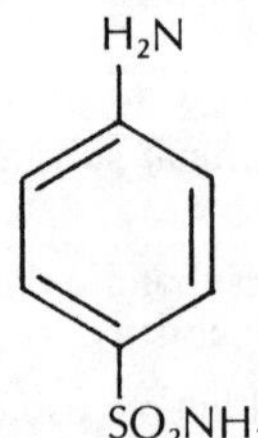

Sulfanilamide

2. Derivatives are made by substitutions in the amide of the sulfonamide group.

B. MECHANISM OF ACTION

1. Sulfonamides are effective against many gram-positive bacteria, including group *A Streptococcus pyogenes* and *Streptococcus pneumoniae.*
2. They prevent the incorporation of PABA into folic acid, a substance which in the reduced form is necessary in the biochemical process for the transfer of certain one-carbon units.
3. Susceptible bacteria are those that need PABA because they are incapable of utilizing folic acid directly.
4. Human cells utilize exogenous folic acid exclusively, however, and thus a lack of PABA does not affect them.

C. SPECTRUM OF ACTIVITY

1. Sulfonamides are effective against many gram-positive bacteria, including group A *Streptococcus pyogenes* and *Streptococcus pneumoniae.*
2. Many gram-negative bacteria are resistant to sulfonamides, but some, such as *Hemophilus influenzae, Escherichia coli* (the organism most often suspect in acute urinary tract infections), and *Proteus mirabilis,* often are sensitive.
3. Other susceptible organisms include *Bacillus anthracis, Nocardia, Actinomyces,* and *Chlamydia trachomatis,* the agent responsible for trachoma, lymphogranuloma venereum, and inclusion conjunctivitis.

D. PHARMACOKINETICS

1. Sulfonamides are absorbed within minutes following oral administration.
2. They are distributed throughout the body water.
3. They diffuse into cerebrospinal fluid.
4. They are metabolized by acetylation of the para-NH_2.
5. Excretion is chiefly via the urine, within 24 hours of administration. The solubility of the various sulfonamides varies widely.

E. THERAPEUTIC USES

1. Sulfonamides are the preferred agents for treatment of:

   a. Acute uncomplicated urinary tract infections.
   b. Nocardiosis.

2. They are effective for treatment of toxoplasmosis when used in combination with pyrimethamine.
3. They are used in trachoma and inclusion conjunctivitis as an alternative to tetracycline.
4. Aside from acute urinary tract infections, the use of sulfonamides alone in many other infections has been replaced by more effective and safer drugs.

F. PREPARATIONS. The most commonly used sulfonamides are:

1. **Trimethoprim-sulfamethoxazole.**
   a. Sulfamethoxazole and trimethoprim inhibit two separate steps in folate metabolism.
   b. Trimethoprim is a highly selective inhibitor of the dihydrofolate reductase of lower organisms.
   c. In combination, the two drugs act synergistically.
2. **Sulfisoxazole.**
3. **Sulfadiazine.**

G. UNTOWARD EFFECTS

1. About 75 percent of untoward effects involve the skin, with sensitization often being responsible. Conditions produced include:
   a. Exfoliative dermatitis.
   b. Stevens-Johnson syndrome (fever, malaise, and erythema multiforme).
2. Drug fever can occur and is probably due to sensitization.
3. Blood dyscrasias are rare but can occur. Sulfonamide therapy is stopped immediately if any of the following hematologic conditions develop to a serious extent:
   a. Acute hemolytic anemia. This is often, but not solely, due to an erythrocytic deficiency of glucose 6-phosphate dehydrogenase activity. Acute hemolytic anemia is particularly likely to develop in blacks and children.
   b. Aplastic anemia.
   c. Agranulocytosis.
   d. Thrombocytopenia.
4. Eosinophilia may accompany other manifestations of hypersensitivity.
5. Crystalluria is a condition that was seen with the older sulfonamides but rarely occurs with the newer, more soluble agents such as sulfisoxazole, although some renal damage is still possible.
6. Hepatitis, causing focal or diffuse necrosis of the liver, occurs rarely and may be caused by either direct drug toxicity or sensitization.
7. Kernicterus can occur in the newborn because of displacement of bilirubin from plasma albumin.

III. THE PENICILLINS

A. CHEMISTRY

1. The structure of the penicillins consists of a thiazolidine ring (marked 1 below) connected to a beta-lactam ring (marked 2), which is attached to a side chain (marked R).

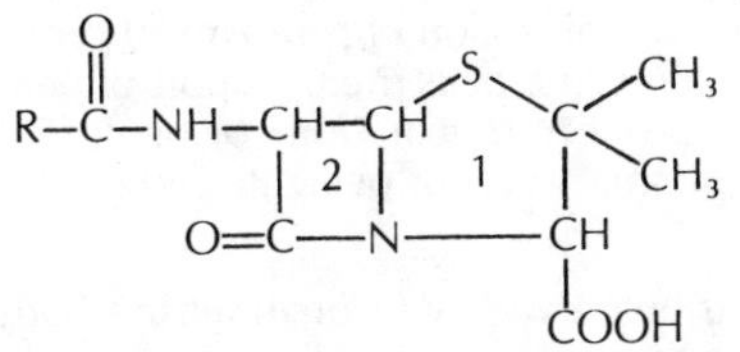

```
       O
       ‖            S
R—C—NH—CH—CH          C  CH3
          | 2 |   1   |  CH3
       O=C—N————————CH
                      |
                     COOH
```

Penicillins

2. All penicillins are derived from 6-aminopenicillanic acid.

B. MECHANISM OF ACTION

1. Penicillins inhibit the synthesis of bacterial cell walls and are considered **bactericidal.**
2. They combine with and inactivate transpeptidase, which, normally, is responsible for cross-linking the linear glycopeptide strands of bacterial cell walls. Loss of cell-wall rigidity in the presence of normal high intracellular osmotic pressure causes lysis of the bacterial membrane.

C. SPECTRUM OF ACTIVITY

1. **Naturally occurring penicillins G and V** are highly effective against gram-positive and gram-negative cocci. Approximately 20 percent of strains of *Staphylococcus aureus,* however, are resistant.
2. The majority of strains of *Corynebacterium diphtheriae* and *Bacillus anthracis* are sensitive to penicillin G.
3. *Treponema pallidum,* the microorganism causing syphilis, is very sensitive to penicillin G.
4. Many gram-negative bacilli strains are sensitive to penicillin G at high drug concentrations only. Gonococci, however, are generally sensitive at a fairly low concentration.
5. In general, microbial sensitivity should be verified whenever possible.

D. BACTERIAL RESISTANCE

1. **Penicillinase** is a beta-lactamase which can hydrolyze the beta-lactam ring of penicillin to form penicilloic acid, a substance that has no antibacterial activity.
2. Microorganisms that are capable of producing penicillinase include:
   a. *S. aureus.*
   b. *Bacillus* species.
   c. *Bacteroides.*
   d. *E. coli.*
   e. *Proteus* species.
   f. *Pseudomonas aeruginosa.*
   g. *Mycobacterium tuberculosis.*
3. Microorganisms can acquire the ability to produce penicillinase through:
   a. Plasmid acquisition via transduction in gram-positive bacteria.
   b. R factor acquisition during conjugation in gram-negative bacteria.

E. PHARMACOKINETICS OF PENICILLIN G

1. **Oral administration**
   a. Because gastric acid inactivates penicillin G, only 30 percent of an oral dose is absorbed from the duodenum.
   b. Because food interferes with its absorption, penicillin G should be administered at least 1 hour before meals and no earlier than 2 to 3 hours after meals.
   c. Peak plasma concentrations occur 30 to 60 minutes after administration.
   d. Penicillin V is more stable in an acidic environment and thus an equivalent oral dose leads to plasma levels two to five times higher than those obtained with penicillin G.
2. **Subcutaneous or intramuscular administration**
   a. Following injection of crystalline penicillin G, peak plasma concentrations occur in 15 minutes.
   b. Sixty to ninety percent of a dose is excreted within one hour.
   c. Up to 99 percent of an intramuscular dose of penicillin G is eliminated via the kidney. Approximately 90 percent is eliminated by tubular secretion and 10 percent by glomerular filtration.
   d. The stimultaneous administration of **probenecid** prolongs the duration of penicillin in the body because probenecid blocks the transport of penicillin in the proximal tubule. However, the use of repository preparations of penicillin provides an alternative means for maintaining high plasma levels of penicillin.
3. **Distribution**
   a. Penicillin G is distributed widely throughout the body, with about 60 percent reversibly bound to plasma albumin.
   b. It penetrates poorly into ocular, pericardial, and cerebrospinal fluids.
   c. Significant amounts of the drug appear in the liver, intestine, and kidney, as well as in bile, semen, and lymph.

F. THERAPEUTIC USES

1. **Infections due to *S. pneumoniae* (pneumococcal infections)**
   a. Penicillin G or V is the drug of first choice for treatment of pneumococcal pneumonia.
   b. For pneumococcal meningitis, penicillin G usually is administered intravenously. Although intrathecal administration sometimes is used, arachnoiditis and encephalopathy can complicate this form of therapy.
   c. Other pneumococcal infections in which penicillin G is the drug of first choice include:
      (1) Suppurative arthritis.
      (2) Mastoiditis.
      (3) Endocarditis.
      (4) Pericarditis.
      (5) Osteomyelitis.

2. **Staphylococcal infections** often are resistant to penicillin therapy, because of penicillinase activity.
   a. **Oxacillin, cloxacillin, dicloxacillin, methicillin,** and **nafcillin** are **penicillinase-resistant penicillins** that are highly effective for this type of infection.
   b. Staphylococcal infections that *are* sensitive to penicillin G should be treated with this form of the drug, since it is more active than the penicillinase-resistant penicillins.

3. **Streptococcal infections,** especially if due to group A *S. pyogenes,* are exquisitely sensitive to penicillin.
   a. Streptococcal pharyngitis and scarlet fever both respond to oral penicillin (penicillin V), with rapid improvement occurring in two to four days.
   b. Otitis media due to *S. pyogenes* also responds to oral penicillin (penicillin V).
   c. Other streptococcal infections (non-pneumococcal) responding favorably to penicillin include:
      (1) Streptococcal endocarditis.
      (2) Streptococcal arthritis.
      (3) Streptococcal meningitis.
   d. α-Hemolytic streptococci often are the cause of subacute endocarditis and, in this case, occasionally are resistant to penicillin, necessitating the use of a semisynthetic penicillin such as nafcillin.

4. **Gonococcal infections.** Penicillin G is the drug of first choice for all types of gonococcal infections, although strains that are more resistant require higher doses.

5. **Syphilis.** Penicillin G is the most effective treatment for all stages of syphilis.

6. **Other microbial infections** responding to penicillin therapy include:
   a. Clostridial infections, including gas gangrene.
   b. In diphtheria, penicillin eliminates the acute and chronic carrier states, whereas specific antitoxin is used for treatment.
   c. Actinomycosis.
   d. Anthrax.
   e. *Listeria* infections.
   f. Salmonellosis and shigellosis, in which sensitive strains respond to ampicillin.
   g. *H. influenzae* infection, in which the drug of choice is ampicillin, provided the strain is sensitive.
   h. *E. coli, Proteus* (indole-positive and -negative) and *Pseudomonas* infections, which respond to broad-spectrum penicillins.
      (1) Ampicillin is effective in the treatment of urinary tract infections caused by *E. coli* and *P. mirabilis.*
      (2) Carbenicillin provides effective therapy for urinary tract infections caused by indole-positive *Proteus* and *Pseudomonas.*
      (3) When a *Pseudomonas* infection is life-threatening, gentamicin often is used in combination with carbenicillin.
      (4) Administration of carbenicillin and gentamicin may be useful in treating pneumonias and burn infections caused by sensitive organisms.

7. Penicillin has been shown to be effective **prophylactically** in the following conditions:
   a. Streptococcal infections.
   b. Rheumatic fever recurrences.
      (1) Oral administration of penicillin V daily or intramuscular injection of benzathine penicillin G monthly reduces the risk of recurrent episodes.
      (2) The duration of therapy is five years after an initial episode in adults, or throughout adolescence when the onset of the disease occurs during childhood.

c. Gonorrheal ophthalmia in neonates, for which conjunctival instillation of penicillin G solution is effective.
d. Surgical procedures in patients who have valvular heart disease.
(1) Such patients, when undergoing dental extractions, tonsillectomy, or genitourinary or intestinal operations, often receive penicillin prophylactically.
(2) Bacteremia is not totally prevented by using prophylactic penicillin.

G. PREPARATIONS AND ADMINISTRATION

1. Soluble forms
a. Penicillin G (benzylpenicillin) sodium and potassium salts are used intramuscularly, intravenously, and orally.
b. Penicillin V (phenoxymethyl penicillin) is a soluble form that is resistant to acid; it is used orally.

2. Repository forms are insoluble salts which allow the slow absorption of penicillin from the site of injection, providing a duration of action lasting 12 to 24 hours. These forms are used intramuscularly only and include:
a. Procaine penicillin G.
b. Benzathine penicillin G. This drug has a low solubility, and effective blood levels often are present for a week.

3. Penicillinase-resistant penicillins
a. Methicillin
(1) The drug has one-twentieth the potency of penicillin G.
(2) It is not administered orally because of poor absorption via this route.
b. Oxacillin
(1) The drug is acid-stable and therefore can be given orally as well as intravenously and intramuscularly.
(2) It is highly protein-bound in the plasma.
(3) It is up to eight times as potent as methicillin.
c. Cloxacillin has pharmacologic and pharmacokinetic properties that are similar to those of oxacillin.
d. Nafcillin can be given orally, intravenously, or intramuscularly.
e. Dicloxacillin. Because it is highly resistant to penicillinase and acid hydrolysis, this agent is very effective when administered orally.

4. Broad-spectrum penicillins
a. Ampicillin is given orally, intravenously, or intramuscularly.
(1) In addition to being effective against gram-positive organisms, ampicillin is effective against *E. coli, H. influenzae, Salmonella, Shigella,* and some *Proteus* species.
(2) It is acid-stable but not penicillinase-resistant.
b. Amoxicillin is given orally only.
(1) It has a spectrum of activity similar to that of ampicillin.
(2) Amoxicillin attains higher blood levels than ampicillin.
(3) The drug is thought to cause a lower incidence of diarrhea than ampicillin.
c. Carbenicillin disodium is given intravenously or intramuscularly. It has a spectrum of activity similar to that of ampicillin and, in addition, is effective against indole-positive *Proteus* and *Pseudomonas.*
d. Carbenicillin indanyl sodium. This indanyl congener is acid-stable and is administered orally.

H. UNTOWARD EFFECTS

1. Hypersensitivity reactions to the penicillins occur in 1 to 10 percent of patients receiving these drugs.
a. All dosage forms of penicillin can cause hypersensitivity reactions.
b. The reaction can range from a mild rash to life-threatening anaphylaxis.
c. A hypersensitivity reaction to one penicillin places the affected patient at a high risk of reaction to any other penicillin.
d. A reaction can occur in the absence of prior therapeutic penicillin administration.
e. The allergic reaction may persist one to two weeks after discontinuation of therapy.
f. Hypersensitivity reactions include:
(1) Skin rashes of all types, including, in severe cases, the Stevens-Johnson syndrome. The highest incidence of skin rash occurs following ampicillin administration and is about 9 percent.
(2) Fever, which disappears within 36 hours after termination of administration.

(3) Eosinophilia.
(4) Angioedema.
(5) Serum sickness.
(6) Anaphylactic reactions.
(a) One in fifty thousand patients treated with penicillin dies from this type of reaction.
(b) It is most common after parenteral administration but it can occur after oral ingestion, and with minute quantities of penicillin.

2. Other untoward effects include:
a. Gastrointestinal upset, which is seen especially with orally administered preparations; for example, ampicillin-associated diarrhea.
b. Nephrotoxicity, which is very rare and which usually occurs only in patients who have compromised renal function.
c. Bone-marrow toxicity (uncommon).
(1) Depression of bone marrow has been reported with methicillin administration.
(2) Agranulocytosis has been reported with ampicillin administration.
(3) Impairment of platelet aggregation has been reported with carbenicillin administration.
d. Superinfection resulting from alterations in intestinal flora.
(1) A low incidence occurs with penicillin G administration.
(2) A higher incidence occurs with broader-spectrum penicillins such as ampicillin and carbenicillin.

IV. THE CEPHALOSPORINS

A. CHEMISTRY

1. These drugs are derivatives of 7-aminocephalosporanic acid and are closely related in structure to penicillin.

2. They have a six-membered sulfur-containing ring (marked 1 below) adjoining a beta-lactam ring (marked 2).

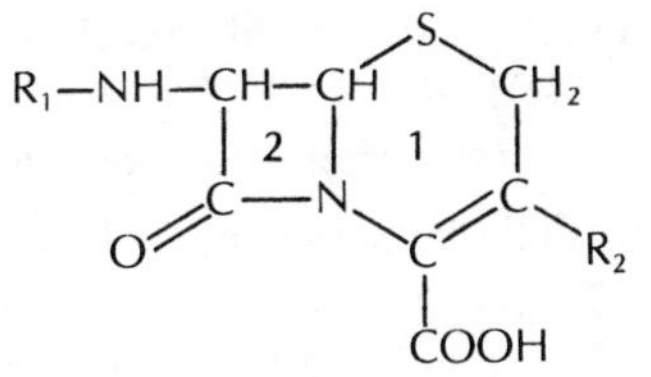

```
                        S
                      /   \
R1—NH—CH—CH            CH2
       |  2 |    1     |
       C——N           C
      //      \     //  \
     O          C         R2
                |
               COOH
```

Cephalosporins

3. They are relatively stable in dilute acid and highly resistant to penicillinase.

B. MECHANISM OF ACTION. Cephalosporins inhibit bacterial cell-wall synthesis in a manner similar to that of penicillin and are considered **bactericidal.**

C. SPECTRUM OF ACTIVITY

1. Cephalosporins are effective against a wide variety of gram-positive and gram-negative microorganisms.

2. The newer, semisynthetic ("third-generation") cephalosporins are more potent than the parent drug.

3. As a group these drugs are now used against:
a. Streptococci, including:
(1) Group A *S. pyogenes.*
(2) The *viridans* group.
(3) Nonhemolytic streptococci.
b. Penicillin-sensitive and penicillin-resistant *S. aureus.*
c. *S. epidermidis.*
d. *Clostridium perfringens.*
e. *B. subtilis.*

f. *C. diphtheriae.*
g. *Neisseria gonorrhoeae.*
h. *N. meningitidis.*
i. *Salmonella typhi.*
j. *Shigella.*
k. Indole-positive and indole-negative *Proteus.*
l. *E. coli.*
m. *H. influenzae.*
n. *Klebsiella.*
o. *P. aeruginosa (the earlier cephalosporins are inactive).*
p. *Bacteroides* species.
q. *Serratia.*

4. The cephalosporins are in general ineffective against enterococci.

5. Some bacteria elaborate a beta-lactamase called **cephalosporinase** that acts on cephalosporin C to destroy its antibacterial activity. Many cephalosporins are, however, resistant to the enzyme.

D. PHARMACOKINETICS

1. Most cephalosporins are administered parenterally; some are, however, well absorbed from the gastrointestinal tract.

2. They become widely distributed throughout body tissues and fluids. The majority do not penetrate the blood–brain barrier and thus are not effective in the treatment of central nervous system infections.

3. The half-life and the degree of serum protein-binding vary widely from agent to agent.

4. Although some cephalosporins are excreted via the bile, most are excreted in the urine via renal tubular secretion. Probenecid blocks the tubular secretion of cephalosporins, often resulting in an increased half-life and elevated plasma concentration.

E. THERAPEUTIC USES

1. Diseases produced by *S. aureus,* both penicillin-sensitive and -resistant, including skin infections, osteomyelitis, and endocarditis, respond favorably to the cephalosporins.

2. Cephalosporins are the drugs of first choice for *Klebsiella pneumoniae* infections.

3. These drugs are used successfully in the treatment of pneumococcal pneumonia and in infections caused by *S. pyogenes.*

4. Some of the parenteral cephalosporins are efficacious in the treatment of gonococcal disease that is resistant to other agents.

5. Diseases caused by a number of gram-negative bacteria, including respiratory and urinary tract infections, respond well.

6. With the expanded-spectrum (third-generation) cephalosporins, susceptible strains of *Bacteroides fragilis, Enterobacter,* and *Serratia* can be treated effectively. In addition, urinary tract infections caused by susceptible strains of *Pseudomonas* can be treated.

7. Third-generation cephalosporins have recently been used to treat bacterial meningitis (see F 3 below.)

8. Prophylactic cephalosporin therapy plays an important role in reducing perioperative infection.

F. PREPARATIONS AND ADMINISTRATION

1. **First-generation cephalosporins** are *not* effective against indole-positive *Proteus, Pseudomonas, Serratia, Enterobacter,* or *B. fragilis.*
   a. **Cephalothin**
      (1) It is not well absorbed from the gastrointestinal tract.
      (2) It is usually given intravenously. Intramuscular injection is painful.
      (3) It is excreted principally via renal tubular secretion.
   b. **Cephapirin** is similar to cephalothin.
   c. **Cefazolin**
      (1) It is not well absorbed from the gastrointestinal tract and is administered intravenously or intramuscularly.

(2) Eighty percent of the drug is reversibly bound to plasma proteins, substantially increasing its half-life.
(3) Cefazolin is eliminated primarily by renal glomerular filtration; renal tubular and biliary secretions play secondary roles.

d. Cephalexin
(1) It is well absorbed from the gastrointestinal tract because of its high acid stability.
(2) It is available in oral capsules, suspensions, and pediatric drops.
(3) More than 90 percent of this drug is excreted unchanged in the urine; it is also excreted into bile.

e. Cephradine is similar to cephalexin. It can be given orally, intravenously, or intramuscularly.

f. Cefaclor is similar to cephalexin but also is effective against beta-lactamase–producing *H. influenzae.* It is given orally.

g. Cephaloridine is no longer used in the United States because of its nephrotoxicity.

2. Second-generation cephalosporins

a. Cefamandole nafate
(1) This expanded-spectrum cephalosporin is effective against indole-positive *Proteus* and beta-lactamase–producing *H. influenzae.*
(2) It is administered parenterally only.

b. Cefoxitin
(1) This expanded-spectrum cephalosporin is effective against indole-positive *Proteus* and *B. fragilis.* It has less activity against the gram-positive organisms.
(2) It is given parenterally.

3. Third-generation cephalosporins—cefotaxime, moxalactam, and ceftizoxime

a. The expanded spectrum of activity of these drugs includes effectiveness against indole-positive *Proteus, B. fragilis, Serratia,* and *Enterobacter,* and some activity against *Pseudomonas.* They are given parenterally.

b. Because of its CSF permeability, moxalactam is effective against meningitis caused by susceptible strains, but its use is restricted because it can cause a bleeding diathesis.

G. UNTOWARD EFFECTS

1. **Hypersensitivity reactions** occur in about 5 percent of patients receiving cephalosporin therapy.
   a. Cephalosporins, like penicillins, elicit a spectrum of reactions that range from mild skin rash to anaphylaxis.
   b. A **cross-sensitivity** reaction to the cephalosporins occurs in about 10 percent of individuals who have experienced an allergic manifestation following the administration of penicillin.
   c. A high incidence of direct positive Coombs' reactions occurs in patients receiving large doses of a cephalosporin.

2. Renal damage, although rare with normal doses of cephalosporins, can occur.

3. Local tissue reactions can occur with parenteral administration. Intravenous administration can cause thrombophlebitis.

4. Superinfections caused by gram-negative bacteria or yeasts can occur following administration of the cephalosporins.

V. AMINOGLYCOSIDES

A. CHEMISTRY

1. The aminoglycosides are compounds containing characteristic amino sugars joined to a hexose nucleus in glycosidic linkage.

2. They are polycations, and their polarity accounts for their pharmacokinetic properties.

B. MECHANISM OF ACTION

1. Aminoglycosides inhibit protein biosynthesis by acting directly on the ribosome and are rapidly **bactericidal.**

2. They interfere with the proper attachment of messenger RNA to ribosomes (initiation), cause misreading of the genetic code, and produce decreased or abnormal protein synthesis.

3. The ability of the aminoglycosides to actually kill bacteria is not, however, adequately explained by any of their known actions.

C. SPECTRUM OF ACTIVITY

1. **Streptomycin**
   a. High concentrations of streptomycin are bactericidal; low concentrations are bacteriostatic.
   b. Streptomycin is effective against the organisms that cause plague (*Yersinia pestis*) and tularemia (*Francisella tularensis*) and (in combination with penicillin; see E 1 a, below) against gram-positive enterococci (streptococci). In vivo, streptomycin suppresses tubercle bacilli.
   c. A major disadvantage of streptomycin therapy is the development of frequent **bacterial resistance** to the drug. Because of this resistance, streptomycin is used *alone* to treat only two infections—tularemia and plague.

2. **Neomycin** is effective against many gram-negative species and is also effective against several gram-positive bacteria (e.g., *S. aureus*). Streptococci are generally resistant to neomycin.

3. **Gentamicin** is bactericidal against a wide variety of gram-negative organisms, including indole-positive *Proteus, Pseudomonas,* and *Serratia* organisms. Some strains of *Staphylococcus* may be sensitive to gentamicin.

4. **Tobramycin** has a spectrum of activity similar to that of gentamicin but may be slightly more effective against *Pseudomonas.*

5. **Amikacin** also has a spectrum of activity similar to that of gentamicin but often is reserved for *Serratia* infections or for cases where resistance to gentamicin has emerged.

6. **Kanamycin** has a more limited spectrum of activity than gentamicin has. It is ineffective against *Pseudomonas* and most gram-positive organisms.

7. Kanamycin, amikacin, streptomycin, and neomycin all have some activity against *M. tuberculosis.*

8. **Cross-resistance** can occur between kanamycin, streptomycin, and neomycin.

9. Anaerobic microorganisms are generally resistant to the aminoglycosides.

D. PHARMACOKINETICS

1. All of the aminoglycosides are poorly absorbed after oral administration because of their polycationic structure.

2. **Streptomycin** is absorbed rapidly after intramuscular or subcutaneous administration.
   a. It is distributed in all the extracellular fluids.
   b. It crosses the blood–brain barrier only if the meninges are inflamed.
   c. It is excreted by glomerular filtration.

3. **Gentamicin, tobramycin, amikacin,** and **kanamycin** have a pharmacokinetic profile similar to that of streptomycin.

4. **Neomycin** is also poorly absorbed following oral administration. It is most often applied topically.

5. All the aminoglycosides are more active in an alkaline environment.

E. THERAPEUTIC USES

1. **Streptomycin**
   a. Subacute bacterial endocarditis caused by the *viridans* group of streptococci or by enterococci is treated with streptomycin, usually in combination with penicillin G.
   b. Tularemia and plague are effectively treated with streptomycin.
   c. Severe cases of brucellosis are treated with a combination of streptomycin and tetracycline.
   d. Urinary and respiratory tract infections, peritonitis, and bacterial meningitis may respond to streptomycin but are more effectively treated with other agents.
   e. Although streptomycin is no longer used alone in the treatment of pulmonary tuberculosis, it is often used in combination with other agents for the treatment of serious forms of tuberculosis (see X D, below).

2. **Gentamicin, tobramycin,** and **amikacin**
   a. Many infections can be treated successfully with these agents, but their toxicity restricts their use to situations involving life-threatening infections caused by:
   (1) *P. aeruginosa, Serratia, Enterobacter,* and *Klebsiella.*

(2) Methicillin-resistant staphylococci that are sensitive to gentamicin.

b. These agents are sometimes used as part of an initial "blind therapy" for serious infections of unknown etiology, in which case a penicillinase-resistant penicillin or a cephalosporin is administered in combination with an aminoglycoside, such as gentamicin.

3. **Neomycin,** because of its serious toxic effects when absorbed systemically, is used most frequently in dermatologic and ophthalmic ointments. In addition, neomycin can be used orally as a bowel preparation for surgery or for the management of hepatic coma.

F. PREPARATIONS AND ADMINISTRATION

1. **Streptomycin**
   a. Intramuscular injection is the most common route of administration.
   b. To avoid the development of bacterial resistance, streptomycin therapy rarely is extended beyond ten days (except in tuberculosis and subacute bacterial endocarditis).

2. **Gentamicin**
   a. This drug can be administered intramuscularly, intravenously, or as an ointment or cream.
   b. When renal function is impaired, peak and trough serum concentrations of gentamicin are measured intermittently to allow optimal guidance for adjusting dosage, and renal function is monitored by means of the serum creatinine level.

3. **Tobramycin** and **amikacin** can be given intramuscularly and intravenously.

4. **Kanamycin** can be given intramuscularly, intravenously, or orally.

5. **Neomycin**
   a. This drug is available in the form of creams, ointments, and sprays, both alone and in combination with polymyxin, bacitracin, other antibiotics, and corticosteroids.
   b. It is also available for oral and parenteral administration, although it is rarely used parenterally.

G. UNTOWARD EFFECTS. All of the aminoglycosides have a narrow therapeutic index that limits their usage.

1. **Streptomycin**
   a. Hypersensitivity reactions can occur.
   b. Labyrinthine damage and vestibular disturbances can occur.
      (1) Permanent damage occurs in a small percentage of patients.
      (2) The incidence is directly related to daily dose and duration of therapy.
      (3) About 7 percent of patients receiving streptomycin for more than one week have a measurable decrease in hearing. The high-frequency sound range is first to be affected.
   c. Dysfunction of the optic nerve can occur, producing scotomas.
   d. Neuromuscular junction blockade may result when streptomycin is given at high doses and in combination with curariform drugs. This results from a decreased sensitivity of the postjunctional membrane to acetylcholine and possibly because of decreased presynaptic release of transmitter.
   e. Renal effects are minimal at normal doses.

2. **Gentamicin, tobramycin,** and **amikacin**
   a. Ototoxicity is the most serious side effect.
      (1) It occurs more commonly when renal failure is present.
      (2) The vestibular division of the eighth cranial nerve is involved.
      (3) Damage to the nerve can occur bilaterally and may be permanent.
      (4) The duration of aminoglycoside treatment may increase the risk.
   b. Nephrotoxicity can occur.
      (1) Gentamicin is the most nephrotoxic of the aminoglycosides. It can produce acute renal insufficiency and tubular necrosis.
      (2) When renal failure of any degree is present, serum creatinine and aminoglycoside levels must be measured and drug dosage adjusted accordingly.

3. **Kanamycin**
   a. Hypersensitivity reactions can occur.
   b. Ototoxicity can occur.
      (1) The cochlear and the vestibular divisions of the auditory nerve may be damaged.
      (2) The simultaneous administration of ethacrynic acid increases the risk of ototoxicity.
   c. Neuromuscular blockade can occur.
   d. Nephrotoxicity can occur.

4. Neomycin

a. Hypersensitivity reactions can occur, with up to 8 percent of patients developing a skin rash when neomycin is applied topically.

b. Renal damage, eighth-nerve damage resulting in nerve deafness, and neuromuscular blockade can occur following oral or parenteral administration.

c. Superinfection and intestinal malabsorption can occur following oral administration.

VI. TETRACYCLINES

A. CHEMISTRY

1. The tetracyclines are derivatives of the polycyclic naphthacenecarboxamide.

2. The structural formula of tetracycline is:

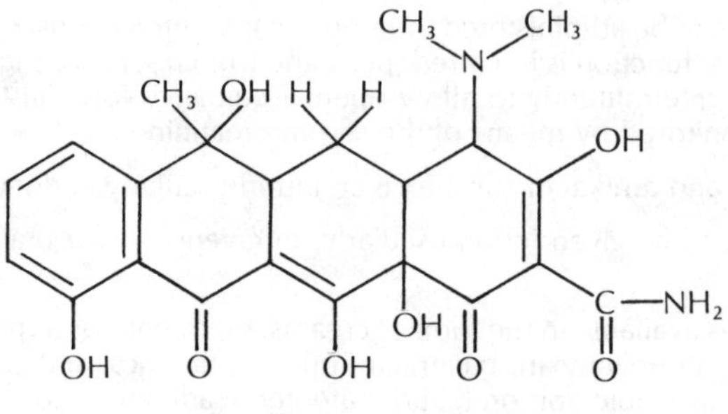

CH_3 CH_3 N CH_3 OH H H OH C—NH_2 OH OH O OH O O

Tetracycline

B. MECHANISM OF ACTION

1. Tetracyclines are primarily **bacteriostatic,** inhibiting protein synthesis by binding to 30S ribosomes.

2. Tetracycline affects both eukaryotic and prokaryotic cells, but apparently penetrates microbial membranes more readily due to the presence of active transport systems in microbes.

3. **Complete cross-resistance** among the tetracycline preparations occurs.

C. SPECTRUM OF ACTIVITY

1. Tetracyclines are effective against many gram-positive and gram-negative bacteria. However, gram-positive bacteria often become resistant to the tetracyclines, limiting the usefulness of these drugs.

2. The tetracyclines are effective against *Mycoplasma, Borrelia, Chlamydia,* and rickettsial species.

3. They are useful secondary drugs against *Leptospira* and *Treponema* species.

4. In high concentrations, the tetracyclines inhibit the growth of the protozoan *Entamoeba histolytica.*

D. PHARMACOKINETICS

1. Tetracyclines are adequately but incompletely absorbed from the gastrointestinal tract, particularly from the stomach and upper small intestine.

2. **Absorption is impaired** by food, milk, milk products, aluminum hydroxide gels, and calcium and magnesium salts. The cations in these substances chelate with tetracycline, preventing gastrointestinal absorption.

3. The tetracyclines diffuse readily into body fluids and bind to plasma proteins to varying degrees, depending on the particular preparation. Concentrations in the cerebrospinal fluid are about 20 percent of serum levels unless the meninges are inflamed.

4. The tetracyclines are removed from the blood by the liver and are excreted into the intestine by way of the bile. They undergo enterohepatic circulation.

5. Excretion occurs primarily via the kidney, although there is some fecal excretion. Renal clearance of these drugs is by glomerular filtration.

E. THERAPEUTIC USES

1. The use of tetracyclines for treatment of infectious disease has declined because of increasing bacterial resistance and the development of newer, more effective antimicrobial agents.

2. Tetracyclines are useful in the following conditions:
   a. **Rickettsial infections.** Tetracyclines are the drugs of first choice for these diseases, which include:
      (1) Rocky Mountain spotted fever.
      (2) Brill's disease.
      (3) Murine and scrub typhus.
      (4) Rickettsialpox.
      (5) Q fever.
   b. **Chlamydial infections.**
      (1) Lymphogranuloma venereum.
      (2) Psittacosis.
      (3) Inclusion conjunctivitis.
      (4) Trachoma.
   c. **Mycoplasma infections.**
   d. **Bacillary infections.**
      (1) Brucellosis.
      (2) Tularemia.
      (3) Cholera.
      (4) Some *Shigella* and *Salmonella* infections.
   e. **Venereal infections.**
      (1) Gonorrhea.
      (2) Syphilis.
      (3) Chancroid.
      (4) Granuloma inguinale.
      (5) Chlamydial urethritis or cervicitis.
   f. **Amebiasis.**

3. Staphylococcal and streptococcal infections may respond to tetracyclines. However, the drugs are "third-line" agents against these infections.

4. In urinary tract infections the use of tetracyclines is limited because of the increasing number of resistant microorganisms.

5. Tetracyclines may be beneficial in the treatment of acne.

F. PREPARATIONS AND ADMINISTRATION

1. Tetracyclines are available for oral, topical, intravenous, and intramuscular administration.
   a. Intramuscular administration of the tetracyclines causes local irritation and results in poor absorption of the drugs.
   b. Tetracyclines are available as ophthalmic solutions for use locally in the eye.

2. The various tetracyclines include:
   a. **Chlortetracycline.**
   b. **Oxytetracycline.**
   c. **Tetracycline.**
   d. **Demeclocycline.** This drug has a greater acid and alkaline stability and slower rate of excretion than most tetracyclines and, therefore, produces higher and more prolonged blood levels of the drug.
   e. **Methacycline.** This drug is absorbed rapidly.
   f. **Minocycline.**
   g. **Doxycycline.**
      (1) Increased absorption of doxycycline allows once-daily administration after the first day.
      (2) As opposed to the other tetracyclines, 90 percent of this drug is excreted in the feces, and therefore it does not accumulate in the blood of patients with compromised renal function. Thus, it is one of the safest tetracyclines for use against extrarenal infections in patients with renal dysfunction.

G. UNTOWARD EFFECTS

1. Hypersensitivity reactions, including skin rash and drug fever, can occur. Cross-sensitivity among the various tetracyclines is common.
2. When tetracyclines are administered orally, gastrointestinal irritation is common.
3. The intravenous administration of tetracyclines often produces thrombophlebitis due to local irritation. Intramuscular injections are painful.
4. Demeclocycline, and less often the other tetracyclines, can produce a phototoxic reaction, resulting in severe skin lesions in patients exposed to sunlight.
5. High doses of tetracyclines can produce hepatic dysfunction. This reaction is exacerbated during pregnancy.
6. Children receiving either short- or long-term tetracycline therapy may develop yellow-brown discolorations of their teeth and suffer depressed bone growth.
   a. The drugs are deposited in the teeth and bones because of their chelating properties and the formation of a tetracycline–calcium orthophosphate complex.
   b. The risk of discoloration is greatest when tetracyclines are given to pregnant women, to neonates, and to babies prior to their first dentition.
   c. Discoloration of the permanent teeth can result, however, from the administration of tetracycline at any time between the ages of two months and five years, the period of tooth calcification.
   d. Tetracycline treatment during pregnancy can produce discoloration of the teeth in the offspring.
7. The ingestion of outdated and degraded tetracycline can result in a form of the Fanconi syndrome.
8. Tetracyclines can cause increased intracranial pressure, especially in infants.
9. Vestibular toxicity can occur following minocycline therapy.
10. Superinfection by strains of resistant bacteria and yeasts is a significant problem that can result in staphylococcal enterocolitis, intestinal candidiasis, and pseudomembranous colitis.

VII. CHLORAMPHENICOL

A. CHEMISTRY.

Chloramphenicol is a nitrobenzene derivative with the following structural formula:

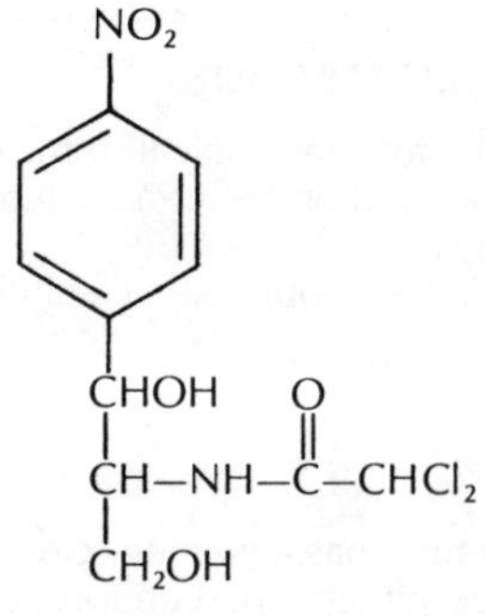

NO_2

CHOH O

CH–NH–C–$CHCl_2$

CH_2OH

Chloramphenicol

B. MECHANISM OF ACTION

1. Chloramphenicol inhibits protein synthesis by acting on the 50S ribosomal subunit, a site of action shared with macrolide antibiotics, lincomycin, and clindamycin.
2. This drug is primarily bacteriostatic, although it may be bactericidal to some strains.

C. SPECTRUM OF ACTIVITY

1. Chloramphenicol has a fairly wide spectrum of antimicrobial activity, including:
   a. Many gram-negative organisms (e.g., it is bactericidal towards *H. influenzae).*
   b. Anaerobic organisms, such as *Bacteroides* species (e.g., *B. fragilis*).
   c. Some strains of *Streptococcus* and *Staphylococcus* (at a high antibiotic concentration).
   d. Species of *Clostridia, Chlamydia,* and *Mycoplasma.*
   e. Rickettsiae, in which it suppresses growth.

2. *P. aeruginosa* is resistant.

D. PHARMACOKINETICS

1. Chloramphenicol is absorbed rapidly from the gastrointestinal tract.
2. It is widely distributed in body fluids and reaches therapeutic levels in cerebrospinal fluid.
3. It also is present in bile, milk, and aqueous humor.
4. Chloramphenicol is metabolized in the liver by glucuronyl transferase.
5. Its metabolites are excreted in the urine.

E. THERAPEUTIC USES

1. Potentially severe toxicity limits the use of chloramphenicol to those infections that cannot be effectively treated with other antibiotic agents. When another agent is as efficacious as chloramphenicol and potentially less toxic, the other agent should be used.
2. Chloramphenicol is the drug of choice for typhoid fever.
3. Bacterial meningitis caused by *H. influenzae* is effectively treated. When children are affected, the combination of penicillin G and chloramphenicol is recommended for initial therapy.
4. Most anaerobic infections respond to chloramphenicol.
5. Rickettsial diseases and brucellosis can be treated with chloramphenicol; however, tetracyclines are the preferred agents.

F. PREPARATIONS AND ADMINISTRATION

1. Chloramphenicol and its palmitate salt are given orally.
2. Chloramphenicol sodium succinate is given intravenously.
3. Ophthalmic solutions and ointments are also available.

G. UNTOWARD EFFECTS

1. Hypersensitivity reactions can occur.
2. The most important effect, which may be related to hypersensitivity, is bone-marrow depression resulting in pancytopenia.
   a. The incidence of this reaction is not dose-related.
   b. It is usually associated with prolonged therapy and more than one episode of treatment with chloramphenicol.
   c. It occurs in 1 in 40,000 patients given chloramphenicol and often is fatal.
3. Dose-dependent, reversible blood dyscrasias may also occur.
4. Superinfections can occur, including oropharyngeal candidiasis and acute staphylococcal enterocolitis.
5. Gastrointestinal upset can occur, and, as with many of the other broad-spectrum antibiotics, the possibility of diarrhea due to superinfection should be differentiated from local irritation effects.
6. **Gray-baby syndrome**
   a. This condition is seen in neonates, especially premature infants who have been given relatively large doses of chloramphenicol.
   b. Cyanosis, respiratory irregularities, vasomotor collapse, abdominal distention, loose green stools, and an ashen-gray color characterize this often fatal syndrome.
   c. The condition develops because of the immature hepatic conjugating mechanism and the inadequate mechanism for renal excretion in neonates.

VIII. ERYTHROMYCIN, LINCOMYCIN, CLINDAMYCIN, AND VANCOMYCIN

A. CHEMISTRY

1. **Erythromycin** is a macrolide antibiotic. Macrolides contain a lactone ring and one or more deoxy sugars.

2. **Clindamycin** is the 7-deoxy,7-chloro derivative of the parent drug, **lincomycin,** which it has essentially replaced.

3. **Vancomycin** is a complex glycopeptide.

B. MECHANISM OF ACTION

1. **Erythromycin** inhibits bacterial protein synthesis by binding to 50S ribosomal subunits of sensitive microorganisms; it is usually bacteriostatic, but can be bactericidal in certain situations.

2. **Clindamycin** and **lincomycin** are similar to erythromycin in their mechanisms of action.

3. **Vancomycin** inhibits bacterial cell-wall synthesis. Thus, unlike erythromycin, lincomycin, and clindamycin, vancomycin is clearly bactericidal.

C. SPECTRUM OF ACTIVITY

1. **Erythromycin**
   - **a.** This drug is effective against gram-positive organisms, including some strains of penicillin G–resistant *S. aureus.*
   - **b.** *Neisseria* species, some strains of *H. influenzae,* and *Bordetella, Legionella, Treponema,* and *Mycoplasma* species are sensitive to erythromycin.
   - **c.** In general, it is not very active against most gram-negative bacilli.

2. **Lincomycin**
   - **a.** This antibiotic has fair activity against gram-positive organisms.
   - **b.** It has good activity against *Corynebacterium diphtheriae, Clostridium tetani,* and *Clostridum perfringens.*
   - **c.** It is active against some strains of *Bacteroides* but *not B. fragilis.*

3. **Clindamycin**
   - **a.** This drug has a broader spectrum of activity than lincomycin has. Clindamycin is effective against:
     - **(1)** Gram-positive organisms, including anaerobic streptococci.
     - **(2)** Many other anaerobic bacteria, especially *B. fragilis.*
   - **b.** Lincomycin and clindamycin are not effective against gonococci, meningococci, or most aerobic gram-negative bacilli.

4. **Vancomycin** is active primarily against gram-positive bacteria.

D. PHARMACOKINETICS

1. **Erythromycin**
   - **a.** The **base** is absorbed from the upper part of the small intestine. It is destroyed by gastric juice.
   - **b.** The **estolate** is resistant to gastric inactivation.
   - **c.** All forms of erythromycin are absorbed following oral administration and diffuse into most body tissues and fluids except cerebrospinal fluid.
   - **d.** Erythromycin is concentrated in the liver and is excreted primarily in bile and feces.

2. **Clindamycin**
   - **a.** Although it is well absorbed following oral administration, clindamycin most often is administered parenterally because pseudomembranous colitis is more likely to occur following oral than parenteral administration.
   - **b.** The drug is widely distributed in body fluids and tissues but does not pass readily into cerebrospinal fluid.
   - **c.** Most of the drug is metabolized to the inactive sulfoxide form, which then is excreted in the urine and bile.

3. **Vancomycin**
   - **a.** This drug is absorbed poorly after oral administration, and, therefore, intravenous administration is preferred.
   - **b.** It is widely distributed and passes into the cerebrospinal fluid when the meninges are inflamed.

c. Most of the compound is excreted via the kidney.

E. THERAPEUTIC USES

1. Erythromycin

a. This drug is useful for patients who are allergic to penicillin when the infecting organism is sensitive to erythromycin, particularly in cases of infection with group A *S. pyogenes* and *S. pneumoniae.*
b. Pneumonia due to *Mycoplasma* organisms is effectively treated.
c. Legionnaires' disease is treated with erythromycin.

2. Clindamycin

a. Although this drug is effective against gram-positive organisms, its toxicity and the availability of more effective agents limit its use to infections where it is clearly superior.
b. Clindamycin is the drug of first choice against *Bacteroides,* especially *B. fragilis,* which often is the cause of anaerobic abdominal infections. Anaerobic infections of the brain are more effectively treated with chloramphenicol because clindamycin shows poor central nervous system penetration.

3. Lincomycin. Its use has generally been superseded by clindamycin.

4. Vancomycin

a. This antibiotic is very effective against penicillin-resistant staphylococci, streptococci of the *viridans* group, and serious enterococcal infections.
b. Toxicity limits its use to serious infections.

F. PREPARATIONS AND ADMINISTRATION

1. Erythromycin

a. Oral erythromycin is supplied as enteric-coated tablets.
b. Erythromycin ethylsuccinate is available as granules or powder for oral suspension.
c. Other available oral salts are erythromycin stearate and erythromycin estolate.
d. Sterile erythromycin gluceptate is available for parenteral administration.

2. Lincomycin is available in oral and parenteral forms.

3. Clindamycin is available in oral as well as parenteral forms.

4. Vancomycin

a. Because it is reserved for severe infections, vancomycin is most often administered intravenously.
b. Oral use is limited to the treatment of staphylococcal enterocolitis and pseudomembranous colitis caused by *Clostridium difficile.*

G. UNTOWARD EFFECTS

1. Erythromycin has a very low incidence of serious side effects.

a. Hypersensitivity reactions include allergic cholestatic hepatitis; this reaction occurs primarily with the estolate form of the drug.
b. Epigastric distress can occur.
c. A high incidence of thrombophlebitis occurs when erythromycin is administered intravenously, even when the drug is dissolved in a large fluid volume.
d. Superinfection can occur.

2. Clindamycin and lincomycin. Pseudomembranous colitis can occur, resulting in diarrhea, abdominal pain, fever, and mucus and blood in the stools. At one time, this condition was often fatal, but now that the causative organism is known to be *C. difficile,* it can be treated with vancomycin.

3. Vancomycin

a. Ototoxicity can lead to deafness.
b. Nephrotoxicity can occur.
c. Hypersensitivity reactions can occur.
d. Thrombophlebitis is frequently observed following prolonged intravenous therapy.

IX. ANTIFUNGAL AGENTS

A. NYSTATIN

1. Chemistry. Nystatin is a polyene antibiotic.

2. **Mechanism of action**
   a. The drug is fungistatic and fungicidal.
   b. It binds to sterols, especially ergosterol, which is enriched in the membrane of fungi and yeasts. As a result of this binding, the drug appears to form channels in the membrane that allow small molecules to leak out of the cell.

3. **Pharmacokinetics**
   a. Nystatin is not absorbed appreciably from the gastrointestinal tract.
   b. It is not absorbed from the skin or mucous membranes.
   c. It is not employed parenterally.
   d. It is poorly soluble and decomposes rapidly in water.

4. **Therapeutic uses**
   a. Nystatin is used to treat *Candida* infections of the skin, mucous membranes, and intestinal tract.
   b. Thrush (oral candidiasis) and vaginitis are treated by topical application, whereas intestinal candidiasis is treated by oral administration.

5. **Preparations.** Nystatin is supplied as an ointment, oral suspension, oral tablets, drops, and powder.

6. **Untoward effects.** Occasional gastrointestinal disturbances occur with oral administration.

B. AMPHOTERICIN B

1. **Chemistry.** This drug is another polyene antibiotic.

2. **Mechanism of action.** The mechanism of action is the same for amphotericin B as for nystatin.

3. **Spectrum of activity**
   a. Amphotericin B is a broad-spectrum antifungal agent.
   b. *Histoplasma capsulatum, Cryptococcus neoformans, Coccidioides immitis, Candida* species, *Blastomyces dermatitidis,* and some strains of *Aspergillus* and *Sporotrichum* are sensitive.
   c. The concentration of amphotericin B determines whether it is fungistatic or fungicidal.

4. **Pharmacokinetics**
   a. Amphotericin B is absorbed poorly from the gastrointestinal tract.
   b. Intravenous administration results in a plasma half-life of about 24 hours.
   c. The drug is excreted very slowly in the urine.

5. **Therapeutic uses**
   a. Amphotericin B is the most effective drug available for systemic fungal infections.
   b. It is used frequently for the treatment of life-threatening fungal infections in patients with impaired defense mechanisms (e.g., patients undergoing immunosuppressive therapy or cancer chemotherapy).
   c. Amphotericin B is used in the treatment of the following infections:
      (1) Pulmonary, cutaneous, and disseminated forms of blastomycosis.
      (2) Acute pulmonary coccidioidomycosis.
      (3) Pulmonary histoplasmosis.
      (4) *C. neoformans* infections.
      (5) Candidiasis, including disseminated forms.
   d. In addition, mucocutaneous lesions of parasitic American leishmaniasis may respond to amphotericin B therapy.
   e. Intrathecal infusion may be helpful in the treatment of fungal meningitis.

6. **Preparations.** Amphotericin B lyophilized powder is available for injection.

7. **Untoward effects**
   a. Hypersensitivity reactions can occur, including anaphylaxis.
   b. Fever, chills, headache, and gastrointestinal disturbances are common with intravenous administration. Patients usually develop tolerance to these adverse effects with continuing administration of amphotericin B.
   c. Decreased renal function occurs in over 80 percent of patients treated with amphotericin B, necessitating close observation. All patients receiving amphotericin B therapy should be hospitalized, at least during the initiation of therapy.
   d. Normochromic normocytic anemia can occur.
   e. Thrombophlebitis can occur.

C. GRISEOFULVIN

1. **Chemistry.** The drug is produced by *Penicillium griseofulvum*. It is poorly soluble in water.

2. **Mechanism of action**
   a. Griseofulvin binds to polymerized microtubules but its exact mechanism of action is undetermined.
   b. It is fungistatic.

3. **Spectrum of activity.** Griseofulvin is active against dermatophytes, including *Microsporum, Epidermophyton,* and *Trichophyton* species. It is ineffective against yeasts.

4. **Pharmacokinetics**
   a. Griseofulvin is absorbed in the upper part of the small intestine following oral administration. Most of the drug is eliminated unchanged in the feces.
   b. Griseofulvin has a particular affinity for keratin.

5. **Therapeutic uses.** Because of its affinity for keratin, griseofulvin is useful for treating mycotic diseases of the skin, hair, and nails such as tinea capitis, pedis (athlete's foot), cruris, and corporis. It is given orally; topical use has little effect.

6. **Preparations.** Griseofulvin is available as tablets, capsules, and an oral suspension.

7. **Untoward effects**
   a. Extensive clinical use of griseofulvin has revealed relatively low toxicity.
   b. Possible side effects include headache, neurologic alterations, hepatotoxicity, leukopenia, neutropenia, gastrointestinal distress, and skin reactions, including urticaria and photosensitivity.

D. FLUCYTOSINE

1. **Chemistry.** This drug is a fluorinated pyrimidine.

2. **Mechanism of action.** Flucytosine is converted within fungal cells (but not in the host's cells) to fluorouracil, a metabolic antagonist that ultimately leads to inhibition of thymidylate synthetase.

3. **Spectrum of activity**
   a. The drug is effective against *C. neoformans.*
   b. It is effective against some strains of *Candida,* including some *C. albicans* strains. However, *C. albicans* can become resistant to flucytosine during therapy.

4. **Pharmacokinetics**
   a. Flucytosine is well absorbed from the gastrointestinal tract and is distributed widely throughout the body, including the cerebrospinal fluid.
   b. It is excreted in the urine, mainly in an unmetabolized form.

5. **Therapeutic uses**
   a. Although flucytosine is not as effective as amphotericin B, it is less toxic and can be administered orally.
   b. It is used for systemic infections caused by *Candida albicans* and *Cryptococcus meningitidis.* It is most often used in combination with amphotericin B.

6. **Preparations.** Flucytosine is available in capsules for oral use.

7. **Untoward effects** have included:
   a. Fatal bone marrow depression.
   b. Gastrointestinal upset.
   c. Rash and hepatic dysfunction.

E. KETOCONAZOLE is a new antifungal drug that is orally active and has low toxicity.

1. It is active in blastomycosis, coccidioidomycosis, histoplasmosis, paracoccidioidomycosis, chronic mucocutaneous candidiasis, and resistant dermatophyte infections.

2. It is slower acting than the other available antifungal agents, requiring long periods of therapy, and thus is less useful for severe or acute systemic infections.

X. AGENTS USED FOR THE TREATMENT OF TUBERCULOSIS AND LEPROSY

A. ISONIAZID

1. **Chemistry.** Isoniazid is the hydrazide of isonicotinic acid and is a pyridine. Its structural formula is:

$$\text{CO—NH—NH}_2$$

(pyridine ring, substituent at position 4)

Isoniazid

2. **Mechanism of action**
   a. Although its mechanism of action is not known, isoniazid probably interferes with cellular metabolism, especially the synthesis of mycolic acid, an important constituent of the mycobacterial cell wall.
   b. Isoniazid is a competitive antagonist in pyridoxine-catalyzed reactions, but this property is not involved in its antituberculous action.
3. **Spectrum of activity**
   a. Isoniazid is effective against most tubercle bacilli.
   b. It is *not* effective against many atypical mycobacteria.
4. **Pharmacokinetics**
   a. The drug is well absorbed from the gastrointestinal tract and diffuses readily into all body tissues and body fluids, including cerebrospinal fluid.
   b. The metabolism of isoniazid is, in part, under genetic control via the activity of acetyltransferase.
      (1) The plasma concentration of the drug is affected by whether a given patient is a **fast or a slow acetylator** of the drugs.
      (2) The acetylation rate has little effect, however, on dosage regimens.
   c. Isoniazid is excreted mainly in the urine. Slow acetylators have a higher concentration of unchanged or free isoniazid than fast acetylators.
5. **Therapeutic uses**
   a. Isoniazid is the most widely used agent in the treatment of tuberculosis.
   b. It is used in conjunction with other agents in active tuberculosis.
   c. It is administered as a single **prophylactic** agent to children and young adults who have skin tests that have converted from tuberculin-negative to -positive. This type of prophylactic therapy also is suggested for very close contacts (especially children) of patients newly identified as having active tuberculosis.
6. **Preparations.** Isoniazid is available as tablets, as syrup, and in injectable form.
7. **Untoward effects**
   a. Fever, jaundice, and skin rash are seen occasionally.
   b. Peripheral and central nervous system toxicity occurs.
      (1) This toxicity probably results from the enhanced excretion of pyridoxine induced by isoniazid, which produces a pyridoxine deficiency.
      (2) Peripheral neuritis, urinary retention, insomnia, and psychotic episodes can occur,
      (3) Concurrent pyridoxine administration with isoniazid prevents most of these complications.
   c. Isoniazid can also exacerbate pyridoxine-deficiency anemia and can produce blood dyscrasias.
   d. Isoniazid can reduce the metabolism of phenytoin, enhancing its toxicity.
   e. Most importantly, severe and potentially fatal hepatic injury can occur, especially in patients over the age of 35.

B. ETHAMBUTOL

1. **Chemistry.** The structural formula of ethambutol is:

```
   CH2OH                          C2H5
     |                              |
H—C—NH—CH2—CH2—HN—C—H
     |                              |
   C2H5                          CH2OH
```

Ethambutol

2. **Mechanism of action.** Ethambutol's mechanism of action is unknown. Resistance to the drug occurs rapidly when it is used alone.

3. **Spectrum of activity.** Ethambutol inhibits many strains of *Mycobacterium,* including *M. tuberculosis.*

4. **Pharmacokinetics**
   a. Ethambutol is well absorbed from the gastrointestinal tract.
   b. It is widely distributed in the body, including the cerebrospinal fluid.
   c. The majority of an ingested dose is excreted in unchanged form in urine and feces.

5. **Therapeutic uses.** Ethambutol is used in combination with other agents for the treatment of tuberculosis.

6. **Preparations.** Ethambutol hydrochloride is available in tablet form for oral use.

7. **Untoward effects**
   a. Visual disturbances, including optic neuritis, occur but are reversible.
   b. Hypersensitivity occurs occasionally, resulting in rash or drug fever.

C. RIFAMPIN

1. **Chemistry**
   a. Rifampin belongs to the group of complex macrocyclic antibiotics.
   b. It is zwitterionic and is soluble in water at low pH.

2. **Mechanism of action**
   a. Rifampin inhibits RNA synthesis in bacteria and chlamydiae by binding to DNA-dependent RNA polymerase.
   b. Prolonged administration of the drug as the single therapeutic agent promotes the emergence of highly resistant organisms.

3. **Spectrum of activity.** Most gram-positive and many gram-negative microorganisms are sensitive to rifampin.

4. **Pharmacokinetics**
   a. Rifampin is well absorbed from the gastrointestinal tract.
   b. It is widely distributed in tissues and is excreted mainly through the liver.

5. **Therapeutic uses**
   a. Rifampin is used in the treatment of:
      (1) Tuberculosis, in combination with other agents, often isoniazid and ethambutol.
      (2) Atypical mycobacterial infections.
      (3) Leprosy.
   b. Rifampin is not used for minor infections because of the emergence of rifampin-resistant mycobacteria.

6. **Preparations.** Rifampin is available for oral use.

7. **Untoward effects**
   a. Urine, sweat, tears, and contact lenses may take on an orange color because of rifampin administration; this effect is harmless.
   b. Light-chain proteinuria and impaired antibody response may occur.
   c. A decrease in the effect of some anticoagulants and increased metabolism of methadone occur when these agents are administered concomitantly with rifampin. Methadone withdrawal symptoms may be induced.
   d. Rashes, gastrointestinal disturbances, and renal damage have been reported.
   e. Jaundice and severe hepatic dysfunction are occasionally produced.

D. STREPTOMYCIN (see V, above)

1. The use of streptomycin as a *single* agent for the treatment of tuberculosis has been obsolete ever since more effective agents became available.

2. When a three-agent combination is used to treat tuberculosis, streptomycin may be one of the drugs used.

E. SULFONES

1. **Chemistry**
   a. The sulfones, the principal class of agents used to treat leprosy, are chemically related to the sulfonamides.

b. The most important derivatives come from **dapsone,** the structure of which is shown below:

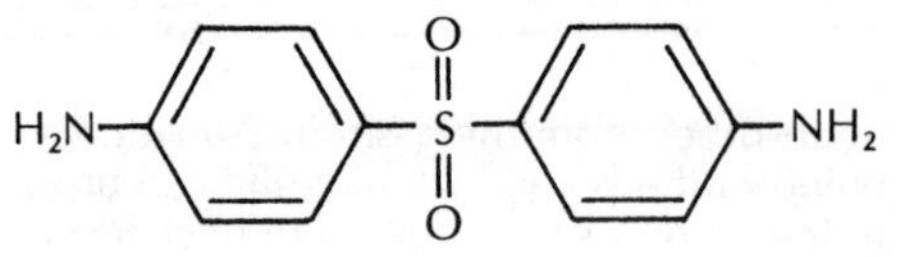

$$H_2N-C_6H_4-\overset{O}{\underset{O}{\overset{\|}{\underset{\|}{S}}}}-C_6H_4-NH_2$$

Dapsone

2. Mechanism of action

a. Dapsone is bacteriostatic for *Mycobacterium leprae.*

b. Its mechanism of action is probably similar to that of the sulfonamides (see II B).

3. Spectrum of activity

a. Dapsone is effective against *M. leprae,* although resistance to the drug can develop.

b. It is bacteriostatic for *M. tuberculosis* in vitro.

4. Pharmacokinetics

a. Dapsone is slowly but completely absorbed from the gastrointestinal tract.

b. It undergoes intestinal reabsorption from the bile, resulting in a sustained level of the drug in the circulation.

c. It is principally excreted in the urine.

5. Therapeutic uses. Dapsone is the most important drug in the treatment of leprosy.

6. Preparations and administration. Dapsone is administered orally. Therapy usually is continued for a minimum of 2 years.

7. Untoward effects

a. The most common untoward effects include hemolysis, methemoglobinemia, nausea, vomiting, rash, transient headache, and anorexia.

b. The sulfones can cause an exacerbation of lepromatous leprosy.

c. A fatal infectious mononucleosis–like syndrome has been reported.

F. CLOFAZIMINE, a phenazine congener, is available from the U.S. Public Health Service for treatment of patients infected with *M. leprae* that is resistant to the sulfones.

XI. ANTHELMINTICS. These drugs are used to treat parasitic infections due to flatworms and roundworms. The major target is usually the nongrowing adult stage of the parasite's life cycle.

A. DIETHYLCARBAMAZINE CITRATE is the drug of choice for filaria worms. It effectively treats *Wuchereria bancrofti, W. malayi, Loa loa,* and *Onchocerca volvulus.*

B. HYCANTHONE MESYLATE is used in the treatment of endemic schistosomiasis. It is administered as a single intramuscular dose.

C. PRAZIQUANTEL is a new broad-spectrum anthelmintic with very good activity against schistosomes.

D. METRIFONATE AND NIRIDAZOLE are effective against *Schistosoma haematobium.*

E. MEBENDAZOLE is the drug of choice in the treatment of *Trichuris trichiura* infestation and is useful in hookworm, pinworm, and *Ascaris* infestations.

F. NICLOSAMIDE is the drug of choice for the treatment of most tapeworms, including *Diphyllobothrium latum, Taenia saginata, Taenia solium,* and *Hymenolepis nana.*

G. PYRANTEL PAMOATE is the drug of choice for the treatment of ascariasis and enterobiasis (pinworms). It produces persistent nicotinic activation, resulting in paralysis of the worms.

H. PIPERAZINE is an alternative drug for the treatment of ascariasis and pinworms. This agent is thought to block the response of *Ascaris* muscle cells to acetylcholine by altering the permeability of the cell membrane to ions that are responsible for the maintenance of the resting potential.

I. THIABENDAZOLE is very effective against cutaneous larva migrans and strongyloidiasis. It is also used in trichinosis.

J. TETRACHLOROETHYLENE is useful for the treatment of hookworm infestations, but more effective and less toxic agents have replaced its use in the United States.

XII. AGENTS USED FOR TREATMENT OF PROTOZOAL INFECTIONS AND MALARIA

A. METRONIDAZOLE

1. This drug is very active in protozoal infections, including trichomoniasis, lambliasis (*Giardia lamblia* infestation), and amebiasis caused by *Entamoeba histolytica*.
2. It is also effective in the treatment of anaerobic bacterial infections (e.g., from *Bacteroides* species).
3. A disulfiram-like (Antabuse-like) reaction can occur when metronidazole is taken in combination with an alcoholic beverage (see Chapter 13, II E 4 c).

B. DILOXANIDE FUROATE

1. This drug is amebicidal.
2. It is used for the treatment of asymptomatic passers of amebic cysts.

C. SURAMIN is a nonmetallic compound employed in the treatment of African trypanosomiasis in the early stage of the disease. **Nifurtimox** is effective in South American trypanosomiasis.

D. STIBOGLUCONATE SODIUM, an antimonial, is the drug of choice for leishmaniasis.

E. PENTAMIDINE ISETHIONATE

1. Although antimonials are considered to be the drugs of choice for the treatment of leishmaniasis, pentamidine can be highly effective in patients who do not respond to antimonial therapy.
2. Pentamidine is effective against early cases of African trypanosomiasis and in the treatment of pneumonia due to *Pneumocystis carinii*.

F. CHLOROQUINE PHOSPHATE is used for the treatment of uncomplicated acute malaria due to any of the *Plasmodium* organisms (except resistant forms). It is also used for prophylaxis during residence in an endemic area.

G. PRIMAQUINE PHOSPHATE is used to prevent relapses of *P. vivax* and *P. ovale* malaria after departure from endemic areas.

H. PYRIMETHAMINE AND SULFADOXINE are used concurrently for prophylaxis and treatment of chloroquine-resistant strains of *P. falciparum*.

I. QUININE

1. Quinine sulfate is effective in the treatment of acute uncomplicated malarial attacks due to chloroquine-resistant *P. falciparum*.
2. Quinine dihydrochloride, administered parenterally, is used in the treatment of severe illness caused by chloroquine-resistant *P. falciparum*.

XIII. ANTIVIRAL AGENTS.

Viruses are obligate intracellular parasites that require the active participation of the metabolic processes of the invaded cell to survive. Thus, agents that are able to kill viruses often injure host cells as well. Because of this interrelationship, there are at present only a few drugs that have substantial therapeutic merit in the treatment of viral infections.

A. AMANTADINE

1. **Chemistry.** Amantadine is a synthetic tricyclic amine with a structure unrelated to that of any of the antimicrobial agents.
2. **Mechanism of action.** Amantadine inhibits the replication of strains of influenza A virus at an early stage, possibly by blocking the uncoating of viral nucleic acids.

3. **Pharmacokinetics.** The drug is well absorbed from the gastrointestinal tract, is not metabolized, and is excreted via the kidneys.

4. **Therapeutic uses**
   a. The major anti-infective use for amantadine is for prophylaxis during influenza A virus epidemics, at which time patients of all ages who are at high risk and who have not been vaccinated are advised to receive the drug.
   b. Amantadine does not alter the immune response to influenza A vaccine; thus, vaccination can be given concurrently with the drug.
   c. Although the antiviral action requires 24 to 48 hours, amantadine may also be useful in shortening the duration of symptoms when administered after the onset of illness.
   d. The use of amantadine in the treatment of some parkinsonian symptoms is discussed in Chapter 3 (IV C).

5. **Preparations and administration.** Amantadine is given orally.

6. **Untoward effects**
   a. These are dose-related and include confusion, hallucinations, seizures, and coma.
   b. Patients with psychiatric disorders or a history of epilepsy require close monitoring when receiving the drug.

B. VIDARABINE (adenine arabinoside, ara-A)

1. **Chemistry.** Vidarabine is an adenosine analog.

2. **Mechanism of action.** Vidarabine acts by inhibiting viral DNA polymerase. Mammalian DNA synthesis is affected to a lesser extent.

3. **Therapeutic uses**
   a. Originally developed for the treatment of leukemia, vidarabine is used in the treatment of herpes simplex encephalitis and keratoconjunctivitis.
   b. It also is effective in the treatment of herpes zoster infections in patients who are immunosuppressed.

4. **Preparations and administration**
   a. Vidarabine is available for intravenous use in the treatment of herpes simplex encephalitis.
   b. For herpes simplex keratoconjunctivitis, vidarabine is administered as an ophthalmic ointment.

5. **Untoward effects**
   a. Gastrointestinal disturbances and dose-related central nervous system toxicity are relatively infrequent.
   b. The drug may be carcinogenic and should not be used to treat insignificant infections.

C. IDOXURIDINE

1. **Chemistry.** Idoxuridine resembles thymidine in structure, being a halogenated pyrimidine.

2. **Mechanism of action.** Idoxuridine is incorporated into both viral and mammalian DNA, producing DNA that is more susceptible to breakage, and ultimately causing production of altered proteins.

3. **Therapeutic uses**
   a. Idoxuridine is used in the treatment of herpes simplex keratitis.
   b. Herpes simplex virus type 2 does *not* respond to idoxuridine.

4. **Preparations.** Idoxuridine is available as an ophthalmic solution or ointment.

D. ACYCLOVIR

1. **Chemistry.** Acyclovir is a synthetic purine nucleoside analog with an acyclic side chain.

2. **Mechanism of action.** After being converted in vivo into the triphosphate form, acyclovir interferes with herpes simplex virus DNA polymerase and inhibits viral DNA replication. It is incorporated into DNA and leads to premature chain termination.

3. **Spectrum of activity.** Acyclovir has inhibitory activity in vitro against herpes simplex virus types 1 and 2, varicella-zoster virus, Epstein-Barr virus, and cytomegalovirus.

4. **Therapeutic uses.** The drug is indicated for primary mucocutaneous herpes simplex infections in immunocompromised patients. It is also useful in herpes genitalis infections.

5. **Preparations and administration.** Acyclovir triphosphate is supplied in ointment form. A finger cot should be used for application.

6. **Untoward effects** include contact sensitivity and pruritus.

E. TRIFLURIDINE (5-Trifluoromethyl-2′-deoxyuridine; F_3-dThd; TFT)

1. **Chemistry.** A halogenated pyrimidine, trifluridine resembles thymidine in structure.

2. **Mechanism of action.** As with idoxuridine, trifluridine is phosphorylated to the triphosphate derivative and, as such, competes with thymidine triphosphate for DNA polymerase for incorporation into viral DNA. Since both drugs are also incorporated into the DNA of uninfected cells, these agents cannot be used systemically.

3. **Therapeutic uses.** Trifluridine is approved for the therapy of herpetic keratitis.

4. **Preparations and administration.** Trifluridine is applied topically.

F. HUMAN INTERFERON

1. This class of glycoproteins inhibits the multiplication of many different viruses.

2. Interferon is produced endogenously by leukocytes in response to viral infection.

3. In patients who have lymphoma, early treatment of a herpes zoster infection with interferon appears to prevent the spread of infection.

4. In addition to its antiviral activity, interferon is also being tested in the treatment of various types of neoplastic disease.

5. A more complete understanding of the clinical usefulness of interferons is limited by the small amounts of material currently available.

6. The Food and Drug Administration has not yet approved interferon for clinical treatment of viral infections.

STUDY QUESTIONS

Directions: Each question below contains five suggested answers. Choose the **one best** response to each question.

1. A known diabetic presents with cough, hemoptysis, and a single shaking chill. His temperature is 101°F, and a chest x-ray demonstrates lobar pneumonia. Gram staining reveals gram-positive diplococci. Correct therapy would be to administer

(A) gentamicin
(B) penicillin G
(C) carbenicillin and gentamicin
(D) ampicillin
(E) nafcillin

2. The following statements about the unwanted effects of orally administered tetracyclines are true EXCEPT that

(A) doxycycline produces frequent gastrointestinal irritation
(B) hepatic dysfunction is most frequently exacerbated during pregnancy
(C) the ingestion of outdated tetracycline can result in a form of the Fanconi syndrome
(D) children receiving short-term as opposed to long-term therapy do not develop discoloration of teeth
(E) staphylococcal enterocolitis may follow tetracycline administration

3. Which of the following statements about aminoglycoside therapy is NOT true?

(A) Aminoglycosides are generally less potent in an acidic environment
(B) Streptomycin therapy is effective against tularemia
(C) Tobramycin is safer than amikacin therapy
(D) Kanamycin has poor activity against *Pseudomonas* species
(E) Amikacin is effective against *Serratia* species

Directions: Each question below contains four suggested answers of which **one or more** is correct. Choose the answer

A if **1, 2, and 3** are correct
B if **1 and 3** are correct
C if **2 and 4** are correct
D if **4** is correct
E if **1, 2, 3, and 4** are correct

4. Isoniazid (INH) is the most widely used agent in the treatment of tuberculosis. Which of the following statements are true regarding this agent?

(1) It is used in conjunction with other agents in the treatment of tuberculosis
(2) Its metabolism partly is under genetic control
(3) It is ineffective against many atypical mycobacteria
(4) It can be administered as a prophylactic agent to children or young adults who have converted from a tuberculin-negative to -positive skin test.

5. The duration of action of which of the following antibiotics would be increased by the concomitant administration of probenecid?

(1) Tobramycin
(2) Erythromycin
(3) Doxycycline
(4) Penicillin G

Questions 6–8

A 57-year-old male with known diverticulitis presents with severe abdominal pain. Examination reveals a "board-like" abdomen, while abdominal x-ray films demonstrate free air under the left diaphragm. The surgeon considers an operation to be mandatory.

6. Correct initial antimicrobial therapy would include

(1) penicillin G
(2) gentamicin
(3) methicillin
(4) clindamycin

7. Postoperatively, the patient develops severe abdominal pain, bloody diarrhea, and fever. Perforation is ruled out. Antimicrobial agents capable of producing this clinical picture include

(1) vancomycin
(2) lincomycin
(3) erythromycin
(4) clindamycin

8. Culture of a stool sample from the patient confirms *Clostridium difficile*. Correct therapy would now include

(1) discontinuation of the clindamycin
(2) instituting erythromycin therapy
(3) instituting vancomycin therapy
(4) discontinuation of the gentamicin

9. Therapy with cephalosporins accounts for a large proportion of inpatient antimicrobial therapy. Reasons for this would include their

(1) broad spectrum of activity
(2) easy passage across the blood–brain barrier
(3) activity against penicillinase-producing staphylococci
(4) uniform ability to be orally administered

10. Which of the following agents are correctly matched with their proposed mechanisms of action?

(1) Sulfadiazine—prevents the incorporation of para-aminobenzoic acid (PABA) into folic acid
(2) Ampicillin—inactivates transpeptidase
(3) Gentamicin—interferes with the function of messenger RNA and ribosomes
(4) Nystatin—acts by competitive inhibition of a metabolic enzyme

Questions 11 and 12

A female patient presents with candidal vaginitis. Her past medical history reveals that she has just completed a course of antibiotic therapy for a urinary tract infection.

11. Antibiotics capable of producing this untoward effect would include

(1) ampicillin
(2) cephalexin
(3) amoxicillin
(4) cefaclor

12. The agent that is most suitable for treating vaginal candidiasis has which of the following characteristics?

(1) It is not employed parenterally
(2) It is a polyene antibiotic
(3) It also effectively treats intestinal candidiasis
(4) It also effectively treats North Amercian blastomycosis

Directions: The group of questions below consist of lettered choices followed by several numbered items. For each numbered item select the **one** lettered choice with which it is **most** closely associated. Each lettered choice may be used once, more than once, or not at all.

Questions 13–16

For each potential untoward effect, select the antimicrobial agent with which it is most likely to be associated.

(A) Cefazolin
(B) Sulfisoxazole
(C) Chloramphenicol
(D) Tobramycin
(E) Ampicillin

13. When administered orally it is likely to cause gastrointestinal upsets and possibly skin rash.

14. The Stevens-Johnson syndrome and an acute hemolytic anemia are sometimes seen with the administration of this agent.

15. Fatal, non–dose-related bone-marrow depression associated with prolonged therapy limits the use of this agent.

16. Cyanosis, vasomotor collapse, abdominal distention, and an ashen-gray color can be seen in neonates who are given this antibiotic.

ANSWERS AND EXPLANATIONS

1. The answer is B. *(III C, F 1, 2, G 4; V C 3, E 2)* The most likely diagnosis is pneumococcal pneumonia, for which the drug of first choice would be penicillin G. Gentamicin is not active against pneumococcal pneumonia, while carbenicillin and ampicillin, although effective, are not the drugs of first choice. Nafcillin use should be reserved for penicillinase-producing staphylococcal infections.

2. The answer is D. *(VI G 2, 5–7, 10)* Children receiving either short- or long-term tetracycline therapy may develop yellow-brown discoloration of the teeth. Tetracyclines are deposited into teeth and bones due to their chelating properties and the formation of a tetracycline–calcium orthophosphate complex. All of the other statements in the question are true.

3. The answer is C. *(V C, D 5, G 2)* Tobramycin and amikacin are similar in their potential for causing untoward effects. These include both ototoxicity and nephrotoxicity.

4. The answer is E (all). *(X A 3, 4, 5)* Isoniazid is the most widely used agent in the treatment of tuberculosis. In order to prevent the development of mycobacterial resistance, isoniazid is used in conjunction with other agents in the treatment of active disease. It can be used alone as prophylaxis in persons who have converted from tuberculin-negative to -positive and in close contacts of patients with newly diagnosed active disease. Isoniazid is not effective against atypical mycobacteria. Its metabolism depends in part on genetically determined acetyl transferase activity.

5. The answer is D (4). *(III E 2 d; V D; VI D; VIII D)* Of the agents listed in the question, only penicillin G is excreted via tubular secretion. Probenecid will block the transport of penicillin G in the proximal tubule, producing elevated blood levels and prolonging the activity of penicillin G.

6. The answer is C (2, 4). *(V C 3, E 2; VIII C 3, E 2)* Gentamicin provides excellent gram-negative coverage, while clindamycin is the drug of first choice against *Bacteroides fragilis,* which would be the offending anaerobic organism in this case. Neither methicillin nor penicillin G provide much if any activity against gram-negative organisms or *B. fragilis.*

7. The answer is C (2, 4). *(VIII G 2)* Clindamycin and lincomycin are capable of producing pseudomembranous colitis due to superinfection. Vancomyin is effective in the treatment of the causative organism of this syndrome, namely *Clostridium difficile.*

8. The answer is B (1, 3). *(VIII G 2)* Since the pseudomembranous colitis is due to superinfection produced as a result of the clindamycin therapy (Questions 6 and 7), clindamycin therapy should be stopped at once. Vancomycin therapy is begun, in order to treat the offending organism, *C. difficile.*

9. The answer is B (1, 3). *(IV A 3, C, D 1, 2)* The two major attractions of cephalosporin therapy are the broad spectrum of therapy and the activity of the cephalosporins against penicillinase-producing staphylococci. Except for some of the newer "third-generation" cephalosporins, they do not pass through the blood–brain barrier, nor are they uniformly capable of action following oral administration.

10. The answer is A (1, 2, 3). *(II B; III B; V B; IX A 2)* Nystatin binds to sterols in the membrane of fungi and yeasts. This interaction results in the formation of channels in the membrane that permit key metabolic intermediates to diffuse out of the cell. All of the other statements regarding the proposed mechanisms of action are true.

11. The answer is E (all). *(I D; III H 2 d; IV G 4)* All of the antibiotics listed are broad-spectrum agents and therefore can produce superinfections, including fungal infections. Local application of an appropriate antifungal agent is often sufficient therapy for the treatment of a fungal vaginitis.

12. The answer is A (1, 2, 3). *(IX A, B 5 c)* Nystatin is the most suitable agent for treating vaginal candidiasis. Like amphotericin B, nystatin is a polyene antibiotic. However, nystatin, unlike amphotericin B, is useful in the topical treatment of vaginal candidiasis but is not useful in the treatment of North American blastomycosis. Nystatin is not employed parenterally, whereas amphotericin B is administered intravenously.

13–16. The answers are: 13-E, 14-B, 15-C, 16-C. *(II G 1, 3; III H 1, 2; VI G 5; VII G 2)* Diarrhea and skin rash can each occur in up to 10 percent of the patients (especially children) who receive ampicillin orally. Amoxicillin, although having a spectrum of activity similar to that of ampicillin, is thought to cause diarrhea less often.

Sulfonamides produce the Stevens-Johnson syndrome only rarely, but fever, respiratory distress, and ulcers in the mouth or anus should serve as important clues. The hemolytic anemia that is sometimes seen with sulfonamides is often due to an erythrocytic deficiency of glucose-6-phosphate dehydrogenase activity.

The irreversible bone marrow depression which can occur with chloramphenicol is probably a hypersensitivity reaction. An acute reversible hemolytic anemia is also sometimes seen, and is due to a toxic effect on the bone marrow.

The gray-baby syndrome is especially likely to occur in premature infants who have been given large doses of chloramphenicol. It is due to the immaturity of the hepatic conjugating and renal excretory mechanisms in neonates.

13 Principles of Drug Interactions

I. INTRODUCTION

A. **A drug interaction** occurs whenever the pharmacologic action of a drug is altered by a second substance.

B. Theoretically, this change may be related to:

1. **Pharmacokinetic interactions**—that is, differences in the plasma levels of a drug, achieved with a given dose of that drug.
2. **Pharmacodynamic interactions**—that is, differences in effects produced by a given plasma level of a drug.

C. Although many examples of drug interactions are known, many are *not* clinically important.

D. Clinically important changes usually are seen with agents having a low therapeutic index (e.g., cardiac glycosides) or a poorly defined therapeutic endpoint (e.g., antipsychotic agents).

E. Often drug interactions can be avoided by employing a different drug having the desired pharmacologic effect but not the unwanted interaction.

II. PHARMACOKINETIC INTERACTIONS

A. The duration and intensity of a drug's action are a function of the plasma level of the drug, which is related directly to the drug's rates of absorption, distribution, metabolism, and excretion. One or more of these rates may be altered by the following:

1. Concomitant or previous drug therapy.
2. Dietary factors.
3. Exposure to environmental chemicals; that is, to chemicals not used for therapeutic purposes.

B. Physical factors, such as the ambient temperature, and effects of disease, for example, fever, can also alter the pharmacokinetic properties of drugs but will not be considered here.

C. DRUG INTERACTIONS AFFECTING SYSTEMIC DELIVERY

1. **Drug interactions in vitro.** Some drugs are **incompatible** with intravenous infusion fluids.
   - **a.** Ampicillin, ascorbic acid, chlorpromazine, barbiturates, or promethazine react with dextran solutions. The drugs break down or form chemical complexes.
   - **b.** Benzylpenicillin, chlorpromazine, erythromycin, gentamicin, hydrocortisone, kanamycin, methicillin, promazine, streptomycin, and tetracyclines react with heparin solutions. Chemical complexes form.
2. **Drug absorption interactions in vivo**
   - **a. Altered parenteral absorption** is not common but can occur.
     - **(1)** For example, a subcutaneous or intramuscular injection of epinephrine or methacholine given concomitantly with another drug will alter the entry of the other drug into nearby capillaries.

(2) This occurs because of the vasoconstricting or vasodilating effects of the accompanying adrenergic or cholinergic agonists.

b. Interactions affecting **absorption after oral administration** are more commonly observed.

(1) **Complexes** can be formed. For example:

(a) Tetracycline and cations such as calcium (e.g., in milk) or aluminum ion (as is found in some antacids) combine to produce an insoluble salt, which results in very poor and erratic tetracycline blood levels.

(b) Cholestyramine binds acidic compounds, cardiac glycosides, and thyroxine, blocking their absorption.

(2) **Intestinal motility** can be altered. The ultimate effect on drug absorption in this case depends upon the site at which the drug is primarily absorbed—e.g., small intestine or stomach.

(a) For example, atropine and opiate-like agents delay gastric emptying and slow the absorption of some drugs, such as acetaminophen, which are absorbed in the intestine.

(b) Stimulation of gastrointestinal motility can reduce drug absorption. For example, metoclopramide decreases absorption of cimetidine, which is absorbed primarily in the stomach.

(3) Absorption can be **blocked**. For example:

(a) Phenytoin and oral contraceptives inhibit the hydrolysis of folic acid (to the monoglutamate) in the gut, and thus they reduce its absorption.

(b) Colchicine produces malabsorption of vitamin B_{12}.

(4) The patient's **diet** may influence drug absorption.

(a) The presence of food in the stomach may exert a nonspecific effect in reducing or slowing the absorption of some drugs.

(b) A fatty meal will increase the absorption of lipid-soluble drugs (e.g., griseofulvin).

(5) Changes in the normal **gastric pH** can alter absorption. For example, weak acids such as salicylates are not absorbed well when the gastric pH is elevated with antacids.

D. DRUG INTERACTIONS AFFECTING DISTRIBUTION

1. Many drugs, especially acidic ones, bind to plasma proteins.

2. Drugs, and also other substances, can **compete for plasma protein binding sites.**

a. The effect is often to release more free drug and thus enhance its pharmacologic effect.

b. This is especially important when a high percentage of the drug (over 90 percent) is normally protein-bound, as is the case with coumarin anticoagulants, sulfonamides, salicylates, indomethacin, and most other nonsteroidal anti-inflammatory agents.

c. For example:

(1) Sulfisoxazole in premature infants increases the likelihood of fatal kernicterus because the sulfonamide displaces bilirubin from protein binding sites.

(2) Phenylbutazone potentiates the anticoagulant actions of warfarin by this mechanism, and may cause excessive bleeding.

3. **Displacement** of a plasma protein–bound drug can result in complex changes in the pharmacologic effects of the drug that can be difficult to predict.

a. There is a transient rise in the plasma levels of free drug, but the plasma half-life is frequently reduced.

b. A marked increase in the pharmacologic effect can occur if the normal route of drug elimination is impaired due to disease (e.g., cirrhosis) or to saturation of metabolizing enzymes required for drug elimination.

E. INTERACTIONS AFFECTING DRUG METABOLISM

1. Probably the most common and most important cause for differences in plasma levels of a drug is a change in the rate of biotransformation of the drug.

2. Variations in a person's plasma drug levels are more common with drugs that undergo extensive gastrointestinal metabolism or first-pass hepatic metabolism (e.g., phenacetin).

3. Many drugs that are inactivated by biotransformation can have a prolonged duration of action if their metabolism is inhibited by other agents.

4. There are a variety of **nonmicrosomal enzymes** (see Chapter 1, VI B) that can be affected. For example:

a. Drugs that can inhibit monoamine oxidase, such as the antitumor agent procarbazine and the antidepressant tranylcypromine, can retard the metabolism of various drugs, such as barbiturates and benzodiazepines, and of amines such as serotonin and norepinephrine.

b. Because 6-mercaptopurine is inactivated in part by xanthine oxidase, the concurrent administration of the xanthine oxidase inhibitor allopurinol can result in an accumulation of 6-mercaptopurine, with a consequent increase in bone marrow depression.

c. Disulfiram inhibits acetaldehyde dehydrogenase and thus prevents acetaldehyde, the oxidation product of ethanol, from being further metabolized. The resulting accumulation of acetaldehyde causes flushing, nausea, vomiting, and tachycardia.

5. The **induction or inhibition of microsomal enzymes (mixed-function oxygenases** or the cytochrome P-450 system) can also affect drug metabolism (see Chapter 1, VI B).

a. More than 200 drugs and a large number of dietary and environmental chemicals are known **inducers** of this enzyme system.

(1) Induction of mixed-function oxygenases results in an accelerated metabolism of substrates.

(2) The induction is due to new protein synthesis. The pattern of the newly synthesized proteins and the rate of appearance of new mixed-function oxygenase activities differ with different inducers.

(3) Some inducers of mixed-function oxygenases are:

(a) Barbiturates, glutethimide, phenytoin.

(b) Polycyclic aromatic hydrocarbons such as benzo[α]pyrene

(c) Halogenated hydrocarbon insecticides (e.g., DDT).

(d) Nicotine.

(e) Ethanol, when ingested chronically.

(4) Some inducers stimulate their own metabolism.

b. There are also a number of **inhibitors** of mixed-function oxygenases, including:

(1) Organophosphorus insecticides.

(2) Carbon tetrachloride.

(3) Ozone.

(4) Carbon monoxide.

F. INTERACTIONS AFFECTING DRUG EXCRETION

1. Many weak organic acids (e.g., aspirin, penicillin, methotrexate) are secreted by a common **transport system** in the proximal tubules.

a. Competition for this transport system by weak acids can result in a reduction in the urinary elimination of the competing drugs.

b. For example:

(1) Probenecid can block the excretion of penicillin, indomethacin, cefazolin, and methotrexate.

(2) Aspirin can block the secretion of methotrexate and thus cause serious untoward effects.

c. Comparable interactions between weak organic bases have not been well characterized in humans.

2. A **change in urinary pH** can influence the elimination of weak acids and bases since their passive reabsorption requires that they be un-ionized. This can be important in the treatment of overdoses of weak acids and bases such as aspirin or amphetamines.

a. Agents that alkalinize the urine (e.g., acetazolamide or sodium bicarbonate) will increase the excretion of weak acids.

b. Agents that acidify the urine (e.g., ammonium chloride) will enhance the elimination of weak bases.

3. Diuretics often can reduce the renal toxicity of chemicals and drugs, presumably by reducing the tubular concentration of the toxin. For example, mannitol reduces cisplatin toxicity.

4. Some drugs can alter the elimination of other drugs by **stimulating biliary excretion.**

a. For example, phenobarbital enhances the biliary excretion of many drugs by increasing both bile flow and the synthesis of proteins that function in the biliary conjugation–excretion mechanism.

b. Activated charcoal and cholestyramine increase the excretion of drugs that undergo extensive enterohepatic recirculation by binding to them in the gastrointestinal tract.

III. PHARMACODYNAMIC INTERACTIONS

A. Drug interactions can occur at the level of the **drug receptor.** For example, the H_2-receptor antagonist cimetidine blocks the action of histamine-like agonists such as betazole by this mechanism.

B. Agents can *reduce* the effect of other drugs by acting via different cellular mechanisms **(physiologic antagonism).** For example, acetylcholine and norepinephrine have opposing effects on heart rate (see Chapter 1, VIII E 3).

C. Agents can *enhance* the actions of other drugs although they act via different cellular mechanisms. For example, ethanol can enhance the CNS depression caused by opioids or tranquilizers.

D. The action of one drug can be influenced by **changes in the intracellular or extracellular environment** that are caused by another drug. For example, diuretic-induced hypokalemia can increase the possibility of digitalis-induced cardiac toxicity.

E. Chemical inactivation can occur systemically to reduce a drug's action. For example, protamine binds to heparin and thereby neutralizes it.

STUDY QUESTIONS

Directions: Each question below contains five suggested answers. Choose the **one best** response to each question.

1. Pharmacokinetic drug interactions can result from all of the following EXCEPT

(A) impaired absorption
(B) induction of the drug microsomal enzyme metabolizing system
(C) inhibition of the drug microsomal enzyme metabolizing system
(D) inhibition of renal secretion
(E) the combination of a bacteriostatic antibiotic with a bactericidal one

2. A classic example of the inhibition of renal secretion of a drug is the interaction between probenecid and

(A) lidocaine
(B) morphine
(C) phenobarbital
(D) cefazolin
(E) furosemide

3. Drug interactions that affect absorption include all of the following EXCEPT

(A) tetracycline—milk
(B) tetracycline—antacids containing aluminum
(C) tetracycline—cimetidine
(D) cholestyramine—cardiac glycosides
(E) cholestyramine—thyroxine

Directions: Each question below contains four suggested answers of which **one or more** is correct. Choose the answer

A if **1, 2, and 3** are correct
B if **1 and 3** are correct
C if **2 and 4** are correct
D if **4** is correct
E if **1, 2, 3, and 4** are correct

4. Which of the following effects are examples of pharmacokinetic drug interactions?

(1) The plasma level of a drug is altered
(2) The responsiveness of the target tissue is altered
(3) Absorption of the drug is impaired
(4) The combined effect of two drugs is greater than either one alone

5. Which of the following drugs are capable of inducing the cytochrome P-450 metabolizing system?

(1) Barbiturates
(2) Glutethimide
(3) Phenytoin
(4) DDT

6. A patient is being treated with 6-mercaptopurine. Which of the following statements apply to the metabolism of this drug?

(1) It is inactivated in part by monoamine oxidase
(2) It is inactivated in part by xanthine oxidase
(3) Its metabolism can be altered by tranylcypromine
(4) Its metabolism can be altered in the presence of allopurinol

7. Probenecid would compete with which of the following drugs for secretion in the proximal tubular transport system?

(1) Penicillin
(2) Cefazolin
(3) Indomethacin
(4) Erythromycin

SUMMARY OF DIRECTIONS

A	B	C	D	E
1, 2, 3 only	1, 3 only	2, 4 only	4 only	All are correct

8. True statements about drug interactions include which of the following?

(1) An interaction occurs whenever the pharmacologic action of a drug is altered by a second substance
(2) Clinically important changes that result from interactions are often seen with agents having a low therapeutic index
(3) Clinically important changes that result from interactions are often seen with agents having a poorly defined therapeutic endpoint
(4) Interactions can often be avoided by using a different drug having the desired pharmacological effect

9. True statements concerning the effects of drugs on gastrointestinal motility, include which of the following?

(1) Atropine delays gastric emptying
(2) Opiates stimulate gastric emptying
(3) Metoclopramide stimulates gastrointestinal motility
(4) Scopolamine stimulates gastrointestinal motility

ANSWERS AND EXPLANATIONS

1. The answer is E. *(II C 2, E 5, F 1)* All of the factors in the question can result in altered plasma levels of a drug after its administration (pharmacokinetic drug interactions) except for the combination of a bacteriostatic antibiotic with a bactericidal one. The latter is a pharmacodynamic type of drug interaction since plasma drug levels are not altered. Instead, the bacteriostatic agent can block the desirable actions of the bactericidal antibiotic by preventing cell replication.

2. The answer is D. *(II F 1 b)* Probenecid is capable of blocking the renal tubular secretion of cefazolin. Since both the penicillins and the cephalosporins are often excreted by renal tubular secretion, probenecid would prolong their half-lives. The renal excretion of lidocaine, morphine, phenobarbital, and furosemide would not be significantly affected by the co-administration of probenecid.

3. The answer is C. *(II C 2 b (1))* Tetracyclines form insoluble complexes with cations such as the calcium in milk and aluminum in antacids. Tetracyclines do not interact with the H_2-receptor antagonist cimetidine. The anion-exchange resin cholestyramine binds both cardiac glycosides and thyroxine, thus blocking their absorption.

4. The answer is B (1, 3). *(I B, II A)* When the delivery of a drug to its site of action is altered (which can be the result of impaired absorption) or when plasma levels are altered, a *pharmacokinetic* drug interaction has occurred. Both a change in the responsiveness of the target tissue and an increase in effect when two drugs are given together are examples of *pharmacodynamic* drug interactions.

5. The answer is E (all). *(II E 5 a)* All of the agents listed in the question are capable of inducing the cytochrome P-450 metabolizing system, so that they all would enhance the metabolism of other agents degraded by this system. The induction of mixed-function oxygenases results from new protein synthesis.

6. The answer is C (2, 4). *(II E 4)* Because 6-mercaptopurine is inactivated in part by xanthine oxidase, the concurrent administration of allopurinol can result in bone marrow depression. This results from accumulated 6-mercaptopurine, which can be toxic to the bone marrow.

7. The answer is A (1, 2, 3). *(II F 1 b)* Probenecid can inhibit the proximal tubular secretion of penicillin, cefazolin, and indomethacin. As a result of this competition for tubular secretion, the systemic blood levels of these agents would be prolonged. Erythromycin is not dependent on proximal tubular secretion for its excretion, and would not be similarly affected.

8. The answer is E (all). *(I A, C, E)* Interactions occur whenever the pharmacologic action of a drug is altered by a second substance. They often can be avoided by using a different drug having the desired pharmacologic effect. Clinically important changes that result from drug interactions usually are seen with agents that have either a low therapeutic index or a poorly defined therapeutic endpoint.

9. The answer is B (1, 3). *(II C 2 b (2))* Both atropine and scopolamine delay gastric emptying and inhibit gastrointestinal activity because of their anticholinergic properties. Opiates delay gastric emptying, while metoclopramide stimulates gastrointestinal motility.

14 Poisons and Antidotes

I. INTRODUCTION

A. DEFINITION. Toxicology is the aspect of pharmacology that deals with the adverse effects of substances on living creatures. These substances may be household, environmental, industrial, or pharmacologic substances.

B. SUBDIVISIONS OF TOXICOLOGY. Several subspecialties have evolved:

1. **Experimental toxicology** involves the investigation of the toxic effects of chemicals on biological systems.
2. **Clinical toxicology** involves the diagnosis and treatment of poisonings.
3. **Environmental toxicology** involves the prevention and reduction of the occurrence of poisoning.

II. GENERAL PRINCIPLES OF TOXICOLOGY

A. POISONS AND THEIR ANTIDOTES

1. A wide variety of industrial solvents, heavy metals, gases, and common household chemicals can be dangerous poisons. Clinically used drugs may also be poisons in high doses.
2. Acute exposure to a toxic substance is likely to produce different symptoms than are seen with chronic exposure to lower concentrations.
3. For some poisons, antidotes have been developed. These act either by preventing absorption or by inactivating or antagonizing the actions of the poisons.

B. QUANTITATIVE TOXICITY

1. The **median lethal dose (LD_{50})** is the smallest dose of a given chemical that will kill 50 percent of a test group of animals. The LD_{50} is used to extrapolate the toxic potential of a compound to the human. It is used with all routes of poisoning except inhalation.
2. The **median lethal concentration (LC_{50})** is the smallest concentration of a given chemical that will kill 50 percent of a test group of animals. It is applicable to chemicals that are inhaled. The LC_{50} is expressed relative to the duration of exposure.
3. The **threshold limit value (TLV)** is the maximal amount of a chemical that is considered safe. Industrial and governmental hygienists provide an official listing of the TLV levels of airborne poisons to which workers may safely be exposed for an 8-hour period.

III. SPECIFIC POISONS. The more important poisons and their antidotes (if available) are presented in this chapter.

A. GASEOUS POISONS

1. **Simple asphyxiants**
   a. Simple asphyxiants are usually inert industrial gases. Examples are **nitrogen** (N_2), **carbon dioxide** (CO_2), and **methane.**
   b. Asphyxiants decrease the oxygen available to the lungs and cause hypoxia.

2. Irritants

a. Irritants affecting the respiratory tract can cause asphyxia.

b. At low concentrations, **water-soluble irritants** affect the eyes and upper respiratory tract. They can affect the lungs and can be corrosive. Examples include **hydrochloric acid** (HCl), **hydrofluoric acid** (HF), **sulfur dioxide** (SO_2), and **ammonia** (NH_3).

c. Water-insoluble irritants can be trapped in nasopharyngeal secretions and can descend into the alveoli, causing pneumonitis and pulmonary edema. Examples include **chlorine gas** and **ozone.**

3. Systemic toxicants. Systemic toxicity occurs because the gas is absorbed by inhalation or percutaneously.

a. Hydrocyanic acid (HCN)

(1) HCN is one of the most rapidly acting poisons.

(2) Cyanide anions form complexes with ferric ions of the cytochrome oxidase system, interfering with electron transfer in the cytochrome a–a_3 complex. This leads to a blockage in oxygen transfer to tissues and causes a cytotoxic hypoxia.

(3) The patient's breath will have the characteristic odor of oil of bitter almond, and this should assist in **diagnosis.**

(4) Treatment must be rapid and is designed to prevent or reverse the cyanide–ferric ion binding in the cytochrome oxidase.

(a) Nitrite oxidizes a limited amount of hemoglobin to methemoglobin, which has a greater affinity for cyanide ion than does the cytochrome a–a_3. The cyanide–cytochrome complex dissociates, and normal oxidative metabolism resumes.

(b) Therefore, amyl nitrite is administered by inhalation, accompanied by intravenous sodium nitrite.

(c) A mitochondrial transsulfurase can convert cyanide to thiocyanate, which is relatively nontoxic. This detoxification can be increased by the intravenous administration of thiosulfate.

(d) If the cyanide has been ingested, gastric lavage should follow the above-mentioned treatment procedures.

b. Carbon monoxide (CO)

(1) Carbon monoxide is an odorless, colorless, and tasteless gas.

(2) Two common sources of carbon monoxide are houses with inadequate ventilation and automobile exhaust systems.

(3) The affinity of hemoglobin for carbon monoxide is 200 times greater than that for oxygen.

(4) Carbon monoxide is absorbed and excreted by the lungs.

(5) Exposure to very high ambient concentrations of carbon monoxide can result in rapid death with no premonitory signs.

(6) Exposure to lower concentrations of carbon monoxide will cause unconsciousness, then coma, followed by convulsions and death.

(7) Usually the circumstances surrounding acute carbon monoxide poisoning, such as a running automobile engine, combined with the patient's "cherry red" cyanosis, will make the **diagnosis** obvious.

(8) Treatment

(a) The patient should be removed from the air containing carbon monoxide.

(b) One hundred percent oxygen should be administered.

(c) When the poisoning is severe, oxygen at 2 to 3 atmospheres pressure is recommended.

4. Organic solvents

a. Organic solvents have an appreciable vapor pressure, are volatile, and can become an inhalation hazard, especially in an industrial environment.

b. They are fat-soluble and can be absorbed through the skin, accumulating in both fat and nervous tissue.

c. Classes of organic solvents that are toxic include:

(1) Saturated hydrocarbons, such as pentane, hexane, heptane, and octane.

(2) Unsaturated hydrocarbons, such as kerosene.

(3) Aromatic compounds, such as benzene and toluene.

(4) Halogenated hydrocarbons, such as methylene dichloride, dichloromethane, chloroform, and carbon tetrachloride.

d. The toxic manifestations of organic solvents vary with the individual substance.

e. In general, the best and only **therapy** is to remove the individual from the exposure to the solvent.

B. HEAVY METAL INTOXICATION

1. Mechanism of action

a. All of the heavy metals bind to a wide variety of macromolecules in membranes and the cytosol.

b. The heavy metals can inactivate important enzyme activities and disrupt membranes.

c. Because of the diverse affinities for the multiple organic ligands, it has been difficult to identify a single molecular target for the toxicity of these substances.

2. Arsenic

a. Arsenic is often used in household plant-spray pesticides as lead arsenate.

b. The trivalent form (As^{3-}) is toxic and binds sulfhydryl groups.

c. In *acute poisoning,* arsenic causes hypotension, capillary transudation, muscle spasms, vertigo, delirium, and interference with kidney function.

d. *Chronic poisoning* results in persistent capillary dilation, malaise, and fatigue. Encephalopathy can occur, as can peripheral neuritis and sensory loss.

e. Tolerance to chronic arsenic poisoning can develop.

f. Sulfhydryl-rich tissues—namely, nails and hair—take up arsenic, and pale bands appear in the finger- and toenails that are useful in **diagnosis.**

g. The **antidote** is dimercaprol (see III B 6 a, below). Dimercaprol contains sulfhydryl groups which compete with sulfhydryl moieties on proteins for the arsenic.

3. Lead

a. Lead is the most common cause of heavy metal poisoning, especially in large urban areas.

b. Acute poisoning is rare. Exposure has been markedly reduced because of stringent regulations on the use of lead in paints and other products.

c. The most common routes of absorption of lead are the gastrointestinal tract and respiratory system.

d. **Signs of lead poisoning**

(1) Wrist-drop and to a lesser extent foot-drop occur as a result of degenerative changes in motor neurons.

(2) An abdominal syndrome consisting of constipation, anorexia, and a persistent metallic taste appears early in the course of lead poisoning.

(3) A black "lead line"can occur on the gums, but may be absent if the intoxicated person practices good dental hygiene.

(4) Since the distribution of lead is similar to that of calcium, lead is deposited in and mobilized from bone.

(5) Lead is a potent inhibitor of hemoglobin synthesis and produces a microcytic hypochromic anemia. A reticulocytosis can also occur.

(6) A characteristic basophilic stippling of red blood cells often occurs.

(7) A coproporphyrinuria occurs and, in addition, δ-aminolevulinic acid is found in the urine.

(8) The most serious manifestation is **lead encephalopathy.**

(a) The patient will often demonstrate clumsiness, irritability, vertigo, and projectile vomiting.

(b) The condition must be differentiated from meningitis.

(c) A fatality rate as high as 25 percent has been reported, with 40 percent of the survivors demonstrating various neurologic abnormalities, including seizures, cerebral palsy, optic atrophy, and mental retardation.

e. **Treatment** consists of intravenous infusions of calcium disodium ethylenediamine tetraacetic acid ($CaNa_2EDTA$).

(1) The calcium disodium derivative of EDTA is recommended rather than Na_2EDTA because $CaNa_2EDTA$ is less likely to cause hypocalcemic tetany.

(2) Initially (for 3 to 5 days), $CaNa_2EDTA$ is given in combination with dimercaprol.

(3) Oral penicillamine, which is a good chelator of lead, can be given as long-term therapy (for 3 to 6 months) after the initial dimercaprol and $CaNa_2EDTA$ therapy.

f. **Organic lead poisoning**

(1) This is rare, except among "gasoline sniffers."

(2) Tetraethyl lead is found in some gasoline and can be absorbed when inhaled.

(3) Penetration can also occur via the skin because tetraethyl lead is fat-soluble.

(4) Eventually, the organic lead is converted in the body to inorganic lead, producing the symptoms of chronic lead poisoning.

4. Mercury

a. Toxicity can occur by inhalation, skin penetration, or ingestion of substances containing mercury:

(1) Mercurial fungicides are present in some latex paints and can be inhaled.
(2) Dermal application of methylmercury ointments can result in absorption through the skin.
(3) Inorganic mercury preparations can be ingested, resulting in acute poisoning, in contrast to the first two instances above, which usually produce chronic poisoning.

b. Mercurous (Hg^{+}) salts are less toxic than mercuric (Hg^{2+}) salts because they are less soluble, resulting in decreased skin penetration.

c. Mercury is capable of attaching to sulfhydryl groups and, in addition, concentrates in the kidney and liver.

d. Signs of intoxication

(1) Acute intoxication can result in cardiovascular collapse and anuria.
(2) Chronic intoxication due to inhalation or skin penetration can result in:
(a) Neurologic manifestations, including irritability, tremors, and psychosis.
(b) Mercuria lentis, a brown discoloration of the anterior portion of the optic lens.
(c) Gingivitis and stomatitis.
(d) Progressive renal damage.

e. Dimercaprol is used in the **treatment** of mercury poisoning.

5. Other metals

a. Antimony produces effects similar to those of arsenic. Chronic poisoning can result in myocardial damage.

b. Gold produces effects similar to those of arsenic.

c. Nickel is a sensitizing agent and causes a dermatitis known as "nickel itch."

d. Beryllium is an industrial hazard capable of causing a chronic granulomatous condition somewhat similar to sarcoid. In some instances lung carcinoma can occur.

e. Zinc intoxication can occur from inhalation of fresh fumes in smelting, causing a condition known as "metal-fume fever." Delayed chills with fever lasting up to 36 hours can occur. Tolerance develops with chronic exposure.

6. Chelating agents as antidotes

a. Dimercaprol (British anti-lewisite; **BAL**; dimercaptopropanol)

(1) Dimercaprol is indicated for the treatment of arsenic, antimony, gold, lead, and mercury poisoning.
(2) Dimercaprol cannot be administered orally. It is administered intramuscularly as a 10 percent solution of dimercaprol in oil.
(3) The dimercaprol–metal complex that forms is less toxic than dimercaprol alone.
(4) Untoward effects include a dose-related rise in blood pressure and a tachycardia. Nausea, vomiting, and headache, as well as a burning sensation of the lips and mouth, have been reported.

b. Calcium disodium EDTA

(1) $CaNa_2EDTA$ is used principally for lead poisoning but has been used for iron, copper, and zinc poisoning as well.
(2) Because of poor oral absorption, it is administered intramuscularly.
(3) It is not metabolized and is rapidly excreted.
(4) Hydropic degeneration of the proximal tubule has been reported, but generally $CaNa_2EDTA$ has a low toxicity potential.

c. Penicillamine and *N*-acetylpenicillamine

(1) These orally administered agents are used for the treatment of heavy-metal poisoning.
(2) D-Penicillamine has caused serious allergic, hematologic, and renal toxicity.
(3) The L isomer is a pyridoxine antagonist.

d. Deferoxamine

(1) Deferoxamine is used to treat acute iron poisoning.
(2) It exhibits a high affinity for the ferric ion.
(3) Deferoxamine competes with the iron of ferritin and hemosiderin, while the iron of transferrin and of cytochromes is not affected.
(4) It can be administered parenterally, orally, or through a nasogastric tube, after which it binds iron, rendering the metal nonabsorbable.
(5) Untoward effects include hypotension, which occurs as a result of histamine release. In addition, skin rashes and gastrointestinal tract irritation after large oral doses have been reported.

C. COMMONLY OCCURRING OVERDOSES

1. Ethanol accounts for approximately one-fourth of all drug poisonings each year.

a. The lethal blood level of ethanol is considered to be 0.5 g per 100 ml; however, it will vary from patient to patient.

b. A microdiffusion test is a simple screening test for the presence of blood ethanol.
c. Gas chromatography, a procedure used to separate out volatile substances, allows one to differentiate between ethanol and methanol. In addition, blood ethanol concentrations can be determined.
d. **Treatment** of ethanol overdosage consists of intensive supportive care with special attention to preventing hypoglycemia and ketoacidosis.

2. **Barbiturate overdosage** is a common form of poisoning in adults.
a. The treatment of barbiturate overdosage is mainly supportive. Maintenance of cardiopulmonary stability is of prime importance.
b. Gastric lavage is contraindicated in the comatose patient.
c. Since most barbiturates are acidic, alkalinization of the urine and the promotion of diuresis is often beneficial.
d. Hemodialysis is the most effective means of treating severe barbiturate overdosage. It tends to be more effective in removing shorter-acting barbiturates rather than longer-acting ones because the degree of protein-binding is considerably less.
e. Analeptic agents are contraindicated.

3. **Salicylate intoxication**
a. Poisoning primarily occurs in children.
b. For the frequently observed signs and symptoms of salicylate intoxication, see Chapter 9, II D.
c. Plasma salicylate levels are often good indicators of the severity of salicylate poisoning.
(1) Plasma levels below 50 mg/100 ml produce no major symptoms, and treatment is to induce emesis or administer gastric lavage.
(2) With plasma levels between 50 and 100 mg/100 ml, the patient often presents with hyperpnea due to salicylate stimulation of the respiratory center. Increased blood glucose levels and hyperpyrexia may be seen.
(a) Treatment is by inducing emesis or using gastric lavage.
(b) The administration of sodium bicarbonate to alkalinize the urine may be advisable, but must be performed with caution.
(c) Correction of hyperthermia with ice blankets is often needed.
(d) The blood salicylate level is rechecked within a few hours.
(3) With plasma levels over 110 mg/100 ml, the same procedures as above are performed; however, hemodialysis or peritoneal dialysis may be needed.
(4) Plasma levels over 160 mg/100 ml are usually lethal, death being due to respiratory arrest.

IV. MANAGEMENT OF POISONING

A. GENERAL PRINCIPLES

1. Separate the patient from the poison.
a. Remove the individual from the contaminated air if the toxic substance is airborne.
b. Remove the person's clothing immediately if the clothing is soaked in the poison.
c. When the poison has been ingested, induce vomiting or use gastric lavage except when this is contraindicated, as in the case of caustic poisons or a comatose patient.

2. Give supportive therapy—provide basic respiratory and cardiovascular support.

3. Give antidotes.
a. Few poisons have specific antidotes.
b. The most common substance that is effective and generally available in a household is **milk.**
(1) Milk is amphoteric, and both acids and bases are compatible.
(2) Both the calcium and protein can serve as chelators.
(3) Milk coats the stomach, thereby protecting it and delaying absorption.

B. INDUCTION OF VOMITING

1. **Syrup of ipecac** is the preferred agent for inducing vomiting.
a. It is an emetic.
b. It is best administered with a glass of warm water because this produces a diluting effect and solubilizes the stomach contents.
c. Syrup of ipecac (or any emetic) must be used with particular caution when central nervous system (CNS) integrity is compromised because of the risk of aspiration pneumonia.

2. Giving salt water or using a finger to provoke emesis are both dangerous.

3. Contraindications to induced emesis include:
   a. Caustic poisons; for example, lye.
   b. Petroleum distillates; for example, lighter fluid or gasoline.
   c. A comatose patient.
   d. A patient in whom convulsions may be imminent, as with ingestion of a large dose of aspirin.

4. Emesis is always indicated in insecticide poisoning.

C. **ALTERNATIVES TO EMESIS.** The major alternatives to emesis include:

1. **Gastric lavage.** This is especially useful in treating poisoning by aromatic substances, such as perfume, or when some contraindication for emesis exists.

2. **Activated charcoal** adsorbs the poison or toxin and delays gastrointestinal absorption. It is especially helpful in the treatment of poisoning from aromatic and alkaloid compounds.

3. **Cathartics** are used to hasten the removal of a toxic substance and are useful for ingestion of hydrocarbons and enteric-coated tablets. Sodium sulfate is a frequently used cathartic.

STUDY QUESTIONS

Directions: Each question below contains five suggested answers. Choose the **one best** response to each question.

1. The therapeutic efficacy of sodium nitrite in the treatment of patients with cyanide poisoning is based upon

(A) the formation of methemoglobin
(B) an increase in oxidative phosphorylation
(C) an increase in coronary arterial blood flow
(D) a decrease in intracranial pressure
(E) relaxation of the nonvascular smooth muscle

2. All of the following statements about carbon monoxide poisoning are true EXCEPT that

(A) it is odorless, colorless, and tasteless
(B) it has slightly less affinity for hemoglobin than does oxygen
(C) death can occur rapidly with no premonitory signs
(D) the diagnosis is often clear from the circumstances
(E) the treatment of choice is 100 percent oxygen

3. Which of the following statements about lead poisoning is correct?

(A) Lead poisoning is the least common cause of heavy metal poisoning
(B) Acute lead poisoning is more common than chronic exposure
(C) The most common route of absorption is through the skin
(D) Foot-drop is the most common sign of lead poisoning
(E) The black "lead line" can often be eliminated from the gums by good dental hygiene

4. The initial disturbance in acute intoxication by salicylates is

(A) respiratory depression causing retention of carbon dioxide
(B) renal loss of fixed cation
(C) respiratory stimulation causing loss of carbon dioxide
(D) inhibition of renal carbonic anhydrase
(E) depression of the brain stem reticular activating system

5. All of the following statements about arsenic poisoning are true EXCEPT that

(A) arsenic is often used in household plant-spray pesticides
(B) the trivalent form is toxic and binds to sulfhydryl groups
(C) the antidote is dimercaprol
(D) a characteristic basophilic stippling of red blood cells often occurs
(E) tolerance to chronic arsenic poisoning can develop

6. All of the following statements about toxicology are true EXCEPT that

(A) certain heavy metals can be considered hazardous poisons
(B) chronic exposure to a toxic substance is likely to produce the same symptoms as acute exposure
(C) antidotes of poisons can act by preventing absorption of the poison
(D) antidotes of poisons can act by antagonizing the actions of poisons
(E) activated charcoal is an alternative to emesis

Directions: Each question below contains four suggested answers of which **one or more** is correct. Choose the answer

A if **1, 2, and 3** are correct
B if **1 and 3** are correct
C if **2 and 4** are correct
D if **4** is correct
E if **1, 2, 3, and 4** are correct

7. Chelating agents matched correctly with the poisons that they are used to treat include

(1) dimercaprol (BAL)—mercury
(2) calcium disodium EDTA—arsenic
(3) penicillamine—copper
(4) deferoxamine—lead

8. A comatose patient is brought to the emergency room after taking an overdose of secobarbital. Proper therapy would include

(1) ventilatory support
(2) amphetamines
(3) placement of an intravenous catheter
(4) an emetic agent

9. True statements about measurements used in quantitative toxicology include which of the following?

(1) The median lethal dose (LD_{50}) is the smallest dose of a chemical that will kill 50 percent of a test group of animals
(2) The LD_{50} of a poison can be determined by using the inhalation route of administration
(3) The threshold limit value (TLV) is the maximal amount of a chemical that is considered safe
(4) The LD_{50} is rarely used to extrapolate the toxic potential of a compound to the human

10. Examples of inert gases which might be considered simple asphyxiants include

(1) nitrogen (N_2)
(2) carbon dioxide (CO_2)
(3) methane (CH_4)
(4) sulfur dioxide (SO_2)

11. Correct statements concerning the systemic toxicant hydrocyanic acid include which of the following?

(1) It is a slow-acting poison
(2) It interferes with the cytochrome oxidase system
(3) It does not affect the odor of the breath
(4) It is treated by preventing or reversing the cyanide–ferric ion binding complex

12. The treatment of carbon monoxide poisoning would include

(1) the administration of 100 percent oxygen
(2) inducing vomiting with syrup of ipecac
(3) administration of oxygen at 2 to 3 atmospheres
(4) hemodialysis

13. Which toxic organic solvents are correctly matched with their chemical class?

(1) Octane—saturated hydrocarbons
(2) Toluene—unsaturated hydrocarbon
(3) Benzene—aromatic compound
(4) Kerosene—halogenated hydrocarbon

ANSWERS AND EXPLANATIONS

1. The answer is A. *(III A 3 a (4))* The inhalation of amyl nitrite and the intravenous administration of sodium nitrite cause the oxidation of hemoglobin to methemoglobin. Methemoglobin competes with cytochrome oxidase for the cyanide ion, allowing the cytochrome oxidase to function in normal oxidative metabolism.

2. The answer is B. *(III A 3 b)* Carbon monoxide has 200 times the affinity for hemoglobin that oxygen has. All of the other statements in the question are correct. If the poisoning is severe, treatment with oxygen at 2 to 3 atmospheres is recommended.

3. The answer is E. *(III B 3)* Lead poisoning is the most common heavy metal poisoning. Chronic exposure is much more common than acute poisoning. The gastrointestinal and respiratory tracts are the most common routes of absorption. Wrist-drop is a more frequently seen physical sign than foot-drop. The black "lead line" often seen on the gums can be eliminated with good dental hygiene.

4. The answer is C. *(III C 3 c (2))* At salicylate plasma levels between 50 and 110 mg per 100 ml, the patient often presents with hyperventilation due to salicylate stimulation of the respiratory center. This respiratory stimulation leads to the loss of carbon dioxide. At plasma doses above 160 mg per 100 ml, respiratory arrest can occur.

5. The answer is D. *(III B 2, 3)* Lead arsenate is often used as a household plant-spray pesticide. The trivalent form is toxic and binds to sulfhydryl groups. Dimercaprol can be used an an antidote because it contains sulfhydryl groups which compete with sulfhydryl moieties on proteins for arsenic. Tolerance to chronic arsenic poisoning can develop, especially in agricultural workers. Basophilic stippling of red blood cells is seen with lead poisoning, not with arsenic.

6. The answer is B. *(II A 2, 3; III B; IV C 2)* Acute exposure to a toxic substance is likely to produce different symptoms than are seen with chronic exposure to lower concentrations. Antidotes act by both preventing the absorption and antagonizing the actions of poisons. Certain heavy metals can be dangerous poisons. Activated charcoal is a useful alternative to inducing vomiting when a person has ingested a poison. It absorbs the poison and delays gastrointestinal absorption.

7. The answer is B (1, 3). *(III B 6)* Dimercaprol (BAL) is useful in the treatment of mercury poisoning, as well as in poisoning by arsenic, antimony, gold, and lead. Penicillamine is an orally effective treatment for copper or lead poisoning. Calcium disodium EDTA ($CaNa_2EDTA$) is useful in the treatment of lead, iron, copper, and zinc poisoning, but not in arsenic poisoning. Deferoxamine exhibits a high affinity for the ferric ion and is used in iron poisoning.

8. The answer is B (1, 3). *(III C 2)* Treatment for an overdose of secobarbital, a barbiturate, would focus on maintaining basic life functions, including placement of an intravenous catheter and ventilatory support if indicated. Maintenance of cardiopulmonary stability is of prime importance. There are no specific antagonists for barbiturates, and generalized CNS stimulants such as amphetamines are not indicated. Hemodialysis is the most effective means of treating severe barbiturate overdosage. If the patient were conscious, emesis would indeed be indicated, but it should not be used in a comatose patient.

9. The answer is B (1, 3). *(II B)* The median lethal dose cannot be calculated for poisons which are inhaled. Instead, the median lethal concentration (LC_{50}) is used and is expressed relative to the duration of exposure. The LD_{50} is the smallest dose of a chemical that will kill 50 percent of a test group of animals and is often used to extrapolate the toxic potential of a compound to the human.

10. The answer is A (1, 2, 3). *(III A 1, 2)* Nitrogen, carbon dioxide, and methane are all examples of simple asphyxiants, which are usually inert gases that cause hypoxia by decreasing the oxygen available to the lungs. Sulfur dioxide can produce asphyxia by irritating the respiratory tract, and can be corrosive to the lungs.

11. The answer is C (2, 4). *(III A 3 a)* Hydrocyanic acid is one of the most rapidly acting poisons. Cyanide anions complex with ferric ions of the cytochrome oxidase system. With systemic toxicity, the patient's breath has a characteristic odor of oil of bitter almond. A combination of inhaled amyl nitrite and intravenous sodium nitrite is used to prevent or reverse the cyanide–ferric ion binding in the cytochrome oxidase.

12. The answer is B (1, 3). *(III A 3 b (8))* Treating a patient poisoned by carbon monoxide involves removing the patient from the contaminated air and giving 100 percent oxygen. If the poisoning is severe, oxygen should be given at 2 to 3 atmospheres of pressure. Inducing vomiting or using hemodialysis would serve no purpose in treating carbon monoxide poisoning.

13. The answer is B (1, 3). *(III A 4 c)* Saturated hydrocarbons include octane, heptane, hexane, and pentane. Toluene, like benzene, is an aromatic organic solvent, while kerosene is an unsaturated hydrocarbon. All of these organic solvents can be quite toxic. Being fat-soluble, they can accumulate in both fat and nervous tissue.

Post-test

QUESTIONS

Directions: Each question below contains five suggested answers. Choose the **one best** response to each question.

1. A useful thrombolytic agent that leads to plasmin activation is

(A) vitamin K
(B) heparin
(C) streptokinase
(D) aminocaproic acid
(E) aspirin

2. A patient is receiving a hypnotic drug that is a chlorinated derivative of ethanol, is converted in the liver to its active form, is irritating to the stomach, and can be administered orally or rectally. These features accurately describe which of the following drugs?

(A) Flurazepam
(B) Ethchlorvynol
(C) Chloral hydrate
(D) Methyprylon
(E) Paraldehyde

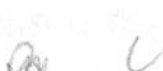

3. All of the following statements about Fick's law as it pertains to simple diffusion are correct EXCEPT that the

(A) greater the concentration gradient, the greater the rate of absorption
(B) smaller the surface area, the greater the drug flux
(C) diffusion constant is directly proportional to the temperature
(D) diffusion constant is directly proportional to the molecular size
(E) greater the lipid–water partition coefficient, the greater the drug flux

4. General principles of the treatment of patients who have been poisoned include all of the following measures EXCEPT

(A) remove the patient from the contaminated air if it is an atmospheric poison
(B) wrap the clothed person in absorbent towels if the poison has soaked into the clothing
(C) induce vomiting but only if the patient is conscious and if the poison has been ingested
(D) provide basic life support whatever the type of poison
(E) administer milk because it is amphoteric if the person has ingested a household poison

5. Which of the following agents used to treat gout could actually increase the frequency of acute gouty attacks during initial therapy?

(A) Sulfinpyrazole
(B) Allopurinol
(C) Colchicine
(D) Probenecid
(E) Indomethacin

6. All of the following statements about triamterene are true EXCEPT that it

(A) inhibits the Na^+–K^+ exchange pump in the distal nephron
(B) inhibits the secretion of K^+ in the distal nephron
(C) produces reversible azotemia relatively commonly
(D) is a weak competitive antagonist of aldosterone
(E) is weakly uricosuric

7. A young child who ingests a fatally toxic dose of dimenhydrinate (Dramamine) will most likely die from

(A) renal dysfunction
(B) general CNS stimulation with convulsions
(C) bronchospasm and suffocation
(D) anaphylactic shock
(E) severe cardiac arrhythmia

8. Allopurinol would be likely to potentiate the pharmacologic action of

(A) 5-fluorouracil
(B) bleomycin
(C) 6-mercaptopurine
(D) doxorubicin
(E) methotrexate

9. A patient with a systemic infection is being treated with an antibiotic whose elimination half-time ($t_{1/2\beta}$) is 8 hours. In order to maintain the patient's total body store at 300 mg of the antibiotic, what should the dosage be?

(A) 100 mg every 8 h
(B) 200 mg every 8 h
(C) 300 mg every 8 h
(D) 400 mg every 8 h
(E) 500 mg every 8 h

10. All of the following statements about digitalis glycosides are correct EXCEPT that

(A) the active moiety of the glycoside molecule is chemically similar to the adrenocorticosteroid molecule
(B) the most important property of the cardiac glycosides is their positive inotropic effect
(C) cardiac glycosides also effect cardiac conductivity
(D) the serum potassium level is related to the therapeutic:toxic ratio of the glycosides
(E) intoxication due to depletion of potassium stores is a common problem with the cardiac glycosides

11. All of the following statements concerning allopurinol are true EXCEPT that

(A) it is an analog of hypoxanthine
(B) its primary metabolite is alloxanthine
(C) it is a noncompetitive inhibitor of xanthine oxidase
(D) it is well tolerated
(E) it is administered orally

12. In the rational prescribing of drugs, one must consider possible interactions when multiple drugs are taken simultaneously. Which of the following drug pairs is *least* likely to produce an adverse interaction?

(A) A barbiturate given for insomnia to an epileptic patient previously stabilized with phenytoin
(B) propranolol given to a hypertensive patient who has periodic attacks of asthma which are relieved by an isoproterenol nebulizer
(C) Chlorothiazide prescribed for hypertension in a patient who is taking digitalis following recovery from a myocardial infarction
(D) Norepinephrine given to a shock victim who has been receiving treatment with phenoxybenzamine for a pheochromocytoma
(E) A barbiturate prescribed to aid sleep for a patient taking aspirin for muscle pain

13. In patients with congestive heart failure, digitalis glycosides are used because they produce a positive inotropic effect that can best be defined as an increase in

(A) the force of myocardial contraction
(B) cardiac filling pressure
(C) in the heart rate
(D) venous pressure
(E) cardiac conduction velocity

14. All of the following statements about efficacy and potency are true EXCEPT that

(A) efficacy is usually a more important clinical consideration than potency
(B) the ED_{50} is a dose that produces a specified effect in 50 percent of the population being tested
(C) the ED_{50} is a measure of a drug's efficacy
(D) drugs that produce a similar pharmacologic effect can have very different levels of efficacy
(E) on a log dose–response curve, two drugs with the same action but with different potencies will usually have parallel curves

15. All of the following untoward effects have been associated with the use of oral contraceptives EXCEPT for

(A) an increased incidence of thromboplebitis and thromboembolism
(B) decreased platelet aggregation leading to "breakthrough" bleeding
(C) reversible hypertension
(D) breast tenderness
(E) weight gain

16. A 62-year-old patient who is known to have glaucoma is scheduled for a cholecystectomy. Which neuromuscular blocking agent is contraindicated?

(A) *d*-Tubocurarine
(B) Pancuronium
(C) Succinylcholine
(D) Gallamine
(E) All neuromuscular blocking agents

17. Which of the following agents would bring a rapid heart rate (120 beats/minute) back to normal?

(A) Isoproterenol
(B) Phentolamine
(C) Propranolol
(D) Phenoxybenzamine
(E) Edrophonium

18. A patient arrives at the emergency room complaining of a severe headache, mental confusion, and visual disturbances. Blood pressure is 240/160 mm Hg, and physical examination is compatible with the the diagnosis of hypertensive encephalopathy. All of the following statements are true EXCEPT that

(A) hydralazine can be used, and its effect is usually noted 15 minutes after administration
(B) diazoxide can be used; its mechanism of action is direct dilation of arterioles
(C) one might see a significant retention of sodium and water if diazoxide is used
(D) nitroprusside can be used; its mechanism of action is direct vasodilation of only arteriolar smooth muscle
(E) methemoglobinemia could develop if nitroprusside is administered for a prolonged period

19. Which of the following statements concerning the pharmacotherapy of petit mal seizures is true?

(A) Drug treatment is similar to that used in grand mal seizures
(B) Trimethadione is the drug of first choice
(C) Trimethadione acts solely by suppressing the seizure focus
(D) Ethosuximide is the drug of first choice
(E) Primidone is the drug of first choice

20. Vitamin B_{12} has all of the following characteristics EXCEPT that

(A) it is a cobalt-containing compound
(B) it is synthesized by the bacterial flora in the colon
(C) it is preferentially stored in the bone marrow
(D) it is obtained from the dietary intake of animal products
(E) it is required for myelin maintenance

21. Monoamine oxidase (MAO) inhibitors and tricyclic antidepressants have which of the following features in common?

(A) Both are useful for the manic phase of manic-depressive psychosis
(B) Both have a considerable lag time before the onset of clinically useful effects
(C) Both can precipitate hypotensive crises if certain foods are ingested
(D) Both act postsynaptically to produce their effect
(E) Both drugs decrease absolute levels of biogenic amines

22. Pharmacologic doses of glucocorticoids can result in all of the following effects EXCEPT

(A) stimulation of leukocyte migration
(B) stabilization of lysosomal membranes
(C) reduced activity of fibroblasts
(D) reversal of a histamine-stimulated increase in capillary permeability
(E) inhibited antibody synthesis

23. All of the following statements about lidocaine are true EXCEPT that

(A) it is a therapeutically useful local anesthetic
(B) it has a rapid onset of activity
(C) it has an esteratic linkage
(D) it is metabolized in the liver
(E) epinephrine is not required when lidocaine is administered

24. Which of the following pairs of hematopoietic substances is INCORRECTLY matched?

(A) Iron—transferrin
(B) Folate—intrinsic factor
(C) Vitamin B_{12}—transcobalamin II
(D) Iron—ferritin
(E) Folate—folate-binding protein

Directions: Each question below contains four suggested answers of which **one or more** is correct. Choose the answer

A if **1, 2, and 3** are correct
B if **1 and 3** are correct
C if **2 and 4** are correct
D if **4** is correct
E if **1, 2, 3, and 4** are correct

25. The inhibition of microsomal enzymes can affect drug metabolism. Which of the following toxic substances would inhibit the mixed-function oxygenase system?

(1) Carbon monoxide
(2) Ozone
(3) Carbon tetrachloride
(4) Organophosphorus insecticides

26. Which of the following points should one bear in mind when considering long-term corticosteroid therapy?

(1) Abrupt withdrawal may cause signs of adrenal insufficiency
(2) Therapy may precipitate peptic ulcers
(3) Patients may become intolerant to severe stressful situations for as long as a year after therapy is stopped
(4) Therapy may lead to increased infections

27. A 22-year-old woman who sustains a severe head injury in an automobile accident is found to have elevated intracranial pressure. Proper therapy for this patient could include the use of which of the following diuretic agents?

(1) Urea
(2) Furosemide
(3) Mannitol
(4) Spironolactone

28. True statements about the use of diuretics in the management of hypertension include which of the following?

(1) The thiazides are the diuretics used most frequently for this purpose
(2) Diuretics are only useful in mild hypertension
(3) Triamterene is used in combination with a thiazide diuretic
(4) Furosemide is a more effective antihypertensive than chlorothiazide

29. Many serious disadvantages hinder the use of general anesthetics. Which of the following disadvantages are correctly matched with the offending drugs?

(1) Explosive—diethyl ether
(2) Poor skeletal muscle relaxation—halothane and ether
(3) Possible liver toxicity—halothane and enflurane
(4) Severe respiratory depression—nitrous oxide and ether

30. A patient presents with a pseudocholinesterase deficiency. A minor procedure requiring local anesthesia is required. Correct statements about the choice of an anesthetic agent in this situation include which of the following?

(1) Procaine may be used, but its duration of action will be shortened
(2) Although cocaine has abuse potential, because it is metabolized in the liver it would be of therapeutic value in this special case
(3) Dibucaine would be contraindicated in this patient if only a topical anesthetic was needed
(4) The chemical structure of lidocaine would most likely explain its therapeutic usefulness in this case

31. Disadvantages of alimentary administration include which of the following?

(1) The rate of absorption is variable
(2) Irritation of the mucosal surfaces can occur
(3) The compliance of the patient is not ensured
(4) It is the least safe route of administration

32. Which of the following are CORRECTLY matched?

(1) Prothrombin—factor II
(2) Vitamin K_1—phytonadione
(3) Heparin—obtained from bovine lung and porcine intestine
(4) Warfarin—coumarin

33. The antianxiety agents (minor tranquilizers) differ from antipsychotic agents in which of the following ways?

(1) There is no parkinsonian tremor
(2) They are better skeletal muscle relaxants
(3) They are good anticonvulsant agents
(4) They are ineffective in treating psychotic symptoms

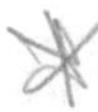

34. Hexamethonium might produce which of the following effects?

(1) Decreased blood pressure
(2) Bronchiolar relaxation
(3) Constipation
(4) Skeletal muscle relaxation

35. Correct statements concerning drug metabolism include which of the following?

(1) Synthesis or conjugation reactions usually follow oxidation reactions
(2) Glucuronides eliminated in the bile can be hydrolyzed and the free drug reabsorbed
(3) Most drug metabolism takes place in the microsomal system of the liver
(4) Conjugation reactions involve linking two or more exogenously administered drug molecules together

36. A patient presents with dyspnea on exertion. After an extensive cardiovascular work-up, the diagnosis of exertional angina is made. Which of the following drugs would be useful in treating this disorder?

(1) Verapamil
(2) Nifedipine
(3) Propranolol
(4) Nitroglycerin

37. Pairs of compounds with opposing effects on blood glucose concentrations include

(1) tolbutamide and diazoxide
(2) insulin and cortisol
(3) insulin and glucagon
(4) glucagon and isoproterenol

38. True statements about drug absorption include which of the following?

(1) The route of administration is an important factor affecting drug absorption
(2) The rate of absorption varies after oral administration
(3) After rectal administration, drug absorption follows first-order kinetics
(4) After intramuscular administration, drug absorption follows first-order kinetics

Questions 39 and 40

A child who has been "sprayed" while walking through an apple orchard was brought to the emergency room. Quick chemical analysis revealed that parathion (an organophosphorus insecticide) was the chemical spray.

39. Which of the following might be presenting signs and symptoms?

(1) Mydriasis
(2) Increased bronchial secretions
(3) Tachycardia
(4) Muscle fasciculations

40. Appropriate therapy for this child would be to administer

(1) neostigmine
(2) atropine
(3) physostigmine
(4) PAM chloride

41. Digitalis glycosides are used in the treatment of

(1) congestive heart failure
(2) atrial fibrillation
(3) paroxysmal atrial tachycardia
(4) atrioventricular block

42. Which of the following factors might influence the absorption of a drug?

(1) Gastric pH
(2) Presence of food in the stomach
(3) A fatty meal
(4) Ingestion of warm water

SUMMARY OF DIRECTIONS

A	B	C	D	E
1, 2, 3 only	1, 3 only	2, 4 only	4 only	All are correct

43. Characteristics of amphetamine include which of the following?

(1) It is a direct-acting sympathomimetic agent
(2) It causes mood elevation
(3) It stimulates monoamine oxidase
(4) It depresses hunger centers in the hypothalamus

44. Colchicine exhibits which of the following properties?

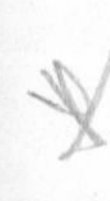

(1) It is a uricosuric agent
(2) It inhibits the migration of polymorphonuclear leukocytes
(3) It can cause constipation
(4) It is capable of producing bone marrow depression

45. Factors affecting drug metabolism include which of the following?

(1) Genetic makeup
(2) Disease
(3) Age
(4) Species

46. True statements about adrenal steroids include which of the following?

(1) "Glucocorticoid activity" implies an effect on electrolyte homeostasis
(2) Corticotropin (ACTH) and cortisol both share the basic steroid nucleus
(3) Pharmacologic doses of glucocorticoids are seldom associated with toxic effects
(4) Steroid receptors mediate the metabolic effects of steroids

47. The action of norepinephrine is terminated by

(1) Re-uptake
(2) Catechol-O-methyltransferase (COMT)
(3) Monoamine oxidase (MAO)
(4) Tyrosine hydroxylase

48. A patient with rheumatoid arthritis, a previous myocardial infarction, and congestive heart failure wants more effective therapy for his arthritis. Agents to be avoided include

(1) aspirin
(2) indomethacin
(3) sulfindac
(4) phenylbutazone

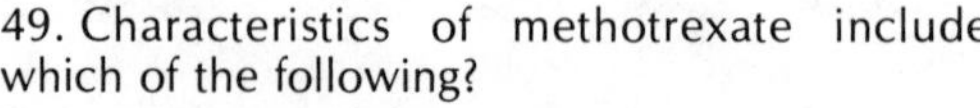

49. Characteristics of methotrexate include which of the following?

(1) It can be used in the treatment of psoriasis
(2) It is metabolized extensively
(3) It is a self-limiting S-phase–specific drug
(4) It penetrates the blood–brain barrier

50. Examples of physiologic antagonists include

(1) acetylcholine
(2) atropine
(3) norepinephrine
(4) phentolamine

51. Areas that often are not readily accessible to drugs include which of the following?

(1) Fetus
(2) Kidneys
(3) Brain
(4) Testes

52. A patient comes to the emergency room with acute substernal chest pain. His electrocardiogram is compatible with an acute lateral myocardial infarction. One hour later the patient develops premature ventricular contractions at a rate of seven per minute. Proper therapy might include

(1) digoxin
(2) oxygen
(3) propranolol
(4) lidocaine

53. Pharmacologic effects of classic antihistamines include which of the following?

(1) Sedation with low doses
(2) Drying of salivary and bronchial secretions
(3) An antipruritic effect
(4) Convulsions with high doses

54. Drugs that are likely to aggravate bronchial asthma include

(1) morphine
(2) tubocurarine
(3) propranolol
(4) amphetamine

55. Characteristics of acetaminophen include which of the following?

(1) It does not inhibit prostaglandin synthesis
(2) It can be used for the treatment of headache in hemophilia
(3) An overdose depletes glucuronide stores
(4) It is capable of reducing pain in arthritis

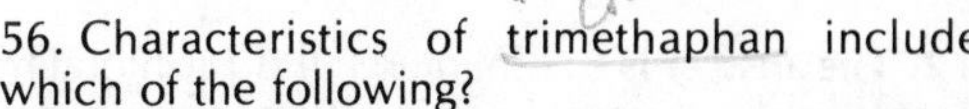

56. Characteristics of trimethaphan include which of the following?

(1) It reduces blood pressure by α-adrenergic blockade
(2) It is rapid-acting
(3) It directly produces tachycardia
(4) It is similar to hexamethonium in its mechanism of action

Directions: The group of questions below consists of lettered choices followed by several numbered items. For each numbered item select the **one** lettered choice with which it is **most** closely associated. Each lettered choice may be used once, more than once, or not at all.

Questions 57–60

For each description of the anti-infective agents listed below, select the untoward effect with which it is most likely to be associated.

(A) Pseudomembranous colitis
(B) Ototoxicity
(C) Peripheral neuritis
(D) Phototoxic reactions
(E) Orange-colored urine

57. This agent is very effective in the treatment of *Chlamydia* infections

58. This agent is often administered along with isoniazid and ethambutol

59. This agent is the drug of first choice for *Bacteroides fragilis* infection

60. This agent consists of organic bases containing characteristic amino sugars

ANSWERS AND EXPLANATIONS

1. The answer is C. *(Chapter 7, III A 1, B 2 a, C 3 a; Chapter 9, II B 6 c)* Vitamin K is required for the synthesis of several coagulation factors; the coumarin-derived anticoagulants act by interfering with this function. Heparin is an anticoagulant, not a thrombolytic; it acts by inhibiting the conversion of prothrombin to thrombin. Aminocaproic acid antagonizes the effects of thrombolytic drugs. Aspirin inhibits platelet aggregation and thereby prevents thrombus formation, presumably through its effects on platelet cyclooxygenase. The value of aspirin as an antithrombotic agent is still under study. Thus, streptokinase is the only drug listed that produces thrombolysis by plasmin activation.

2. The answer is C. *(Chapter 3, II B 1)* Chloral hydrate is a chlorinated derivate of ethanol. It is administered orally or rectally, is irritating to the gastrointestinal tract, and is quite bad tasting.

3. The answer is B. *(Chapter 1, III D 1 a)* Fick's law is expressed as

$$dQ/dt = (-D)(A)(dc/dx)$$

where dQ/dt is the rate of drug flux, D is the temperature-dependent diffusion constant of the molecule, A is the area of the absorbing surface, and dc/dx is the concentration gradient. Thus, the larger the surface area, the greater the drug flux. All of the other statements in the question are true.

4. The answer is B. *(Chapter 14, IV A)* If the poison has soaked into the person's clothing, the clothing should be immediately removed, in order to reduce the duration of contact between the poison and the skin surface. All of the other statements in the question are correct.

5. The answer is B. *(Chapter 9, X E 6)* Acute attacks of gout occur more frequently during initial therapy with allopurinol. This effect may be explained by the active dissolution of microcrystalline deposits of sodium urate (tophi) in subcutaneous tissue, which results in brief episodes of hyperuricemia and crystal deposition in joints. Simultaneous administration of colchicine decreases the frequency of these attacks.

6. The answer is D. *(Chapter 6, IX A 1, 4)* Triamterene is not a competitive antagonist of aldosterone. All of the other statements in the question are true. Unlike spironolactone, triamterene acts independently of aldosterone. It does inhibit the Na^+-K^+ exhange pump in the distal nephron, and it causes a slight increase in uric acid excretion.

7. The answer is B. *(Chapter 8, III A 1 f)* Dimenhydrinate is a "classic" antihistaminic agent—a H_1 receptor antagonist. A toxic dose of dimenhydrinate would result in generalized CNS stimulation with convulsions. Renal dysfunction is not a side effect of H_1 receptor antagonists. Bronchospasm, suffocation, and cardiac arrhythmias are also not untoward effects seen with acute poisoning. Allergic manifestations may be observed with topical application of the drug, but these are not severe enough to constitute anaphylactic shock, and would not be lethal.

8. The answer is C. *(Chapter 11, III C 1 f 4)* Attempts to inhibit the degradation of 6-mercaptopurine (and thus enhance its effects) led to the development of the xanthine oxidase inhibitor allopurinol. Allopurinol blocks not only the metabolism of 6-mercaptopurine but also the formation of uric acid from hypoxanthine and xanthine. The dose of 6-mercaptopurine must be reduced when a patient is being treated with allopurinol.

9. The answer is B. *(Chapter 1, VII D)* A drug accumulates in the body if the time interval between doses is less than four half-times, in which case the total body store of the drug increases exponentially to a plateau. The average total body store of a drug at the plateau is a function of the dose, the interval between doses, and the elimination half-time of the drug. When the drug is administered at the half-time of elimination, the average total body store of the drug is approximately equal to 1.5 times the amount administered.

10. The answer is D. *(Chapter 5, II A 1, B 1, 2, H 2, 3)* The therapeutic:toxic ratio is an inherent property of a drug, and would not be altered by the serum potassium level. However, the serum potassium level does affect the serum glycoside level, and glycoside intoxication is frequently precipitated by depletion of potassium stores. Hypokalemia and consequent digitalis intoxication are most often due to diuretic administration, but can also result from prolonged administration of corticosteroids, protracted vomiting, diarrhea, or other causes. Intoxication can also be due to the accumulation of maintenance doses of a glycoside. The other statements in the question are correct.

11. The answer is C. *(Chapter 9, X E 1-3, 5, 7)* Allopurinol is an analog of hypoxanthine. Together with its primary metabolite alloxanthine, allopurinol prevents the final step in uric acid formation by inhibiting the enzyme xanthine oxidase. Allopurinol acts as a competitive inhibitor, and alloxanthine acts noncompetitively. Administered orally, allopurinol is well tolerated; the most common untoward effects of allopurinol are hypersensitivity reactions.

12. The answer is E. *(Chapter 13, II E 5; III B, D)* Barbiturates stimulate the drug microsomal metabolizing system; therefore, the metabolism of phenytoin would be increased. The metabolism of aspirin would not be affected by this microsomal enzyme induction. Propranolol would counteract the beneficial effects of the β-adrenergic agonist isoproterenol. Chlorothiazide could produce hypokalemia, which increases the potential of digitalis toxicity. The α-blocker phenoxybenzamine, when administered to a shock victim, would produce a decreased response to norepinephrine.

13. The answer is A. *(Chapter 5, II B 1, C 1, 2)* The most important property of the cardiac glycosides is to increase the force of myocardial contraction (positive inotropic effect). In patients with congestive heart failure, this leads to an increase in cardiac output, a decrease in cardiac filling pressures, and decreases in heart size and venous and capillary pressures. Digitalis also tends to slow the heart rate in patients with congestive heart failure; this negative chronotropic effect is the result of a decrease in sympathetic activity brought about by increased cardiac output. Digitalis also decreases conduction velocity through the A–V node; this effect is unrelated to the positive inotropic effect.

14. The answer is C. *(Chapter 1, VIII B 3, C)* The ED_{50} is a measure of a drug's potency, not its efficacy. The smaller the ED_{50}, the greater the potency of the drug. All of the other statements in the question are true.

15. The answer is B. *(Chapter 10, II C 6)* Estrogens increase platelet aggregation. Although "breakthrough" vaginal bleeding can occur at the start of oral contraceptive use, this is unrelated to platelet function. All of the other untoward effects listed in the question have been associated with oral contraceptive use.

16. The answer is C. *(Chapter 2, VIII E 1)* Because succinylcholine can depolarize cholinergic skeletal muscle receptors, it affects the extraocular muscles and therefore can cause an increase in intraocular pressure. This effect would be contraindicated in glaucoma.

17. The answer is C. *(Chapter 2, III B 1)* Propranolol is an effective agent for treating an abnormal tachycardia. Its mechanism of action is β-adrenergic blockade. Propanolol decreases the heart rate and cardiac output and prolongs systole. It reduces total coronary blood flow to most tissues (except the brain) and lowers oxygen consumption.

18. The answer is D. *(Chapter 5, V A 3 c, C 1 a, 3 a, b, e, D 1)* Nitroprusside will directly dilate both arteriolar and venous smooth muscle. It will decrease blood pressure in both the supine and upright positions. The increased venous capacitance produces a decreased cardiac preload, thus decreasing myocardial oxygen demand.

19. The answer is D. *(Chapter 3, III C–F)* Phenytoin is used in the treatment of grand mal seizures but may exacerbate petit mal epilepsy. Trimethadione is effective but not the drug of first choice; it acts by both suppressing the epileptic focus and inhibiting the spread of the seizure discharge. Primidone may exacerbate petit mal epilepsy. Ethosuximide is the drug of first choice.

20. The answer is C. *(Chapter 7, II C 1 a, d, e)* Vitamin B_{12} is a cobalt-containing compound that is synthesized by the bacterial flora in the colon. However, because it cannot be absorbed there, humans must obtain vitamin B_{12} from the dietary intake of animal products. The liver, not the bone marrow, preferentially stores vitamin B_{12}. A portion of the stored vitamin is secreted into the bile each day and is absorbed in the ileum. Vitamin B_{12} is essential for cell growth and for the maintenance of normal myelin. It is also important for the normal metabolic functions of folate.

21. The answer is B. *(Chapter 3, VII B, C)* Monoamine oxidase (MAO) inhibitors are not useful in the manic phase of bipolar manic-depressive illness. They can precipitate a *hyper*tensive crisis if certain foods are ingested. Tricyclic antidepressants act presynaptically by preventing the re-uptake of biogenic amines. Both groups of antidepressants produce an absolute increase in biogenic amine levels. In addition, they have a considerable lag time prior to the onset of clinically useful effects.

22. The answer is A. *(Chapter 10, I C 4 b)* Leukocyte migration is suppressed by glucocorticoids, an effect that is thought to be one component of the overall anti-inflammatory effect of corticosteroids. Pharmacologic doses of glucocorticoids can result in all of the other effects listed.

23. The answer is C. *(Chapter 4, II C 4)* All of the statements listed in the question are true except that lidocaine has an amide, not an esteratic linkage. Possessing an amide linkage gives it a greater duration of action than procaine has. The latter drug is metabolized by ester hydrolysis.

24. The answer is B. *(Chapter 7, I A 4, B 2; II B 4, C 1 b, c)* Intrinsic factor, a glycoprotein, is necessary for the gastrointestinal absorption of vitamin B_{12}, not of folate. Once in the circulation, vitamin B_{12} is transported to the tissues by a plasma β-globulin, transcobalamin II. Folate deficiency can result from a decrease in the amount of folate-binding proteins in the plasma, as well as from an inadequate dietary supply, diseases involving the small intestine, and defects in the folate enterohepatic cycle. About 1 gram of iron is stored as ferritin in the bone marrow, liver, and spleen. This stored iron is available for the synthesis of hemoglobin in cases of blood loss. The serum iron carrier is transferrin. In iron-deficiency anemia, the ratio of serum iron to serum-binding capacity is less than 10 percent—that is, the serum transferrin is less than 10 percent saturated with iron.

25. The answer is E (all). *(Chapter 13, II E 5 b)* Inhibitors of the mixed-function oxygenase system include carbon monoxide, ozone, carbon tetrachloride, and organophosphorus insecticides. Inhibiting the microsomal enzymes causes the metabolism of certain drugs to be reduced, resulting in higher systemic levels of the drug. Thus, poisoning by any of these toxic substances might cause an increased drug effect, as well as the effects of the poison itself.

26. The answer is E (all). *(Chapter 10, I C 4, 9, 10)* Because corticosteroids alter the mucosal defense mechanisms, peptic ulceration can result from prolonged therapy. The immunosuppressive effects of corticosteroids increase susceptibility to infection. Sudden withdrawal of corticosteroids can result in signs of adrenal insufficiency. The patient may have to be protected during stressful situations for a year or more after withdrawal.

27. The answer is A (1, 2, 3). *(Chapter 6, VII B 4; VIII B 1)* Cerebral edema resulting in increased intracranial pressure is helped by diuretic therapy. The osmotic diuretics mannitol and urea reduce cerebrospinal fluid pressure. Furosemide, due to its potent edema-reducing ability, is also being used in the treatment of elevated intracranial pressure.

28. The answer is B (1, 3). *(Chapter 5, V A 3, B)* Thiazides are the diuretics used most frequently in the management of hypertension, and are used for mild, moderate, and severe hypertension. If a thiazide is ineffective alone in the treatment of mild hypertension, it is usually combined with a β-adrenergic blocking agent or with another type of antihypertensive agent. Triamterene and spironolactone have only modest hypotensive effects, but they potentiate the effects of the thiazides and minimize the potassium loss that thiazides can cause. Furosemide and ethacrynic acid produce greater diuresis than the thiazides, but they have a weaker antihypertensive effect.

29. The answer is B (1, 3). *(Chapter 4, III A 2, 3, 5, 6)* Diethyl ether is a highly explosive general anesthetic and has a limited use in the United States. Ether and halothane are good skeletal muscle relaxants having both central and peripheral mechanisms. Both halothane and enflurane have hepatic toxicity potential. Nitrous oxide has only minimal effects on respiration when used alone, although response to carbon dioxide is depressed in the presence of thiopental. Ether, due to an enhanced sympathetic activity, produces some bronchodilation but no severe respiratory depression.

30. The answer is D (4). *(Chapter 4, II B 2, C 1 c, 4 a, 5)* With a pseudocholinesterase deficiency procaine's duration of action would be lengthened. Cocaine is also degraded by plasma esterases. Dibucaine would not be contraindicated since it is a "surface" anesthetic. Lidocaine, being an amide anesthetic, is not dependent on pseudocholintesterase for its metabolism.

31. The answer is A (1, 2, 3). *(Chapter 1, II B 1 c)* Drugs that are orally administered will have variable rates of absorption. Compliance is not ensured, and irritation of the mucosal surfaces can occur with some drugs (e.g., nonsteroidal anti-inflammatory drugs). The oral route of administration is considered to be a relatively safe route.

32. The answer is E (all). *(Chapter 7, III A 1 b, B 1, 2, 7)* Heparin prolongs the clotting time of blood, both in vivo and in vitro. It is prepared commerically from bovine lung and porcine intestinal mucosa. Warfarin is considered the prototype of the coumarin-derived anticoagulants. The coumarin-derived anticoagulants interfere with vitamin K synthesis of active coagulation factors II (prothrombin), VII, IX, and X. Careful monitoring of the prothrombin time is essential with oral anticoagulant therapy, to reduce the risk of hemorrhage. Should the prothrombin time fall too low, anticoagulant therapy is stopped. Following discontinuation of oral anticoagulants, the prothrombin time gradually returns to normal. Oral administration of vitamin K_1 (phytonadione) will enhance recovery.

33. The answer is E (all). *(Chapter 3, V, VI)* Antianxiety agents such as diazepam do not produce parkinsonian tremors, are better skeletal muscle relaxants, and are good anticonvulsant agents compared to antipsychotic agents such as the phenothiazines. Antianxiety agents are not used in the treatment of psychosis.

34. The answer is B (1, 3). *(Chapter 2, VII B 3)* The ganglionic blocker hexamethonium can decrease blood pressure (sympathetic ganglionic blockade) and cause constipation (parasympathetic ganglionic blockade). It does not cause bronchiolar relaxation or skeletal muscle relaxation.

35. The answer is A (1, 2, 3). *(Chapter 1, VI A, B)* Synthetic or conjugation reactions frequently follow oxidation reactions. Glucuronides that are eliminated in the bile can be hydrolyzed by β-glucuronidases and the free drug will then be reabsorbed into the blood. This "enterohepatic recirculation" can be very important in increasing the half-time of a drug. Most drug metabolism occurs in the hepatic microsomal metabolizing system. In conjugation reactions exogenous compounds react with endogenous functional groups to produce a more polar compound.

36. The answer is E (all). *(Chapter 5, IV A, B, C)* Verapamil and nifedipine are "calcium channel blockers": they inhibit Ca^+ influx into vascular smooth muscle cells. This results in vasodilation, which exerts an antianginal effect. Propranolol, a β-adrenergic blocking agent, decreases sympathetic stimulation and thus reduces the heart rate, especially during exertion, and decreases myocardial contractility. These effects in turn decrease the oxygen requirements of the myocardium. Nitrates such as nitroglycerin relax all vascular smooth muscle, resulting in an increased peripheral pooling of blood and a decreased preload. Myocardial oxygen requirements are therefore reduced.

37. The answer is A (1, 2, 3). *(Chapter 10, I C 4, IV A 1; Chapter 5, V C 3 e (3))* The oral hypoglycemic agent tolbutamide decreases blood glucose concentrations, while the antihypertensive agent diazoxide increases them. Insulin decreases blood glucose concentrations, while cortisol, glucagon, and isoproterenol all increase blood glucose concentrations.

38. The answer is E (all). *(Chapter 1, II B; VII A)* The route of administration is an important determinant of the rate and efficiency of absorption of a drug. Delivery of the drug into the circulation is relatively slow after oral administration, and the rate of absorption is variable. Parenteral routes of administration bypass the alimentary canal and result in rapid, direct drug absorption. After intravenous administration, the absorption of a drug follows zero-order kinetics; thus a constant *amount* (i.e., 100 percent) of the drug is absorbed. After any other route of administration, the absorption of most drugs follows first-order (exponential) kinetics; thus, a constant *fraction* of the drug is absorbed.

39–40. The answers are: 39-C (2, 4); 40-C (2, 4). *(Chapter 2, V D 4, 5)* Since parathion is an irreversible cholinesterase inhibitor, signs of cholinergic toxicity should be present. These would include increased bronchial secretions and muscle fasciculations. Mydriasis and tachycardia are adrenergic effects.

Appropriate therapy would be to administer the muscarinic blocker atropine and the cholinesterase reactivator PAM chloride.

41. The answer is A (1, 2, 3). *(Chapter 5, II E, H 5 f)* Cardiac glycosides are of greatest value for treating low-output cardiac failure. They are also of great value in the control of atrial fibrillation and flutter because of their ability to reduce the ventricular rate by prolonging the refractory period of conduction tissue. Paroxysmal atrial tachycardia frequently responds to digitalis therapy, presumably as a result of reflex vagal stimulation. A–V dissociation and block are the consequences of digitalis toxicity, not indications for digitalis use. Paroxysmal atrial tachycardia can also result from digitalis intoxication; determining whether this cardiac arrhythmia is a sign of too much or too little digitalis can be a worrisome problem for the physician.

42. The answer is A (1, 2, 3). *(Chapter 13, II c 2 b (4), (5))* The ingestion of warm water will not usually influence the absorption of a drug. Alterations in gastric pH and the presence of food in the stomach can inversely influence the absorption of a drug, while the ingestion of a fatty meal can increase the absorption of lipid-soluble drugs.

43. The answer is C (2, 4). *(Chapter 2, II G)* Amphetamine is a mixed-acting sympathomimetic agent that causes mood elevation. It does not stimulate monoamine oxidase, but blocks it. Amphetamine has been used in the treatment of obesity because of its effects on the lateral hypothalamic feeding center.

44. The answer is C (2, 4). *(Chapter 9, X D 2, 4–6)* Colchicine is not a uricosuric agent. It appears to attach to microtubular proteins, thus preventing the migration of granulocytes. Diarrhea, not constipation, is a characteristic untoward effect and is an indicator for discontinuation of the drug. Chronic administration can lead to agranulocytosis.

45. The answer is E (all). *(Chapter 1, VI C)* The genetic makeup, the presence or absence of disease, the age of the subject, and species differences can all affect metabolism. Likewise, the chemical properties of the drug, its route of administration, and the dosage given are also important factors. Circadian rhythm should also be taken into account.

46. The answer is D (4). *(Chapter 10, I B 1, C 2–4, 9)* Glucocorticoid activity results in the stimulation of the liver glycogen deposition system. Mineralocorticoids, not glucocorticoids, affect electrolyte homeostasis. Corticotropin (ACTH) does not have a basic steroid nucleus but contains 39 amino acids. Pharmacologic doses of glucocorticoids are often associated with untoward effects. Steroid receptors do indeed mediate the metabolic effects of steroids.

47. The answer is A (1, 2, 3). *(Chapter 2, II A 5)* The principal mechanism by which the action of norepinephrine is terminated is by re-uptake. The enzymes monoamine oxidase (MAO) and catechol-O-methyltransferase (COMT) also play an important role. Tyrosine hydroxylase is the rate-limiting enzyme necessary for the synthesis of norepinephrine.

48. The answer is D (4). *(Chapter 9, IV B 1)* Although all nonsteroidal anti-inflammatory agents have salt-retaining properties, phenylbutazone has the greatest liability and should be avoided. This drug exerts a direct effect on renal tubules which can cause cardiac decompensation and acute pulmonary edema. Thus, it should not be used in a patient already experiencing decreased cardiac function.

49. The answer is B (1, 3). *(Chapter 11, III B 1, 2, 4)* Methotrexate has been used in the treatment of psoriasis to suppress the proliferation of epidermal cells. It is a folic acid antagonist which is eliminated unmetabolized, primarily via the kidneys. It slows the rate of entry of cells into S phase but kills cells in S phase. Thus, it can be labeled a self-limiting S-phase–specific drug. Methotrexate does not cross the blood–brain barrier well, but it can be administered intrathecally.

50. The answer is B (1, 3). *(Chapter 1, VIII E)* Physiologic antagonists are agonists producing opposite effects by interacting with two different types of receptors. Acetycholine and norepinephrine would be examples of such physiologic antagonists.

51. The answer is B (1, 3). *(Chapter 1, IV B, C)* Drugs frequently cannot readily enter the brain because of the blood–brain barrier. This is due primarily to the continuous layer of endothelial cells with tight gap junctions that line the cerebral capillaries. The fetus is also protected from many drugs because the fetal circulation is separated from the maternal circulation by several placental layers. Both the kidneys and the testes are exposed to circulating drugs.

52. The answer is C (2, 4). *(Chapter 5, III E 6)* This patient has an irritable cardiac focus secondary to his myocardial infarction. Oxygen and lidocaine would be the appropriate remedies in this acute situation. Unless the patient has heart failure, digoxin is not indicated. Propranolol is not indicated because of its negative inotropic effect.

53. The answer is E (all). *(Chapter 8, III A 1 d)* All of the pharmacologic effects listed in the question are associated with antihistamines. The drying of salivary and bronchial secretions is one of the anticholinergic properties of the classic antihistamines. Overdosage can lead to convulsions, while low (therapeutic) doses cause sedation.

54. The answer is A (1, 2, 3). *(Chapter 2, III B 1 d (3); VIII D 3; Chapter 3, VIII A; IX C)* Both morphine and tubocurarine are capable of releasing histamine and thus aggravate bronchial asthma. Since propranolol is a nonselective β-adrenergic blocker it too can aggravate bronchial asthma. Amphetamine, being a sympathomimetic, does not aggravate bronchial asthma.

55. The answer is C (2, 4). *(Chapter 9, III B 1–3, D 3)* Acetaminophen does inhibit prostaglandin synthesis centrally. It is capable of reducing the pain, but not the inflammation, associated with arthritis. Due to its lack of effect on hemostasis, it can be used for the treatment of headache in hemophilia. An overdose depletes glutathione stores, not glucuronide.

56. The answer is C (2, 4). *(Chapter 2, VIII C)* Trimethaphan is a ganglionic blocker with a short duration of action. It acts rapidly and is similar to hexamethonium in its mechanism of action. It does not directly produce tachycardia.

57–60. The answers are: 57-D, 58-E, 59-A, 60-B. *(Chapter 12, V A G; VI C, G 4, VIII E 2, G 2; X C 5, 7 a)* Tetracyclines are effective in the treatment of *Chlamydia* infections. Agents such as demeclocycline can produce a severe phototoxic skin reaction in treated individuals exposed to sunlight.

Rifampin, which is used in combination with isoniazid and ethambutol for the treatment of tuberculosis may cause urine, sweat, tears, and contact lenses to have a harmless orange color.

Clindamycin is the drug of first choice for *Bacteroides fragilis* infections. It can produce pseudomembranous colitis as an untoward effect.

The aminoglycosides have this characteristic chemical structure. These agents have a predilection for causing both ototoxicity and nephrotoxicity.

Appendix

Drug Interactions

The list in this appendix is an index to the drug interactions that are mentioned in the text of this book. Page numbers followed by a (t) denote tables.

A
Acetaminophen
 and atropine, 230
 and opiates, 230
Acetazolamide
 and weak acids, 231
Acids
 and cholestyramine, 230
Acids, organic
 and probenecid, 152
Acids, weak
 and acetazolamide, 231
 and antacids, 230
Adrenergic agents
 and halothane, 81
β-Adrenergic blocking agents
 and nifedipine, 102
 and verapamil, 102
Allpurinol
 and 6-mercaptopurine, 10, 184, 231, 233, 235, 248, 254
Aluminum salts
 and tetracycline, 210, 230
Aminoglycoside antibiotics
 and ethacrynic acid, 119
 and ether, 83
 and furosemide, 119
 and neuromuscular blocking agents, 45
Amphetamine
 and guanethidine, 35
 and monoamine oxidase inhibitors, 35
Anesthetics, general
 and monoamine oxidase inhibitors, 63
Anesthetics, inhalation
 and neuromuscular blocking agents, 45
Antacids
 and salicylates, 230
 and tetracyclines, 4, 10, 230, 233, 235
 and weak acids, 230
Antibiotics, aminoglycoside, *see* Aminoglycoside antibiotics
Antibiotics, bacteriostatic
 and bactericidal antibiotics, 235
Anticholinergic agents
 and levodopa, 56
Anticoagulants, oral
 and aspirin, 127(t), 130, 131, 132
 and barbiturates, 51, 127(t), 131, 132
 and cholestyramine, 127(t)
 and cimetidine, 127(t)
 and clofibrate, 127(t)
 and disulfiram, 127(t), 131
 and glutethimide, 127(t), 130, 131, 132
 and metronidazole, 127(t)
 and oxyphenbutazone, 127(t)
 and phenobarbital, 130, 132
 and phenylbutazone, 127(t), 130, 131, 132
 and rifampin, 127(t), 219
 and trimethoprim-sulfamethoxazole, 127(t)
Anticonvulsants
 and valproic acid, 55
Antihistamines
 and ethanol, 139
Aspirin
 and methotrexate, 231
 and oral anticoagulants, 127(t), 130, 131, 132
 and probenecid, 152, 154
 and sulfinpyrazone, 154
Atropine
 and acetaminophen, 230
Atropine-like drugs
 and monoamine oxidase inhibitors, 63

B
Barbiturates
 and diazepam, 55
 and digitoxin, 51
 and glucocorticoids, 51
 and monoamine oxidase inhibitors, 230–231
 and oral anticoagulants, 51, 127(t), 130, 131, 132
 and phenothiazines, 59
 and phenytoin, 51, 248, 255
 and procarbazine, 230–231
 and warfarin, 131
Benzodiazepines
 and CNS depressants, 61

and monoamine oxidase inhibitors, 230–231
and procarbazine, 230–231
and tranylcypromine, 230–231
Betazole
and cimetidine, 231
Butyrophenones
and levodopa, 56

C
Calcium salts
and tetracyclines, 210, 230, 235
Cardiac glycosides
and cholestyramine, 230, 233, 235
and corticosteroids, 92
and diuretics, 92, 232, 254
Central nervous system depressants
and benzodiazepines, 61
Cefazolin
and probenecid, 231, 233, 235
Cephalosporins
and probenecid, 206, 235
Chloramphenicol
and phenytoin, 54
Chlorothiazide
and digitalis, 248, 255
Cholestyramine
and acidic compounds, 230
and cardiac glycosides, 230, 233, 235
and oral anticoagulants, 127(t)
and thyroxine, 230, 233, 235
Cimetidine
and betazole, 231
and metoclopramide, 230
and oral anticoagulants, 127(t)
and propranolol, 141
Clofibrate
and oral anticoagulants, 127(t)
Cocaine
and guanethidine, 108
Codeine
and methaqualone, 53
Colchicine
and vitamin B_{12}, 230
Contraceptives, oral
and folic acid, 230
Corticosteroids
and cardiac glycosides, 92
Curariform drugs
and streptomycin, 209

D
Diazepam
and barbiturates, 55
Dicumarol
and phenytoin, 54
Digitalis
and chlorothiazide, 248, 255
and ethacrynic acid, 119
and furosemide, 119, 122
and thiazide diuretics, 118
and verapamil, 102
Digitoxin
and barbiturates, 51
Disulfiram
and ethanol, 231
and oral anticoagulants, 127(t), 131
and paraldehyde, 52
and phenytoin, 54
and warfarin, 130, 131
Diuretics
and digitalis, 92, 232, 254

E
Echothiophate
and succinylcholine, 45
Ethacrynic acid
and aminoglycoside antibiotics, 119
and digitalis, 119
Ethanol
and antihistamines, 139
and disulfiram, 231
and methaqualone, 53
and metronidazole, 221
and opioids, 232
and phenothiazines, 59
and tranquilizers, 232
Ether
and aminoglycoside antibiotics, 83

F
Folic acid
and oral contraceptives, 230
and phenobarbital, 125
and phenytoin, 125, 230
and primidone, 125
Furosemide
and aminoglycoside antibiotics, 119
and digitalis, 119, 122

G
Glucocorticoids
and barbiturates, 51
Glutethimide
and oral anticoagulants, 127(t), 130, 131, 132
and warfarin, 131
Guanethidine
and amphetamine, 35
and cocaine, 108
and tricyclic antidepressants, 108
and tyramine, 108

H
Halothane
and adrenergic agonists, 81
and norepinephrine, 80
and succinylcholine, 45
Heparin
and protamine, 232

I
Indomethacin
and probenecid, 154, 231, 233, 235

Insulin
and propranolol, 38
Isoniazid
and phenytoin, 54, 218
Isoproterenol
and propranolol, 248, 255

L
Levodopa
and anticholinergic agents, 56
and butyrophenones, 56
and monoamine oxidase inhibitors, 56
and phenothiazines, 56
and pyridoxine, 56
and reserpine, 56
Lincomycin
and neuromuscular blocking agents, 45

M
Magnesium salts
and tetracyclines, 210
Meperidine
and monoamine oxidase inhibitors, 63
6-Mercaptopurine
and allopurinol, 10, 184, 231, 233, 235, 248, 254
Methadone
and rifampin, 219
Methaqualone
and codeine, 53
and ethanol, 53
Methotrexate
and aspirin, 231
and probenecid, 231
and salicylates, 183
and sulfonamides, 183
Metoclopramide
and cimetidine, 230
Metronidazole
and ethanol, 221
and oral anticoagulants, 127(t)
Milk
and tetracyclines, 210, 230, 233, 235
Monoamine oxidase inhibitors
and amphetamine, 35
and atropine-like drugs, 63
and barbiturates, 230–231
and benzodiazepines, 230–231
and general anesthetics, 63
and levodopa, 56
and meperidine, 63
and narcotics, 63
and sedatives, 63
and serotonin, 230–231
and sympathomimetic agents, 32, 230–231
and tricyclic antidepressants, 63, 64, 71, 74
and tyramine, 62–63, 74
Morphine
and phenothiazines, 67

N
Narcotics
and monoamine oxidase inhibitors, 63
and phenothiazines, 59
Neuromuscular blocking agents
and aminoglycoside antibiotics, 45
and inhalation anesthetics, 45
and lincomycin, 45
Nifedipine
and β-adrenergic blocking agents, 102
Norepinephrine
and halothane, 80
and phenoxybenzamine, 248, 255
and procarbazine, 230–231
and tranylcypromine, 230–231

O
Opiates
and acetaminophen, 230
Opioids
and ethanol, 232
Oxyphenbutazone
and oral anticoagulants, 127(t)

P
Paraldehyde
and disulfiram, 52
Penicillin
and probenecid, 152, 157, 202, 224, 227, 231, 233, 235
Phenobarbital
and folic acid, 125
and oral anticoagulants, 130, 132
and valproic acid, 56
Phenothiazines
and barbiturates, 59
and ethanol, 59
and levodopa, 56
and morphine, 67
and narcotics, 59
Phenoxybenzamine
and norepinephrine, 248, 255
Phenylbutazone
and oral anticoagulants, 127(t), 130, 131, 132, 150, 230
Phenytoin
and barbiturates, 51, 248, 255
and chloramphenicol, 54
and dicumarol, 54
and disulfiram, 54
and folic acid, 125, 230
and isoniazid, 54, 218
and sulfonamides, 54
Primidone
and folic acid, 125
Probenecid
and aspirin, 152, 154
and cefazolin, 231, 233, 235
and cephalosporins, 206, 235
and indomethacin, 154, 231, 233, 235
and methotrexate, 231
and organic acids, 152
and penicillin, 152, 157, 202, 224, 227, 231, 233, 235
and salicylates, 154, 157

Procaine
and sulfonamides, 78
Procarbazine
and barbiturates, 230–231
and benzodiazepines, 230–231
and norepinephrine, 230–231
and serotonin, 230–231
and sympathomimetics, 193
and tricyclic antidepressants, 193
and tyramine, 193
Propranolol
and cimetidine, 141
and insulin, 38
and isoproterenol, 248, 255
Protamine
and heparin, 232
Pyridoxine
and levodopa, 56

R
Reserpine
and levodopa, 56
Rifampin
and methadone, 219
and oral anticoagulants, 127(t), 219

S
Salicylates
and antacids, 230
and methotrexate, 183
and probenecid, 154, 157
and sulfinpyrazone, 154
and uricosuric agents, 147
Sedatives
and monoamine oxidase inhibitors, 63
Serotonin
and monoamine oxidase inhibitors, 230–231
and procarbazine, 230–231
and tranylcypromine, 230–231
Streptomycin
and curariform drugs, 209
Succinylcholine
and echothiophate, 45
and halothane, 45
Sulfinpyrazone
and salicylates, 154
Sulfonamides
and methotrexate, 183
and phenytoin, 54
and procaine, 78
Sympathomimetic amines
and monoamine oxidase inhibitors, 32, 230–231
and procarbazine, 193
and tricyclic antidepressants, 32

T
Tetracyclines
and antacids, 4, 10, 230, 233, 235
and cations (calcium, aluminum, magnesium), 210, 230, 233, 235
and milk, 210, 230, 233, 235
Thiazide diuretics
and digitalis, 118
Thyroxine
and cholestyramine, 230, 233, 235
Tranquilizers
and ethanol, 59, 232
Tranylcypromine
and barbiturates, 230–231
and benzodiazepines, 230–231
and norepinephrine, 230–231
and serotonin, 230–231
Tricyclic antidepressants
and guanethidine, 108
and monoamine oxidase inhibitors, 63, 64, 71, 74
and procarbazine, 193
and sympathomimetic agents, 32
Trimethoprim-sulfamethoxazole
and oral anticoagulants, 127(t)
Tyramine
and guanethidine, 108
and monoamine oxidase inhibitors, 62–63, 74
and procarbazine, 193

U
Uricosuric agents
and salicylates, 147

V
Valproic acid
and other anticonvulsants, 55
and phenobarbital, 56
Verapamil
and β-adrenergic blocking agents, 102
and digitalis, 102
Vitamin B_{12}
and colchicine, 230

W
Warfarin
and aspirin, 130, 131, 132
and barbiturates, 131
and disulfiram, 130, 131
and glutethimide, 131
and phenylbutazone, 130, 131, 132, 230

Index

Note: Page numbers in *italics* denote illustrations; those followed by (t) denote tables.

A

Absorption of drugs, *see* Drug absorption
Acetaminophen, 145, 148–149, *148,* 156, 157, 253, 258
Acetaminophen overdosage, 149
Acetazolamide, 7, 9, 12, 115, 117, 121, 122
 effect on drug excretion, 231
Acetohexamide, 168
Acetylcholine, 29, 39–40, *39,* 46, 48
Acetylcholine receptors, 30
N-Acetylpenicillamine, 240
Acetylsalicylic acid, *see* Aspirin
Acidifying salts as diuretics, 115, 117–118
ACTH, *see* Corticotropin
Actinomycin D, *see* Dactinomycin
Action potential, 49
Activated charcoal, 242
 effect on drug excretion, 231
Active transport, 14, 15
Acyclovir, 222–223
Additive drug effects, 22, 26
Adenine arabinoside, *see* Vidarabine
Adenohypophysis, *see* Anterior pituitary gland
Adrenal corticosteroids, 159, *159,* 160, 160–163, 252, 258
 see also Glucocorticoids, Mineralocorticoids
 as anticancer agents, 191
 anti-inflammatory effects, 6, 11, 161
 endogenous, 160, 162, 172, 174
 glucocorticoid activity, 6, 11, 161
 mechanism of action, 161
 mineralocorticoid activity, 161
 pharmacokinetics, 161
 principles of use, 162, 250
 structure, *160*
 structure–activity relationships, 160
 therapeutic uses, 162
 untoward effects, 4, 10, 162–163, 250, 256
Adrenal corticosteroid inhibitors, 163
Adrenal insufficiency, diagnosis with corticotropin, 160
Adrenal physiology, 159–160, *159*
Adrenergic(sympathomimetic) agents, 31–36
α-Adrenergic agonists, 30
β-Adrenergic agonists, 30
α-Adrenergic antagonists, *see* α-, β-Adrenergic blocking agents
α-Adrenergic blocking agents (α-blockers), 36–37, 46, 48
β-Adrenergic blocking agents (β-blockers), 37–38, 46, 48
Adrenergic nerve inhibitors, 38–39, 107–108
Adrenergic receptors, 30, 47, 48
α-Adrenergic receptor agonists, use as antihypertensives, 106–107
Adrenocorticotropic hormone (ACTH), *see* Corticotropin
Adriamycin, *see* Doxorubicin
Agonist, 21
Alcohol, *see* Ethanol
Aldomet, *see* Methyldopa
Aldosterone, 11, 160, 161
 biosynthesis (release), 108, 161
 daily secretion, 162
 and renin-angiotensin system antagonists, 141
Aldosterone antagonists, *see* Spironolactone
Alimentary routes of administration, 13, 250, 256
Alkyl sulfonates, 182
Alkylating agents, 178–182
 mechanism of action, 178–179, 195, 197
 untoward effects, 197
Allopurinol, 153–154, 155, 157, 248, 254, 255
 use in cancer chemotherapy, 2, 8
  with 6-mercaptopurine, 10, 184, 231, 233, 235, 248, 254
  with 6-thioguanine, 185
 use in gout, 153–154, 155, 157
Amantadine, 221–222
 use in parkinsonism, 57
Amikacin, 208, 209, 227
γ-Aminobutyric acid (GABA), and barbiturates, 50
Aminocaproic acid, 128, 254
Aminoglycosides, 207–210, 219 , 224, 227
 chemistry, 207
 mechanism of action, 207
 pharmacokinetics, 208
 susceptible organisms, 208
 therapeutic uses, 208–209
 untoward effects, 209–210
Amitriptyline, 63, 64, 74
Ammonia poisoning, 238
Ammonium chloride, 117–118, 231
Amobarbital, 50, 51, 51(t)

Amoxicillin, 204, 225, 227
Amphetamine, 34–35, 47, 48, 64–65, 252, 257
Amphetamine overdosage, 64–65
treatment of, 35, 65
urinary pH and, 231
Amphotericin B, 10, 216, 227
Ampicillin, 203, 204, 225, 226, 227
Amyl nitrite, as antianginal agent, 100
for cyanide poisoning, 238, 245
Analgesia definition, 65
Analgesics, *see* Narcotic analgesics, Nonsteroidal anti-inflammatory agents
Androgens, 164, 191
Anemias, drugs for, 123–125
Anesthetic agents, 77–85
general, 7, 12, 80–84, 250, 256
inhalation, 80–83, 86, 88
blood:gas partition coefficient, 80, 86, 88
minimum alveolar concentration (MAC), 80, 88
tissue:blood partition coefficient, 80, 88
intravenous, 84–85
local, 5, 11, 77–80, 87, 88, 250, 256
adverse effects, 80
chemistry, 78
mechanism of action, 77
relative duration of action, 86, 88
structure–activity relationship, 78, 78(t)
structure–metabolism relationship, 78
Angina pectoris drugs for, 99–102
Angiotensins, 135–136, 144, 161
Angiotensin II, 11, 109, 135–136
biosynthesis, 135–136, 144, 161
drugs inhibiting, 108–109
mechanism of action, 136
metabolism, 135–136
physiologic effects, 136
therapeutic uses, 136
Angiotensin II receptor antagonists, 109, 141
Ankylosing spondylitis drugs for, 157
Antabuse, *see* Disulfiram
Antacids, effect on drug absorption, 230
Antagonisms between drugs, 21–22
see also Drug interactions
competitive, 21, *21*, 25, 27
by neutralization, 22
noncompetitive, 22, *22*, 27
partial, 26
pharmacologic, 1, 8, 21–22
physiologic, 1, 8, 22, 232, 252, 258
Antagonist, 21
Anterior pituitary gland, role in adrenal physiology, 159, *159*
Anthelmintics, 3, 9, 199, 220–221
Anthracyclines, 187–188
Antiadrenergic antihypertensive agents, 106–107
Antianginal agents, 89, 99–102, 251, 257
Antianxiety agents, 60–61
effects of ethanol on, 232
vs antipsychotic agents, 251, 257
Antiarrhythmic agents, 89, 92–99, 94(t)
Antibacterial agents, categories of, 199
Antibiotics, definition, 199
Anticancer agents, 1, 2, 5, 8, 177–194
classification, 178, 195, 197
combination therapy, 2, 8
rationale, 11, 177
dosage calculations, 178
mechanism of action, 5, 11, 177–178
role of cell cycle in, 177–178
principles of use, 5, 11, 177
toxicity, 178
Anticholinergic agents, *see also* Parasympathetic antagonists
before anesthesia, 85
in parkinsonism, 57
Anticholinesterase agents, 40–42
Anticoagulants, 126–128, 250, 256
see also Oral anticoagulants
effect on insulin requirements, 167
Anticonvulsants, *see* Antiseizure agents
Antidepressant agents, 62–64, 72, 74
Antidotes, mechanism of action, 237, 243, 245
Antifungal agents, 4, 10, 215–217
Antihistamines, 142, 144
see also H_2 receptor antagonists
chemistry, 139, *139*, 139(t)
classification, 139, 139(t)
pharmacokinetics, 139
pharmacologic effects, 139–140, 144, 253, 258
therapeutic uses, 57, 140, 142, 144
untoward effects, 140
Antihistamine overdosage, 140
Antihypertensive agents, 89, 102–109
classes of, 102
Anti-infective agents, 199–223, 253, 258
Antimalarial agents, 221
use in rheumatoid arthritis, 145
Antimetabolites, 183–186
mechanism of action, 182
Antimicrobial agents, *see* Anti-infective agents
Antimony poisoning, 240
Antineoplastic agents, *see* Anticancer agents, Cancer chemotherapy
Antiparkinsonian agents, 56–57
Antipsychotic agents, 57–59, 72, 74
Antiseizure agents, 53–56, 72, 75, 249, 255
Antithrombotic agents, 128, 132
Antithyroid agents, 169–170
Antitussives, nonopioid, 70
Apparent volume of distribution, 18
Ara-A, *see* Vidarabine
1-3-D-Arabino-furanosylcytosine, *see* Cytarabine
Ara-C, *see* Cytarabin
Arachidonic acid, 137
Arsenic poisoning, 239, 243, 245
Arterial (white) thrombi, 126
drugs used for, 128, 130, 132
Arteriolar vasodilators, 103–104
Arthritis, *see* Rheumatoid arthritis
Ascariasis, drugs for 3, 9, 220–221
Asphyxiant gases, 237–238, 244, 245
Aspirin, 5, 11, 145–148, 156, 157
see also Salicylates
as antithrombotic agent, 132, 254

chemistry, 145, *145*
effects on blood, 146–147
effects on oral anticoagulants, 127(t), 130, 131, 132
effects on platelet aggregation, 146–147, 254
Aspirin poisoning, *see* Salicylate intoxication
Asthma, *see* Bronchial asthma
Atenolol, 38
Atropine, 42–43
actions, 42, 46, 48
effect on intestinal drug absorption, 230, 234, 235
mechanism of action, 9, 42
pharmacokinetics, 42
therapeutic uses, 42
in digitalis intoxication, 92
with diphenoxylate, 68
for poisoning by anticholinesterase agents, 42
as preanesthetic medication, 85
for untoward effects of parasympathetic agonists, 40
untoward effects, 43
Atropine poisoning, drugs for, 41, 43
Autacoid antagonists, 133, 139–141
Autacoids, 5, 6, 11, 133–139, 142, 144
classification, 133
clinical uses, 143, 144
physiologic roles, 133
Automaticity of heart, 93, 94(t)
Autonomic nervous system, 29
drugs affecting, 29–45
Autoreceptors, *see* Presynaptic receptors
Azathioprine in rheumatoid arthritis, 145

B

Bacterial infections, drugs for, 199, 200–215, 217–220
Bacterial resistance, 202
Bacteriostatic antibiotic, effect on bactericidal antibiotic, 235
BAL (Bristish antilewisite, *see* Dimercaprol
Barbital, 51(t)
Barbiturates, 50–52, 53
chemistry, 50, *50,* 51(t)
classification, 50, 51(t)
duration of action, 50, 51, 51(t), 72, 74
mechanism of action , 50
pharmacokinetics, 51
pharmacologic actions, 50–51
role in drug interactions, 50–51
effect on oral anticoagulants, 127(t), 131
effect of monoamine oxidase inhibitors on, 230–231
effect on phenytoin, 248, 255
therapeutic uses, 51
as antiseizure agents, 53
as sedative–hypnotics, 50–52
as general anesthetics, 84–85
as preoperative sedatives, 85
in regional anesthesia, 85
untoward effects, 74
Barbiturate dependence, 51
withdrawal symptoms, 51, 71, 74, 75
Barbiturate intoxication, 51–52, 241, 244, 245
treatment of, 52
Barbituric acid, 50, *50*
BCNU, *see* Carmustine
Beclomethasone, 161, 174
Benzathine penicillin G, 203, 204
Benzene toxicity, 238, 244, 246
Benzodiazepines, 60–61
central nervous system effects, 53, 60–61
effect of monoamine oxidase inhibitors on, 230–231
pharmacokinetics, 61
therapeutic uses, 61
as anticonvulsants, 61
as antiseizure agents, 55
untoward effects, 5, 11, 61
Benzodiazepine habituation, 61
withdrawal effects, 61
Benzothiadiazides, *see* Thiazide diuretics
Benzylpenicillin, *see* Penicillin G
Beryllium toxicity, 240
Beta-lactam ring, *201, 205*
Beta-lactamases, 202, 206
Betamethasone, 161, 162(t), 163(t)
Betazole, 135, 144
Bethanechol, 40
Biliary tract, role in drug excretion, 16
Binding of drugs, *see* Drug binding
Bioavailability, 14, 26
Biogenic amines, effects of monoamine oxidase inhibitors on, 62, 230–231
Bleomycin, 1, 6, 8, 11, 188–189, 190, 194
"Blind therapy, " for serious infections, 209
α-, β-Blockers, *see* α-, β-Adrenergic blocking agents
Blood–brain barrier, 49
Blood:gas partition coefficient of inhalation anesthetics, 80, 86, 88
Blood glucose, effects of drugs on, 251, 257
Blood:tissue partition coefficient of inhalation anesthetics, 80, 88
Bradykinin, 11, 109, 136, 141
Breast carcinoma, drugs for 1, 8
Bretylium, 39, 99, 110, 112
Bromocriptine, 57
Bronchial asthma, 86, 139–140, 253, 258
Bupivacaine, 78(t), 79–80
Busulfan, 182, *182*
Butabarbital, 51(t)
Butorphanol, 69
Butyrophenones, 59

C

Calcitonin, 171, 173, 175
Calcium channel blockers (calcium antagonists), 101–102, 257

effects on the heart, 101
mechanism of action, 101
Calcium disodium ethylenediamine tetraacetate ($CaNa_2$EDTA), 239, 240
Cancer chemotherapy, 177–194
see also Anticancer agents
Captopril 109, 110, 112, 141
Carbachol (carbamylcholine), 5, 11, 40
Carbamazepine, 55
Carbamylcholine, *see* Carbachol
Carbenicillin, 10, 203, 204, 227
Carbidopa, 56
Carbinoxamine, 139(t)
Carbon dioxide poisoning, 237
Carbon monoxide poisoning, 238, 243, 244, 245, 246
Carbon tetrachloride poisoning, 238
Carbonic anhydrase inhibitors, 115, 117, 122
Carcinoma of breast, drugs for 1, 8
Cardiac arrhythmias, 92–93
drugs for, 92–99, 249, 252, 255, 258
Cardiac automaticity, 93, 94(t)
Cardiac conduction velocity, 93
Cardiac effective refractory period (ERP), 93, 94(t)
Cardiac glycosides, 89–92, 248, 255
chemistry, 89
digitalizing and maintenance dosage, 91
effects on the heart, 89–90, 90(t)
extracardiac effects, 90
mechanism of action, 90
pharmacodynamics, 89
pharmacokinetics, 91, 91(t)
therapeutic uses, 90–91, 95(t), 251, 257
untoward effects, 2, 9, 91–92
Cardiac glycoside intoxication, *see* Digitalis intoxication
Cardiovascular agents, 89–109
Carmustine (BCNU), 181
Carrier-mediated facilitated diffusion, 6, 11, 14, 15
Catapres, *see* Clonidine
Catecholamines, 31–33
Cathartics, use in poisoning, 242
CCNU, *see* Lomustine
Cefaclor, 107, 225
Cefamandole naftate, 207
Cefazolin, 206–207, 226, 231, 233, 235
Cefotaxime, 207
Cefoxitin, 207
Ceftizoxime, 207
Ceiling effect, 19
Cell cycle, 177, *178*
and cancer chemotherapy, 177–178, 195, 197
Cell-cycle phase-nonspecific anticancer agents, 178
Cell-cycle phase-specific anticancer agents, 177
Central nervous system, agents acting on, 49–70
mechanism of action, 49
Central nervous system stimulants, 64–65
Centrally acting antiadrenergic antihypertensive agents, 106–107
Cephalexin, 207, 225
Cephaloridine, 207
Cephalosporinase, 206
Cephalosporins, 205–207, 225, 227
chemistry, 205, *205*
first-generation, 206–207
mechanism of action, 205
pharmacokinetics, 206, 235
second-generation, 207
susceptible organisms, 205–206
therapeutic uses, 206, 209
third-generation, 207
untoward effects, 207, 225, 227
Cephalothin, 206
Cephapirin, 206
Cephradine, 207
Cerubidine, *see* Daunorubicin
Chelating agents as antidotes for heavy metals, 240, 244, 245
Chemical inactivation (neutralization) of drugs, 22, 232
Chemoreceptor trigger zone, 65
Chloramphenicol, 212–213, *212*, 226, 228
Chloral hydrate, 52, 75, 247, 254
Chlorambucil, 180, *180*
Chlordiazepoxide, 60–61, *60*
Chlorine gas poisoning, 238
Chloroform poisoning, 238
Chloroquine, 145, 221
Chlorothiazide, 7, 12, 118, 121, 122, 248, 255
Chlorpheniramine, 139(t)
Chlorpromazine, 35, 58, 58(t), 59, 73, 74, 75
Chlorpropamide, 168, 172, 174
Chlorprothixene, 59
Chlortetracycline, 211
Cholestyramine, effect on oral anticoagulants, 127(t)
effect on drug absorption, 230, 233, 235
effect on drug excretion, 231
use in digitalis intoxication, 92
Cholinergic (parasympathetic) agonists, 39–40
Cholinergic receptors, 30
Cholinesterase inhibitors, 45, 46, 48, 257
see also Organophosphate cholinesterase inhibitors
Chronotropic effect, 30
Cimetidine, 140–141, 143, 144, 213
effect on oral anticoagulants, 127(t)
Cisplatin, 2, 8, 189, 190, 193–194, *193*, 197
Citrovorum factor, *see* Leucovorin
Clindamycin, 214–215, 225, 227
Clofazimine, 220
Clofibrate, effect on oral anticoagulants, 127(t)
Clonazepam, 55
Clonidine, 106, 110, 111, 112
Clorazepate, 55, 60
Cloxacillin, 203, 204
Cocaine, 65, 78, 87, 88
Codeine, 65, 67
Colchicine, 153, 157, 252, 254, 258
effect on vitamin B_{12} absorption, 230
"Combination pill' contraceptive, 163
Compazine, *see* Prochlorperazine
Competitive antagonism, 21, *21*, 25, 27
Competitive neuromuscular blocking agents, *see* Neuromuscular blocking agents
Conduction velocity of heart, 93

Conjugation of drugs, role in drug metabolism, 17
Contraceptives, *see* Oral contraceptives
Corticosteroids, *see* Adrenal corticosteroids, Glucocorticoids, Mineralocorticoids
Corticosterone, 160
  daily secretion, 162
Corticotropin (adrenocorticotropic hormone, ACTH), 6, 11, 159–160, *159,* 172, 173, 174
Cortisol, 11, 160
Cortisol hemisuccinate, 162
Cortisone, 160, 161, 162(t), 163(t), 173, 174
Cough center, 65
Coumarin-derived anticoagulants, 127–128, 132, 254
Cromolyn sodium, 140
Crystalline zinc (regular) insulin, 166, 173, 174
Curare, *see* Neuromuscular blocking agents
Cyanide poisoning, 8, 238, 243, 244, 245
  from nitroprusside, 105
Cyanocobalamin, *see* Vitamin B_{12}
Cyclizine, 139(t)
Cyclooxygenase, 137
  inactivation of, 145
  and platelet aggregation, 145, 146–147
Cyclophosphamide, 179–180, *180,* 195, 197
  in rheumatoid arthritis, 145
Cyproheptadine, 141
Cytarabine (cytosine arabinoside, ara-C), 186–187, *187,* 196, 197
Cytochrome P-450, *see* Mixed-function oxygenase system
Cytosine arabinoside, *see* Cytarabine

D

Dacarbazine (DTIC), 1, 8, 182, *183*
Dactinomycin (actinomycin D), 187
Dapsone, 220, *220*
Daunorubicin, 188
o,p′-DDD, *see* Mitotane
Decamethonium, *see* Neuromuscular blocking agents
Deferoxamine, 240
Demeclocycline, 211, 212
Deoxybarbiturates, 53–54
Depolarizing agents, *see* Neuromuscular blocking agents
Depression, 62
Desipramine, 63, 74
Desoxycoticosterone, 11, 160, 161, 173, 174
Dexamethasone, 162(t), 163(t)
Dextran solutions, incompatibilities, 229
Dextroamphetamine, 65
Dextromethorphan, 70
DFP, *see* Diisopropyl fluorophosphate
Diabetes mellitus, 165, 166, 172, 174
  see also Insulin deficiency
  juvenile-onset (insulin-dependent), 165, 166
  maturity-onset (non-insulin-dependent), 166
Diazepam, 55, 60–61, 85
Diazoxide, 104, 111
Dibenamine, 36
Dibucaine, 78(t), 79, 87, 88
Dichloromethane poisoning, 238
Dicloxacillin, 203, 204
Dicyclomine, 43
Diethyl ether, 7, 12, 80, 83
Diethylcarbamazine citrate, 220
Diffusion of drugs, *see* Drug diffusion
Digitalis, *see* Cardiac glycosides
Digitalis intoxication, 91–92, 95(t), 110, 112
  and diuretics, 3, 4, 9, 92, 232, 254
  and hypokalemia, 4, 9, 10, 92, 118, 232, 254
Digitalizing dosage, 91
Digitoxin, 89, 91, 91(t)
Digoxin 89, 91, 91(t), 110, 111, 112
Digoxin-induced arrhythmia *see,* Digitalis intoxication
Diisopropyl fluorophosphate (DFP), 6, 12, 41, 47, 48
Dilantin, *see* Phenytoin
Diloxanide furoate, 221
Dimenhydrinate, 139(t)
Dimenhydrinate intoxication, 248, 254
Dimercaprol (BAL), 240
Diphenhydramine, 57, 139(t)
Diphenoxylate, 68, 75
Diphenylhydantoin, *see* Phenytoin
Dipyridamole, 102
Disopyramide, 94(t), 95(t), 96–97, 110
Dissociative anesthesia, 84
Distribution of drugs in body, *see* Drug distribution
Disulfiram, 127(t), 131, 231
Diuretic agents, 115–120
  classification, 115–116
  definition, 115
  and digitalis intoxication, 3, 4, 9, 92, 232, 254
  relative efficacy, 115
  "self-limiting," 115
  sites of action, 7, 12, 115
  therapeutic uses, 3, 9, 115, 250, 256
    in hypertension, 103, 111, 112, 250, 256
    to reduce nephrotoxicity, 2, 8, 115, 119, 194, 231
Dobutamine, 33–34
Dopa, 31
Dopamine, 31, 33, 56
Dosage, *see* Drug dosage, Dose–response relationships
Dose–response curve, 27
Dose–response relationships, 13, 19–23
  ceiling effect, 19
  graded dose–response, 19
  graded dose–response curve, 19–20, *20*
  log dose–response curve, 20, *20, 21,* 25, 27
  quantal dose–response curve, 19, *19*
  quantal response, 19, *19,* 26
Doxepin, 63
Doxorubicin, 187–188, 197
Doxycycline, 10, 211
Dramamine, *see* Dimenhydrinate
Dromostanolone, 191

Droperidol, 59, 84
Drug absorption, 18
drug interactions affecting, 229–230, 233, 235
factors affecting, 13–14, 25, 26, 230, 251, 257
Drug administration routes, 13–14
alimentary, 13, 250, 256
inhalation, 14
oral, 13, 24, 26
parenteral, 13–14
topical, 14
Drug antagonism, *see* Antagonism between, drugs, Drug interactions
Drug binding, to plasma proteins, 15, 26
role in drug interactions, 230
to receptors, 20–21, 24, 26
Drug bioavailability, 14, 26
factors affecting, 14
Drug diffusion, carrier-mediated, 6, 11, 14, 15
Fick's law, 14, 247, 254
passive, 14–15, 25, 26, 27
simple, 14–15, 25, 26, 27
Drug distribution, 15–16, 18, 25, 26, 252, 258
alpha and beta half-times, 18
drug interactions affecting, 230
effect of repeated doses, 18, 254
multicompartment model, 18
one-compartment model, 18
two-compartment model, 18
Drug dosage, and absorption, 13
effect of repeating, 18, 248, 254
Drug efficacy, 19, 20, 25, 26, 27, 248, 255
Drug elimination from blood, 18
Drug excretion, 16, 25, 26
effects of drug interactions, 231, 233, 235
effect of urinary pH, 231
Drug incompatibilities, 229
Drug interactions, 229–232, 233–235, 248, 255
see also Antagonisms between drugs
additive drug effects, 22, 26
affecting drug absorption, 229–230, 233, 235
affecting drug distribution, 230
affecting drug excretion, 231, 233, 235
affecting drug metabolism, 230–231
chemical inactivation (neutralization), 22, 232
competitive antagonism, 21, *21*, 25, 27
definition, 229
enhancement of drug effects, 22
due to incompatibilities, 229
involving barbiturates, 51, 127(t), 131, 248, 255
involving levodopa, 56
involving monoamine oxidase (MAO) inhibitors 62–63, 71, 74, 230–231
involving oral anticoagulants, 127(t), 130, 131, 132
involving phenytoin, 54
noncompetitive antagonism, 22, *22*, 27
pharmacodynamic, 229, 231–232, 235
pharmacokinetic, 229–231, 233, 235
factors influencing, 229
potentiation, 22, 24, 26
principles of, 229–232, 234, 235
synergism, 22, 26
Drug metabolism, 16–18, 25, 26, 251, 257
see also Mixed-function oxygenase system
biochemical reactions, 16–17
conjugation reactions, 17
effects of drug interactions, 230–231
enzyme systemic involved, 16–17
factors affecting, 4, 10, 17–18, 252, 258
first-pass effect, 3, 9, 13, 17, 26
glucuronide conjugation, 17
microsomal, 16
nonmicrosomal, 16–17
by oxidation of drugs, 16–17, 27
by reduction of drugs, 17
Drug pharmacokinetics, 13, 18
Drug potency, 20, 25, 26, 27, 248, 255
Drug receptors, *see* Receptors
Drug–receptor complex, 20–21, 26
Drug–receptor interactions, 20–21, 26
Drug safety, measurements of, 22–23, 24, 26
Drug transport, 14–15, 25
active, 14, 15
carrier-mediated facilitated diffusion, 6, 11, 14, 15
endocytosis, 14, 15
filtration, 15
passive diffusion, 14–15, 25, 26, 27
DTIC, *see* Dacarbazine
Dystonic reactions, 59

E

E_{max}, 19, 20, *20*, *22*, 24, 25, 26, 27
Eating, effect on drug absorption, 230
Echothiophate, 41
ED_{50} (median effective dose), 20, *20*, 23, 26, 248, 255
Edrophonium, 41, 45
Effective refractory period (ERP) of heart, 93, 94(t)
Efficacy, 19, 20, 25, 26, 27, 248, 255
Electrocardiogram, effects of antiarrhythmic drugs on, 94(t)
Elimination of drugs from blood, 18
Emesis, in poisoning, 241–242
Endocrine function, agents affecting, 159–171
Endocytosis, 14, 15
Endorphins, 65
Enflurane, 81–82, 86, 88
Enhancement of drug effects, 22
Enkephalins, 65
Enterohepatic recirculation of drugs, 17
Enzyme systems in drug metabolism, 16–17
see also Mixed-function oxygenase system
Ephedrine, 34
Epilespy drugs for, *see* Antiseizure agents
Epinephrine, 31–33, 46, 48
actions, 31–32
biosynthesis, 31
chemistry, *31*
effects on insulin requirements, 167
effects on local anesthetics, 78, 80
effects on parenteral absorption, 229–230
pharmacokinetics, 32

therapeutic uses, 32
untoward effects, 32–33
Epinephrine receptors, 30
Ergonovine, 37
Ergot alkaloid derivatives, as serotonin antagonists, 141
Ergot alkaloids, 4, 10, 37
Ergotamine, 37
Erithrityl tertranitrate, 100
ERP (effective refractory period), 93, 94(t)
Erythromycin, 10, 11, 214–215
Estrogen, 163–164, 172, 174
Estrogen receptors, in breast carcinoma, 1, 8, 190–191
Ethacrynic acid, 103, 112, 119, 121, 122
Ethambutol, 218–219, *218*
Ethanol overdosage, 240–241
Ethanolamines, 139(t), 140
Ethchlorvynol, 53
Ether, *see* Diethyl ether
Ethinyl estradiol, 163
Ethosuximide, 55
Ethynodiol, 163
Etidocaine, 78(t), 79
Etidronate, 171
Excretion of drugs, *see* Drug excretion
Exponential (first-order) kinetics, 18
Extended insulin zinc suspension (ultralente insulin), 167
Extrapyramidal symptoms, 57

F

Facilitated diffusion, 6, 11, 15
Fecal excretion of drugs, 16
Fentanyl, 59, 68, 84, 85
Ferritin, 249, 256
Ferrous choline citrate, 124
Ferrous fumarate, 124
Ferrous gluconate, 124
Ferrous sulfate, 123, 129, 131
Fever, 146, 148
Fick's law, 14, 247, 254
Filtration, as form of drug transport, 15
First-order (exponential) kinetics, 18
First-pass effect, 3, 9, 13, 17, 26
Flucytosine, 10, 217
Fludrocortisone, 161
5-Fluorouracil, 185–186, *186*, 195, 197
Fluoxymesterone, 164, 191
Fluphenazine, 58(t)
Flurazepam, 53
Folate-binding protein, 249, 256
Folate-deficiency, 2, 8, 124–125, 129, 130, 131, 132, 256
Folic acid (folate), 124–125, 129, 249, 256
effects on anticonvulsant agents, 125
Folinic acid, *see* Leucovorin
Food in stomach, effect on drug absorption, 230
Fungal infections, drugs for, 199, 215–217
Furosemide, 2, 7, 9, 12, 103, 112, 119, 121, 122

G

G_1, G_2, G_0 phases of cell cycle, 177, *178*
GABA, *see* γ-Aminobutyric acid
Gallamine, 44
see also Neuromuscular blocking agents
Ganglionic blocking agents, 43–44
Ganglionic nicotinic receptors, 30
Ganglionic stimulators, 43–44
Gaseous poisons, 237–238
systemic toxicants, 238
Gastric lavage, 242
Gastric pH, effect on drug absorption, 230
General anesthetics, *see under* Anesthetics
Gentamicin, 10, 203, 208, 209, 225, 227
Glucagon, 166, 167
Glucocorticoids, 145, 160–162, 162(t), 163(t), 249, 256
see also Adrenal corticosteroids
anti-inflammatory activity, 6, 11, 161, 162(t)
duration of action, 163(t)
endogenous, 160
mineralocorticoid activity, 162(t)
pharmacologic effects, 249, 256
physiologic effects, 1, 2, 8, 161, 173, 174
relative potency, 162(t)
Glucuronide conjugation of drugs, 17
Glutethimide, 52, 74
effect on oral anticoagulants, 127(t), 130, 131, 132
Glutethimide intoxication, 52
Glyceryl trinitrate, *see* Nitroglycerin, Nitrates
Glycopyrrolate, 85
Gold, 151–152, 156, 157
Gold toxicity, 240
Gout, 152
drugs for, 145, 152–154, 155, 157, 247, 254
Gouty inflammation, pathogenesis, 152
Graded dose-response curve, 19–20, *20*
Gray-baby syndrome, from chloramphenicol, 213, 226, 228
Griseofulvin, 10, 217
Growth hormone, effect on insulin requirements, 167
Guanethidine, 39, 108, 112

H

H_1 and H_2 (histamine) receptors, 134
H_1 (histamine) receptor antagonists (H_1 receptor blockers), 4, 9–10, 139–140
see also Antihistamines
H_2 (histamine) receptor antagonists (H_2 receptor blockers), 140–141, 142, 144
Half-times, of drug elimination and distribution, 18
Haloperidol, 59
Halothane, 7, 12, 80–81

hepatotoxic potential, 81, 86, 88
Heavy metal intoxication, 239–240
Helminthiasis, drugs for, 199, 220–221
Hematopoietic agents, 123–125
Hematopoietic substances, 249, 256
Hemostasis, drugs affecting, 126–128
Henderson-Hasselbalch equation, 14–15, 25, 26, 27
Heparin, 126–127, 129, 130, 131, 254
incompatible drugs, 229
mechanism of action, 129
pharmacokinetics, 126
pharmacologic properties, 126
in pregnancy, 127
therapeutic uses, 126, 132
untoward effects, 126, 130, 132
reversal of, 126–127
Hepatic microsomal enzyme metabolizing system, *see* Mixed-function oxygenase system
Heptane poisoning, 238, 246
Heroin, 9, 67
Hexamethonium, 44, 251, 257
Hexane poisoning, 238, 246
Hexobarbital, 51(t)
High-ceiling diuretics, 119
mechanism of action, 119
site of action, 115, 119
therapeutic uses, 119
untoward effects, 119
Histamine, 11, 133–135
biosynthesis, 133
cardiovascular effects, 134
chemistry, *133,* 142, 144
clinical uses, 134–135, 144
effects on exocrine glands, 134
effects on smooth muscle, 134
mechanism of action, 11, 134
metabolism, 133
pathologic roles, 134
physiologic roles, 134
storage sites, 133–134
triple response to, 134
untoward effects, 135
Histamine antagonists, 139–141, 142, 144
see also Antihistamines, H_1 receptor antagonists, H_2 receptor antagonists
Histamine overdose, 142, 144
Histamine receptors, *see* H_1 and H_2 (histamine) receptors
Hormones, 159–171
adrenocortical 159–163
androgenic, 164
as anticancer agents, 190–191
insulin, 165–168
of menstrual cycle, 163
parathyroid, 170–171
thyroid, 169
Hycanthone mesylate, 220
Hycodan, 67
Hydantoins, 54
Hydralazine, 103, 111
Hydrochloric acid poisoning, 238
Hydrochlorothiazide, 118
Hydrocodone, 67
Hydrocortisone, 161, 162, 162(t), 163(t)
Hydrocyanic acid, *see* Cyanide
Hydrofluoric acid poisoning, 238
Hydrolysis of drugs, role in drug metabolism, 17
Hydromorphone, 67, 75
Hydroxychloroquines, 145
5-Hydroxytryptamine, *see* Serotonin
Hydroxyurea, 191–192, *192,* 197
Hydroxyzine, 85
Hyoscine (scopolamine), 43
dl-Hyoscyamine, 42
Hyperparathyroidism, 171
Hypertension, drugs for, 89, 102–109
principles of drug therapy, 1, 102–103, 256
Hypertensive emergencies, drugs for, 103, 249, 255
Hyperthyroidism, drugs for, 169–170
Hyperuricemia, 152
Hypnotics, *see* Sedative-hypnotics
Hypokalemia, and digitalis intoxication, 4, 9, 10, 92, 118, 232, 254
Hypoparathyroidism, 171
Hypothalamus in adrenal physiology, 159, *159*
Hypothyroidism, drugs for, 169, 173

I

Ibuprofen, 151, 156, 157
Idoxuridine, 222
Imipramine, 63, 64, 74
Indomethacin, 9, 150, 154, 155, 156, 157
effect of probenecid on, 231, 233, 235
Inhalation anesthetics, *see under* Anesthetics
Inhalation route of administration, 14
Innovar, 59, 84
Inotropic effect, 30, 89, 248, 255
Insecticides, *see* Organophosphate cholinesterase inhibitors, Organophosphate poisoning
Insulin, 165–168
chemistry, 165
distribution and fate, 165
mechanism of action, 166
physiologic role, 173, 174
regulation of secretion, 165
Insulin deficiency, *see also* Diabetes mellitus
metabolic effects, 166
Insulin preparations, 166–167, 172, 174
administration, 167
factors affecting requirements, 38, 167–168
untoward effects, 167
Insulin shock, 6, 12, 167
Insulin zinc suspension (lente insulin), 167
Interferon, 223
Interphase, of cell cycle, 177
Intestinal motility, 234, 235
effects on drug absorption, 230
Intracranial pressure, elevated, diuretics for, 250, 256
Intravenous anesthetic, *see under* Anesthetics
Intrinsic activity of a drug, 21
Intrinsic factor, 125, 249, 256

Intrinsic factor deficiency, 8
Iodide, 169, 170
Iodine, 169, 170
Iodism, 170
Ionic thyroid inhibitors, 169
Ipecac, 241
Iproniazid, 62
Iron, 249, 256
Iron-deficiency anemia, 8, 123, 129, 131
 drugs for, 123–124
Iron dextran, 124, 129, 131
Iron preparations, 123–124, 129, 131
Irritant gases, 238
Ischemic heart disease, *see* Angina pectoris
Isoflurane, hepatotoxic potential, 86, 88
Isoniazid, 217–218, *218,* 224, 227
Isosorbide, 120
Isosorbide dinitrate, 100
Isocarboxazid, 62
Isoflurane, 82
Isophane (NPH) insulin, 166–167
Isoproterenol, 33

K

Kallidin, 136
Kallikreins, 136
Kanamycin, 208, 209
Kerosene poisoning, 238, 244, 246
Ketamine, 77, 84
Ketoconazole, 217
Kininogen, 136
Kinins, 136–137
 mechanism of action, 136–137
 physiologic effects, 11, 136
 synthesis and degradation, 136

L

LC_{50} (median lethal concentration), 237, 245
LD_{50} (median lethal dose), 26, 237, 244, 245
Lead poisoning, 239, 243, 245
Legionnaires' disease, 5, 11
Lente insulin (insulin zinc suspension), 167
Lente insulins, 167
Leprosy, drugs for, 199, 219–220
Leucovorin (citrovorum factor, folinic acid), 125, 183
Leucovorin "rescue," 183
Leukemia, acute lymphoblastic, drugs for, 2, 8
 lymphocytic, drugs for, 8
Leukotrienes, 137–139
Levamisole, 145
Levodopa (L-dopa), 56
Levorphanol, 67
Levothyroxine, 169, 173, 175
Lidocaine, 5, 10, 11, 78(t), 79, 86, 87, 88, 249, 256
 as antiarrhythmic agent, 5, 10, 92, 94(t), 95(t), 97–98, 110, 112
Lincomycin, 214–215, 225, 227
Liothyronine, 169
Lipoxygenases, 137
Lithium, 61–62, 71, 74
Local anesthetics, *see under* Anesthetic agents
Log dose-response curve, 20, *20, 21,* 25, 27
Lomotil, 68
Lomustine (CCNU), 181–182
Lorazepam, 60–61
Lugol's solution, 170

M

M phase, of cell cycle, 177, *178*
MAC, *see* Minimum alveolar concentration
"Major tranquilizers," *see* Antipsychotic agents
Malaria, drugs for, 221
Malignant hyperthermia, from inhalation anesthetics, 81
Mannitol, 119, 120
 use with nephrotoxic therapy, 2, 8, 115, 119, 194, 231
MAO inhibitors, *see* Monoamine oxidase inhibitors
Margin of safety, 23
Mebendazole, 220
Mechlorethamine, 179, 195, 197
 see also MOPP regimen
Meclizine, 139(t), 142, 144
Median effective dose (ED_{50}), 20, *20,* 23, 26, 248, 255
Median lethal concentration (LC_{50}), 237, 245
Median lethal dose (LD_{50}), 26, 237, 244, 245
Medroxyprogesterone, 191
Megaloblastic anemia, causes, 124, 131
 drugs for, 124–125
Megestrol, 191
Mellaril, *see* Thioridazine
Melphalan, 180, *180*
Menstrual cycle, 163
Meperidine, 67–68, 75
Mephentermine, 35
Mephenytoin, 54
Mepivacaine, 5, 11, 78(t), 79, 87, 88
Meprobamate, 60
Mercaptomerin, 116
6-Mercaptopurine, 5, 10, 184, *184,* 231, 233, 235
Mercurial diuretics, 115, 116, 121, 122
Mercury poisoning, 2, 8, 239–240
Mestranol, 163
Metabolism of drugs, *see* Drug metabolism, Mixed-function oxygenase system
Metaproterenol, 35–36
Metaraminol, 35
Methacholine, 40, 47, 48
 effect on parenteral absorption, 229–230
Methacycline, 211
Methadone, 68, *68*
Methadone maintenance, 68
Methamphetamine, 35, 65
Methane poisoning, 237
Methaqualone, 53, 74
Methicillin, 203, 204, 227

Methotrexate, 178, 183–184, 195, 197, 252, 258
effect of aspirin on, 231
effect of probenecid on, 231
Methoxamine, 35
Methsuximide, 55
Methyldopa, 106–107, 111, 113
Methylene dichloride poisoning, 238
Methylprednisolone, 161, 162(t), 163(t)
Methyltestosterone, 164
Methyprylon, 53, 74
Methysergide, 141
Metoclopramide, 40
effect on drug absorption, 230, 234, 235
Metoprolol, 38
Metrifonate, 220
Metronidazole, 9, 200, 221
effect on oral anticoagulants, 127(t)
Metyrapone, 163
"Mickey Finn," 52
Microsomal enzymes, role in drug metabolism, 16–17
Microsomal oxidation of drugs, 16
Milk, as antidote, 241
Mineralocorticoids, 161, 172, 174
endogenous, 160
physiologic effects, 161
Minimum alveolar concentration (MAC), of inhalation
anesthetics, 80, 88
"Minipill" contraceptive, 163, 174
Mini-Press, *see* Prazosin
Minocycline, 211
"Minor tranquilizers," *see* Antianxiety agents
Minoxidil, 8, 104
Mitomycin, 1, 8, 189, 196, 197
Mitotane (o,p′-DDD), 193, *193*
Mixed-acting sympathomimetic agents, 34, 46, 48
Mixed-function oxygenase (hepatic microsomal, cytochrome P-450) system of drug metabolism, 16, 25, 26–27
barbiturates and, 50–51
inducers of, 231, 233, 235
inhibitors of 231, 250, 256
role in drug interactions, 231, 255
Monoamine oxidase (MAO) inhibitors, 62–63, 249, 255
chemistry, 62, *62*
mechanism of action, 62
pharmacokinetics, 63
pharmacologic effects, 62–63
role in drug interactions, 62–63, 63, 71, 74, 230–231
therapeutic uses, 63
untoward effects, 62–63, 63, 72, 74
Mood-altering drugs, 61–64
MOPP regimen of cancer chemotherapy, 11, 177, 179, 190, 191, 192
Morphine, 3, 9, 65–67, *66*, 75, 85
pharmacokinetics, 66
pharmacologic effects, 65–66
therapeutic uses, 66–67, 85
tolerance, 66
untoward effects, 67
Morphine addiction (dependence), 66, 67
Moxalactam, 207
Muscarinic receptors, 30
Mushroom poisoning, 42
Mycobacterial infections, drugs for, 199, 217–220
Mycoplasmal pneumonia, drugs for, 5, 11
Myxedema, *see* Hypothyroidism

N

Nadolol, 38
Nafcillin, 203, 204, 227
Nalbuphine, 69
Nalorphine, 12, 70
Naloxone, 12, 69
Naproxen, 151
Narcotic analgesics, 65–70, 73, 75
mechanism of action, 65
untoward effects, 74
Natural products as anticancer agents, 187–190
Neomycin, 208, 209, 210
Neostigmine, 40, 41, 45, 47, 48
Nephrotoxicity, prophylactic diuretics for, 2, 8, 115, 119, 194, 231
Nerve impulse transmission, 49
methods of altering, 49
Neuroleptanalgesia, 84
Neuroleptanesthesia, 84
Neuromuscular blocking agents, 44–45, 48, 83, 249, 255
factors affecting, 45
mechanism of action, 44, 46, 48
metabolism, 44
pharmacokinetics, 44
reversal of blockade, 41, 45
therapeutic uses, 44–45
untoward effects, 45
Neurotransmitter–receptor complex, 49
Neurotransmitters, 29, 30–31, 32, 49
mechanism of action, 49
methods of altering, 49
Nickel toxicity, 240
Niclosamide, 220
Nicotine, 43–44
Nicotinic receptors, 30
Nifedipine, 101–102
Nifurtimox, 221
Niridazole, 220
Nitrates, 99–101
chemistry, 99–100
effects on the heart, 100
extracardiac effects, 100
mechanism of action, 100
pharmacokinetics, 100
route of administration, 100
therapeutic uses, 100
untoward effects, 8, 100–101
Nitrate poisoning, 101
Nitrites, 2, 8–9, 99
use in cyanide poisoning, 238, 243, 245
Nitrogen mustards, 179–180, *179*, 195, 197
mechanism of action, 179

Nitrogen poisoning, 237
Nitroglycerin (glyceryl trinitrate), 100, 110, 112
Nitroprusside, 104–105, 255
Nitrosoureas, 181–182, *181*
 mechanism of action, 181
Nitrous oxide, 7, 12, 80, 82–83, 87, 88
Nonbarbiturate sedative-hypnotics, 52–53, 71, 72, 74
Noncompetitive antagonism, 22, *22*, 27
Nonmicrosomal enzymes, role in drug interactions, 230–231
 role in drug metabolism, 16–17
Nonmicrosomal oxidation of drugs, 16–17
Non-narcotic analgesics, 145–152, 154
Nonopioid antitussives, 70
Nonsteroidal anti-inflammatory drugs (NSAIDs), 145–152, 154
 effect of monoamine oxidase inhibitors on, 62, 230–231
 mechanism of action, 145
 untoward effects, 3, 9
 use in gout, 154
Norepinephrine, 29, *31*, 31–33, 252, 258
Norethindrone, 4, 163
Norethynodrel, 163
Nortriptyline, 63, 74
NPH (isophane) insulin, 166–167, 172, 174
NSAIDs *see* Nonsteroidal anti-inflammatory drugs
Nylidrin, 102
Nystatin, 215–216, 225, 227

O

Octane poisoning, 238, 244, 246
Oncovin, *see* Vincristine, MOPP regimen
o,p′-DDD, *see* Mitotane
Opiate receptors, 65
Opiates, 65–67, 230, 234, 235
Opioid agonist-antagonists, 69–70
Opioid antagonists, 6, 12, 69–70
Opioids, 3, 9, 65–69, 83, 85, 232
Oral administration, 13, 24, 26
Oral anticoagulants, 127–128
 factors affecting activity, 127
 pharmacokinetics, 128
 pharmacologic properties, 127
 reversal of effects, 128
 therapeutic uses, 128
 untoward effects, 128
  drug interactions, 127(t), 130, 131, 132
Oral contraceptives, 163–164, 172, 174
 effect on folic acid absorption, 230
 mechanism of action, 4, 10, 163
 types of, 163
 untoward effects, 163–164, 172, 174, 174, 248, 255
Oral hypoglycemic agents, *see* Sulfonylureas
Organic lead poisoning, 239
Organic solvents as poisons, 238, 244, 246
Organomercurial diuretics, *see* Mercurial diuretics
Organophosphate cholinesterase inhibitors, 41–42
Organophosphate poisoning, 3, 251, 257
Osmotic diuretics, 115, 119–120
Ouabain, 89
 see also Cardiac glycosides
Oxacillin, 203, 204
Oxazepam, 60–61
Oxidation of drugs, role in drug metabolism, 16–17, 27
Oxycodone, 67
Oxyphenbutazone, effect on oral anticoagulants, 127(t)
Oxytetracycline, 211
Ozone poisoning, 238

P

PAM (pralidoxime), 42
Pancuronium, 45, 47, 48
 see also Neuromuscular blocking agents
Papaverine, 65, 102, 110, 112
Paraldehyde, 52, *52*
Parasympathetic (cholinergic) agonists, 39–40
Parasympathetic antagonists, 42–43
 see also Anticholinergic agents
Parasympathetic nervous system, 29
 organs innervated by, 29
Parasympathetic neurotransmitter, 29
Parasympathetic stimulation, effects, 30
Parathion, 42, 251, 257
Parathormone, *see* Parathyroid hormone
Parathyroid gland, agents affecting, 170–171
Parathyroid hormone (PTH, parathormone), 170–171
Parenteral routes of administration, 13–14
Parkinson's disease, drugs for, 56–57
Partial antagonism between drugs, 26
Partial antagonist, 21
Partial thromboplastin time, for monitoring heparin therapy, 126
Passive diffusion, 14–15, 25, 26, 27
Penicillamine, 145, 240
Penicillin G, 202, 204, 208, 213, 224, 227
Penicillin V, 202, 203, 204
Penicillinase, 202
 microorganisms producing, 202
Penicillinase-resistant penicillins, 203, 204, 209
Penicillins, 201–205, *201*
 bacterial resistance, 202
 broad-spectrum forms, 204
 chemistry, 201, *201*
 effect of probenecid on, 202, 224, 227, 231, 233, 235
 mechanism of action, 202
 penicillinase-resistant forms, 203, 204, 209
 repository forms, 204
 susceptible organisms, 202
 therapeutic uses, 203–204
 untoward effects, 203, 204–205
  hypersensitivity reactions, 204–205
Pentaerythritol tetranitrate, 100
Pentagastrin, 135, 144
Pentamidine isethionate, 221
Pentane poisoning, 238, 246

Pentazocine, 3, 9, 69
Pentobarbital, 50, 51, 51(t), 85
Peptidyl dipeptidase inhibitors, 109, 141
Peripheral efferent nervous system, 29
Peripheral neurohumoral transmission, drugs affecting, 29–45
Pharmacodynamic drug interactions, 229, 231–232, 235
Pharmacokinetic drug interactions, 229–231, 233, 235
Pharmacokinetics, 13, 18
Pharmacologic antagonism, 1, 8, 21–22
Pharmacology, definition, 13
Phase-nonspecific anticancer agents, 178
Phase-specific anticancer agents, 177
Phenacetin, 148–149
Phencyclidine, 84
Phenelzine, 62
Phenergan, *see* Promethazine
Phenobarbital, 50, 51, 51(t), 53
  effect on biliary excretion of drugs, 231
  effect on oral anticoagulants, 127(t), 130, 132
Phenothiazine derivatives, as preanesthetic medications, 85
  as serotonin antagonists, 141
Phenothiazines, 57–59, 58(t)
  chemistry, 57, *58*
  pharmacokinetics, 59
  pharmacologic effects, 57, 58–59
  therapeutic uses, 59
  untoward effects, 59, 71, 74, 75
    extrapyramidal symptoms, 57–58, 58(t), 59, 71, 74, 75
    orthostatic hypertension, 58(t), 59
Phenoxybenzamine, 36, 248, 255
Phenoxymethyl penicillin, *see* Penicillin V
Phensuximide, 55
Phentolamine, 36–37
Phenylbutazone, 9, 149–150, 154, 156, 157
  effect on oral anticoagulants, 127(t), 130, 131, 132, 230
Phenylephrine, 34, 47, 48
  actions on the heart, 94(t), 98
Phenytoin, 2, 9, 54
  as antiarrhythmic drug, 94(t), 95(t), 98
  effect on folic acid absorption, 230
  pharmacokinetics, 98
  use in digitalis intoxication, 92, 95(t), 98
Physiologic antagonism, 1, 8, 22, 232, 252, 258
Physostigmine, 40–41, 43, 64
Phytonadione, 128
Pilocarpine, 40, 47, 48
Piperazine, 9, 220
Piperazine antihistamines, 139(t), 140
Pituitary-adrenal axis, suppression by corticosteroids, 162
Pituitary gland, anterior, *see* Anterior pituitary gland
Plasma-protein binding by drugs, 15, 26
  role in drug interactions, 230
Platelet aggregation, effects of aspirin on, 127(t), 130, 132, 146–147, 254
  inhibition of, 127(t), 130, 132, 138, 146–147, 157, 254
  see also Antithrombotic agents
  role of prostaglandins and thromboxanes, 138, 146–147
Platelet cyclooxygenase, 145, 146–147
Plummer-Vinson syndrome, 123, 131
Pneumococcal infections, penicillin for, 203, 224, 227
Poisoning, 237–242
  commonly occurring overdoses, 240–241
  principles of management, 241–242, 247, 254
Postganglionic adrenergic neuron blockers, *see* Adrenergic nerve inhibitors
Potassium iodide, 170
Potassium-sparing diuretics, 9, 115, 120
Potency, 20, 25, 26, 27, 248, 255
Potentiation of drug effects, 22, 24, 26
Pralidoxime (PAM), 42
Prazepam, 60
Praziquantel, 220
Prazosin, 37, 105–106, 112
Preanesthetic medications, 85
Prednisolone, 161, 162(t), 163(t), 173, 174
Prednisone, 161, 162(t), 163(t)
  as anticancer agent, 8, 190, 191, 197
  see also MOPP regimen
Prekallikrein, 136
Presynaptic receptors (autoreceptors), and release of neurotransmitter, 49
Prilocaine, 79
Primaquine, 221
Primary atypical pneumonia, drugs for, 11
Primidone, 53–54, *54*
Probenecid, 152–153, 155, 156, 157
  effect on drug excretion, 152, 157, 231, 233, 235
  use with penicillin, 202, 224, 227
Procaine, 4, 5, 10, 11, 78, 78(t), 86, 87, 88
Procaine penicillin G, 204
Procainamide, 94(t), 95(t), 95–96, 110, 112
Procarbazine, 192–193, *192*
  see also MOPP regimen
  as monoamine oxidase inhibitor, drug interactions from, 230–231
Prochlorperazine, 58(t)
Prodrugs, 16
Progesterone, 163
Progestins, 163, 172, 174, 191
Proinsulin, 165
Proliferation-independent anticancer agents, 177, 195, 197
Prolixin, *see* Fluphenazine
Promethazine, 58(t), 85, 139(t)
Prompt insulin zinc suspension (semilente insulin), 167
Propantheline, 43
Propoxyphene, 68–69, 71, 74
Propranolol, 37–38, 248, 249, 255
  actions, 37
  effects on the heart, 94(t), 98
  pharmacokinetics, 37

precautions, 38
therapeutic uses, 37–38
as antianginal agent, 101
as antiarrhythmic drug, 94(t), 95(t), 98–99, 111, 112
in digitalis intoxication, 92, 95(t), 98, 112
untoward effects, 38
Propylthiouracil, 169, 170, 173, 175
Prostacyclin, *see* Prostaglandins
Prostaglandin inhibitors, 145
salicylates as, 145, 146–147, 157
Prostaglandins, 137–139, 144
cardiovascular effects, 137–138
effects on central nervous system, 137
effects on platelet aggregation, 138, 146–147
effects on smooth muscle, 138
gastrointestinal effects, 138
hormonal effects, 137, 138
mechanism of action, 139
physiologic roles, 137–138
in fever, 146
synthesis, 137
therapeutic uses, 139, 144
Protamine sulfate, 126–127, 131
Protamine zinc insulin, 166
Prothrombin activity, for monitoring warfarin therapy, 128
Protozoal infections, drugs for, 200, 221
Pseudomembranous colitis, from clindamycin and lincomycin, 215, 225, 227
PTH, *see* Parathyroid hormone
Purine analogs, 184–185
Pyrantel pamoate, 9, 220
Pyridostigmine, 45
Pyridoxine deficiency, from isoniazid, 218
Pyrilamine, 139(t)
Pyrimethamine, 201, 221
Pyrimidine analogs, 185–187

Q

Quaalude, *see* Methaqualone
Quantal dose-response curve, 19, *19*
Quantal response, 19, *19*, 26
Quantitative toxicology, 237, 244, 245
Quinidine, 6, 11, 93–95, 94(t), 95(t), 110, 112
Quinine, 221

R

Radioactive iodine, 169, 170, 173, 175
Ranitidine, 141
Rate constant, of drug elimination, 18
Receptors, 13, 20–21, 24, 26
adrenergic, 30, 47, 48
cholinergic, 30
drug interactions involving, 231
for estrogen, 1, 8, 190–191
for histamine, *see* H_1 and H_2 receptors
for neurotransmitters, 30
nicotinic, 30
for opiates, 65
presynaptic, 49
Reduction of drugs, role in drug metabolism, 17
Regular (crystalline zinc) insulin, 166, 173, 174
Renal dysfunction, anti-infective agents in, 5, 10
Renal excretion of drugs, 16
Renin-angiotensin system, 108, 136, 161
drugs interfering with, 108–109, 141
Reserpine, 38–39, 107–108, 111, 112
Respiratory irritants, *see* Irritant gases
Reye's syndrome, 148
Rheumatoid arthritis, drugs used in, 3, 145, 252
corticosteroids, 162
gold therapy, 152, 157
salicylates, 148
Rifampin, 219
effect on oral anticoagulants, 127(t)
Routes of administration, *see* Drug administration routes

S

S phase of cell cycle, 177, *178*
Salicylate intoxication, 146, 147–148, 241, 243, 245
see also Salicylism
treatment, 148
urinary pH and, 231
Salicylates, 145–148, 155, 157
analgesic action, 146
antipyretic action, 146
cardiovascular effects, 146
effect on insulin requirements, 167
effect on kidney, 147
effect on prostaglandin synthesis, 145, 146, 146–147, 157
effect on respiration, 146
endocrine effects, 147
gastrointestinal effects, 146
metabolic effects, 147
pharmacokinetics, 147
therapeutic uses, 148, 154
Salicylism, 147, 157
see also Salicylate intoxication
Saralasin, 109, 141
Scopolamine (hyoscine), 1, 8, 43, 48, 85, 142, 144
effect on gastrointestinal motility, 234, 235
Secobarbital, 51(t), 85
Sedative-hypnotics, 50–53, 71, 72, 74, 85, 247
Self-limiting anticancer agents, 178
Semilente insulin (prompt insulin zinc suspension), 167
effect of monoamine oxidase inhibitors on, 62, 230–231
Serotonin (5-hydroxytryptamine), 11, 135, *135*, 142, 144
Serotonin antagonists, 141, 144
Simple diffusion, 14–15, 25, 26, 27
Sinemet, 56

Skeletal muscle nicotinic receptors, 30
Sodium bicarbonate, effect on drug excretion, 231
Sodium iodide (I 131; I 125), see Radioactive iodine
Sodium salicylate, 148
Somatic nervous system, 29
Spironolactone, 7, 10, 12, 103, 120, 121, 122
Stabilizing neuromuscular blocking agents, *see* Neuromuscular blocking agents
Staphylococcal infections, use of penicillins in, 203
Steroids, adrenal, *see* Adrenal corticosteroids
Stibogluconate, 221
Streptococcal infections, use of penicillin in, 203
Streptokinase, 128, 129, 131, 254
Streptomycin, 11, 208, 209, 219
Substance P, 133, 137
Succinimides, 55
Succinylcholine, 45, 48, 255
  see also Neuromuscular blocking agents
Sulfadiazine, 201, 225, 227
Sulfadoxine, 221
Sulfamethoxazole, *see* Trimethoprim-sulfamethoxazole
Sulfanilamide, *200*
Sulfinpyrazone, 153, 157
Sulfisoxazole, 201, 226, 230
Sulfonamides, 200–201
  mechanism of action, 200, 225, 227
  pharmacokinetics, 200
  susceptible organisms, 200
  therapeutic uses, 4, 10, 200–201
  untoward effects, 201, 228
Sulfones, 219–220
Sulfonylureas, 168, 172, 174
Sulfur dioxide poisoning, 238
Sulindac, 9, 150–151, 156, 157
Suramin, 9, 221
Sympathetic antagonists, 36–39
Sympathetic nervous system, 29
  organs innervated by, 29
Sympathetic neurotransmitter, 29
Sympathetic stimulation, effects, 30
Sympathomimetic (adrenergic) agents, 31–36, 46, 47, 48
  mixed-acting, 34
Synapse, 49
Synaptic transmission of nerve impulses, methods of altering, 49
Synergism, 22, 26
Syrup of ipecac, 241

T

Tamoxifen, 1, 8, 190–191
Tardive dyskinesia, 59
Terbutaline, 36
Testosterone, 164, 191
Testosterone cypionate, 164
Testosterone propionate, 164
Tetracaine, 5, 11, 78–79, 78(t)
Tetrachloroethylene, 221
Tetracycline, 211
Tetracyclines, 210–212
  binding by cations, 4, 10, 210, 230, 233, 235
  chemistry, 210, *210*
  mechanism of action, 210
  pharmacokinetics, 210–211
  susceptible organisms, 210
  therapeutic uses, 11, 211
  untoward effects, 212, 224, 227
Tetraethyl lead poisoning, 239
Thebaine, 65
Therapeutic index, 22–23, 24, 26, 27
Thiabendazole, 221
Thiazide diuretics, 118
  mechanism of action, 118
  site of action, 115, 118
  therapeutic uses, 118, 121, 122
    in hypertension, 103, 112
  untoward effects, 118
Thiobarbiturates, 50, 51
Thiocyanate, 105, 238
6-Thioguanine, 185, *185*, 186
Thiopental, 7, 12, 50, 51, 51(t), 74, 77, 83, 84–85, 86, 88
Thioridazine, 58(t)
Thiothixene, 59
Thioxanthene derivatives, 59
Thorazine, *see* Chlorpromazine
Threshold limit value, 237, 244
Thrombi, arterial (white), 126
    drugs used for, 128
  venous (red), 126
    drugs used for, 126–128
Thrombolytic agents, 128, 247
  antagonists for, 128
Thromboxanes, 137–139, 145, 146–147
Thyroglobulin, 169
Thyroid gland, agents affecting, 169–170
Thyroid hormones, 169
Thyroid inhibitors, 169–170
Thyroxine (T_4), 169, *169*
  effect of cholestyramine on, 230, 233, 235
Timolol, 38
Tissue: blood partition coefficient, of inhalation anesthetics, 80, 88
Tobramycin, 208, 209, 226, 227
Tolazamide, 168
Tolazoline, 36–37
Tolbutamide, 168, 172, 174
Tolmetin, 151
Toluene poisoning, 238, 244, 246
Tooth discoloration from tetracyclines, 212, 224, 227
Topical administration, 14
Total body clearance, 18
Total body stores of drug, 18, 248, 254
Toxicology, definition, 237
  subspecialties, 237
Tranquilizers, *see also* Antianxiety agents
  use as preanesthetic medication, 85
Transcobalamin II, 125, 249, 256
Transferrin, 123, 249, 256
Transmission of nerve impulses, 49
  methods of altering, 49

Transport of drugs, *see* Drug transport
Tranylcypromine, 62, *62*, 74
 drug interactions from, 230–231
Triamcinolone, 161, 162(t), 163(t), 173, 174
Triamterene, 10, 103, 112, 120, 121, 122, 247, 254
Triazenes, 182, *183*
Tricyclic antidepressants, 63–64, 249, 255
 autonomic effects, 64
 cardiovascular effects, 64
 central nervous system effects, 63–64
 chemistry, 63, *63*
 interaction with monoamine oxidase (MAO) inhibitors, 64, 74
 mechanism of action, 63
 pharmacokinetics, 64
 therapeutic uses, 64
 untoward effects, 64, 74
Triflupromazine, 58(t)
Trihexyphenidyl, 57
Triiodothyronine (T_3), 169, *169*
 see also Thyroid hormones
Trimethaphan, 44, 253, 258
Trimethoprim-sulfamethoxazole, 201
 effect on oral anticoagulants, 127(t)
Tripelennamine, 139(t)
Triple response to histamine, 11, 134
Tuberculosis, drugs for, 199, 217–219
Tubocurarine, 45, 48
 see also Neuromuscular blocking agents

U

Ultralente insulin (extended insulin zinc suspension), 167
University Group Diabetes Program, and sulfonylurea use, 168
Urea, 120
Uric acid, role in gout, 152
Urinary pH, effect on drug excretion, 231
Urinary tract infections, drugs for, 4, 10
Urokinase, 128, 129, 132

V

Valproic acid (valproate), 55
Vancomycin, 214–215, 225, 227
Vasoactive intestinal polypeptide (VIP), 133, 137
Vasodilators, 99, 102, 104–106
 as antianginal agents, 99, 102
 as antihypertensive agents, 104–106
Venous (red) thrombi, 126
Venous thrombosis, drugs used for, 126–128
Verapamil, 101–102
Vesprin, *see* Triflupromazine
Vidarabine (ara-A, adenine arabinoside), 222
Vinblastine, 1, 8, 189–190, 194, 195, 197
Vinca alkaloids, 189–190, 197
Vincristine, 8, 189–190, 196, 197
 see also MOPP regimen
Viral infections, drugs for, 200, 221–223
Vitamin B_{12}, 125, 131, 249, 255
Vitamin B_{12} deficiency, 8, 125, 129, 130, 131
Vomiting, inducing, in poisoning, 241–242

W

Warfarin, 127–128, 127(t), 129, 130, 131, 132, 230

X

Xanthine diuretics, 115, 116, 121, 122

Z

Zero-order kinetics, 18
Zinc intoxication, 240

7/13 – 4, 7-27, 8/4

7/27

MICROBIOLOGY

#24 causative organisms are initially introduced into hosts in the form of spores in all of the following diseases EXCEPT:

A) tetanus

B) gas gangrene

C) anthrax

* D) diphtheria

E) pseudomembranous colitis (antibiotic associated)